W9-DDA-920

REVIEW COPY

Please submit two tear sheets of review.

U.S. list price: $125.00

With the compliments of
FUTURA PUBLISHING COMPANY, INC.
135 Bedford Road, PO Box 418,
Armonk, NY 10504-0418
Web Site: www.futuraco.com

Dispersion of Ventricular Repolarization:

State of the Art

Edited by

S. Bertil Olsson, MD, PhD
Professor of Cardiology
Department of Cardiology
University Hospital
Lund, Sweden

Jan P. Amlie, MD, PhD
Professor of Cardiology
Medical Department
Rikshospitalet
Oslo, Norway

and

Shiwen Yuan, MD, PhD
Cardiologist
Department of Cardiology
University Hospital
Lund, Sweden

**Futura Publishing
Company, Inc.
Armonk, NY**

Library of Congress Cataloging-in-Publication Data

Dispersion of ventricular repolarization: state of the art / edited by S. Bertil Olsson, Jan P. Amlie, and Shiwen Yuan.
    p. ; cm.
  Includes bibliographical references and index.
  ISBN 0-87993-458-1
  1. Arrhythmia—Pathophysiology. 2. Ventricular fibrillation—Pathophysiology. 3. Myocardial depressants. I. Olsson, S. Bertil. II. Amlie, Jan P. III. Yuan, Shiwen.
  [DNLM: 1. Arrhythmia—physiopathology. 2. Cardiovascular Diseases—physiopathology. 3. Electrophysiology. 4. Ventricular Dysfunction—physiopathology. WG 330 D612 2000]
  RC685.A65 D56 2000
  616.1′28—dc21
                                          00–037552

Preface

The understanding of the mechanisms involved in the development and perpetuation of different cardiac arrhythmias has expanded rapidly over the past decades. The role of spatial differences in the repolarization of the ventricles is only one such example. Not only has the knowledge of basic cellular electrophysiology expanded considerably, this knowledge has also had a direct clinical impact. Furthermore, invasive and noninvasive methods have been further developed, allowing a more precise interpretation of the role of dispersion of ventricular repolarization (DVR) concerning the pathophysiology of malignant ventricular arrhythmias and its prognostic role in several patient groups.

A rapidly expanding field of knowledge within any area will always benefit from a state-of-the-art review from time to time. A few years ago, it was the feeling of the editors that the further progress of knowledge concerning DVR could be promoted by a comprehensive scientific meeting specifically devoted to this topic, gathering the true global expertise. Our efforts turned out to be inadequate in order to reach the economy necessary for this goal. This book became the alternative, thus being the result of the joint efforts of scientists actively working with different aspects of DVR. After having had the pleasure of editing this book, we believe that it may in fact be an even better way to promote the further acquisition of knowledge within this specific field. As always, the interpretations of recent scientific findings can differ. In order to maintain these important differences, the editing of the different chapters has been limited to correction of apparent spelling and typing errors, thereby minimizing any unwanted influence on the authors' original messages.

We extend our sincere thanks to Astra Hässle AB, Biosense, Boehringer Ingelheim, CPI/Guidant Scandinavia AB, Hoechst Marion Roussel, Medtronic Vingmed, and Pfizer AB. Their ongoing support of our clinical research has been a main source of inspiration for us to gather today's knowledge about the DVR and its role in ventricular arrhythmias in the present publication.

S. Bertil Olsson
Jan P. Amlie
Shiwen Yuan
Lund, Sweden and Oslo, Norway

Contributors

Fadi G. Akar, MS   Research Associate, Heart and Vascular Research Center, Case Western Reserve University, Department of Biomedical Engineering, Cleveland, OH

Jan P. Amlie, MD, PhD   Professor of Cardiology, Medical Department, Rikshospitalet, Oslo, Norway

Charles Antzelevitch, PhD   Executive Director and Director of Research, Masonic Medical Research Laboratory, Utica, NY

Fabio Badilini, PhD   ECG Laboratory, Service de Cardiologie, Hôpital Lariboisière, Paris, France

Shlomo A. Ben-Haim, MD, DSc   Cardiovascular Laboratory, The Bruce Rappaport Faculty of Medicine, Technion-Israel Institute of Technology, Haifa, Israel

Lennart Bergfeldt, MD, PhD   Associate Professor, Department of Cardiology, Karolinska Institutet at Karolinska Hospital, Stockholm, Sweden

Jean-Paul Bounhoure, MD, PhD   Department of Cardiology, Rangueil University Hospital, Toulouse, France

Serge Boveda, MD   Department of Cardiology, Rangueil University Hospital, Toulouse, France

Günter Breithardt, MD, FESC, FACC   Hospital of the Westfälische Wilhelms-Universität Münster; Department of Cardiology and Angiology and Institute of Arteriosclerosis Research, Münster, Germany

A. John Camm, MD, FRCP, FESC, FACC   Professor of Clinical Cardiology, Head, Department of Cardiological Sciences, St. George's Hospital Medical School, London, United Kingdom

Jean Philippe Couderc, PhD   Assistant Professor of Medicine, Cardiology Unit, University of Rochester Medical Center, Rochester, NY

Philippe Coumel, MD   Professor of Medicine, Head, Service de Cardiologie, Hôpital Lariboisière, Paris, France

Daniel Curnier, PhD   Department of Cardiology, Rangueil University Hospital; INSERM U 317, Department of Pharmacology, Faculty of Medicine, Toulouse, France

C.P. Day, MD   Professor of Liver Medicine, Centre for Liver Research, University of Newcastle, Newcastle upon Tyne, United Kingdom

Bruno Dongay, MD   Department of Cardiology, Rangueil University Hospital, Toulouse, France

Lars Eckardt, MD   Hospital of the Westfälische Wilhelms-Universität Münster; Department of Cardiology and Angiology and Institute of Arteriosclerosis Research, Münster, Germany

Nabil El-Sherif, MD   Professor of Medicine and Physiology, Director, Clinical Electrophysiology Program, State University of New York Health Science Center; Chief, Cardiology Division, DVA New York Harbor Healthcare System, Brooklyn, NY

C. Larissa Fabritz, MD   Assistentin und Wissenschaftliche Mitarbeiterin der Klinik und Poliklinik für Kinderheilkunde, Allgemeine Kinderheilkunde, Westfälische Wilhelms-Universität Münster, Münster, Germany

Jocelyne Fayn, PhD   Institut National de Statistique et de la Recherche Medicale, Lyon, France

Joelle Fourcade, MD   Department of Cardiology, Rangueil University Hospital, Toulouse, France

Michael R. Franz, MD, PhD, FACC   Professor of Medicine and Pharmacology, Georgetown University Medical Center; Director of Cardiac Electrophysiology, Veterans Affairs Medical Center, Washington, DC

Michel Galinier, MD, PhD   Department of Cardiology, Rangueil University Hospital; INSERM U 317, Department of Pharmacology, Faculty of Medicine, Toulouse, France

Lior Gepstein, MD, PhD   Senior Lecturer, Physiology Department, The Bruce Rappaport Faculty of Medicine, Technion-Israel Institute of Technology; Cardiology Department, Rambam Medical Center, Haifa, Israel

Wolfram Grimm, MD   Assistant Professor of Medicine, Director, Electrophysiology Laboratory, Department of Cardiology, Philipps-University Marburg, Marburg, Germany

Wilhelm Haverkamp, MD   Hospital of the Westfälische Wilhelms-Universität Münster; Department of Cardiology and Angiology and Institute of Arteriosclerosis Research, Münster, Germany

Gal Hayam, BSc   Cardiovascular Laboratory, The Bruce Rappaport Faculty of Medicine, Technion-Israel Institute of Technology, Haifa, Israel

Eva Hertervig, MD   Cardiologist, Chief of Staff, Department of Cardiology, University Hospital, Lund, Sweden

Stefan H. Hohnloser, MD, FACC, FESC   Director of Electrophysiology, Department of Medicine, Division of Cardiology, J.W. Goethe University, Frankfurt, Germany

Magnus Holm, MS, PhD   Business Manager, Biosense Webser, Waterloo, Belgium

Michiel J. Janse, MD, PhD, FRCP, FESC Professor Emeritus of Experimental Cardiology, University of Amsterdam; Editor-in-Chief, *Cardiovascular Research,* Academic Medical Center, Amsterdam, The Netherlands

Paulus Kirchhof, MD Hospital of the Westfälische Wilhelms-Universität Münster; Department of Cardiology and Angiology and Institute of Arteriosclerosis Research, Münster, Germany

Ole Kongstad, MD Cardiologist, Department of Cardiology, University Hospital, Lund, Sweden

Dmitry O. Kozhevnikov, MD Research Associate, Cardiology Research Program, DVA New York Harbor Healthcare System, Brooklyn, NY

Kenneth R. Laurita, PhD Assistant Professor of Medicine and Biomedical Engineering, Heart and Vascular Research Center, Case Western Reserve University, Department of Biomedical Engineering, Cleveland, OH

Katrin Leuchtenberger, MD Research Fellow, Department of Cardiology, Philipps-University Marburg, Marburg, Germany

Bernhard Maisch, MD Professor of Medicine, Director, Department of Cardiology, Philipps-University Marburg, Marburg, Germany

Pierre Maison-Blanche, MD Cardiologist, Head of ECG Laboratory, Service de Cardiologie, Hôpital Lariboisière, Paris, France

Arthur J. Moss, MD Professor of Medicine, Cardiology Unit, University of Rochester Medical Center, Rochester, NY

Carlo Napolitano, MD, PhD Molecular Cardiology Laboratories, Fondazione Salvatore Maugeri IRCCS, Pavia, Italy

S. Bertil Olsson, MD, PhD Professor of Cardiology, Department of Cardiology, University Hospital, Lund, Sweden

Joseph M. Pastore, MS Research Associate, Heart and Vascular Research Center, Case Western Reserve University, Department of Biomedical Engineering, Cleveland, OH

Atul Pathak, MD Department of Cardiology, Rangueil University Hospital; INSERM U 317, Department of Pharmacology, Faculty of Medicine, Toulouse, France

Juha S. Perkiömäki, MD Division of Cardiology, Department of Medicine, University of Oulu, Oulu, Finland

Silvia G. Priori, MD, PhD Molecular Cardiology Laboratories, Fondazione Salvatore Maugeri IRCCS, Pavia, Italy

Mark Restivo, PhD Senior Scientist, Research Department, DVA New York Harbor Healthcare System; Research Associate Professor, Department of Medicine, State University of New York Health Science Center, Brooklyn, NY

David S. Rosenbaum, MD   Director, Heart and Vascular Research Center, Associate Professor of Medicine, Biomedical Engineering, Physiology, and Biophysics, Case Western Reserve University, MetroHealth Medical Center, Cleveland, OH

Peter J. Schwartz, MD   Department of Cardiology, Policlinico San Matteo, IRCCS, Pavia, Italy

Wataru Shimizu, MD, PhD   Research Scientist, Masonic Medical Research Laboratory, Utica, NY; Codirector, Clinical Cardiac Electrophysiology Laboratory, National Cardiovascular Center, Osaka, Japan

Peter Sutton, MD   Senior Lecturer and Assistant Director, The Hatter Institute; Department of Cardiology, University College London Hospitals and Medical School, London, United Kingdom

Peter Taggart, MD   Reader in Medicine and Cardiology, The Hatter Institute; Department of Cardiology, University College London Hospitals and Medical School, London, United Kingdom

Gioia Turitto, MD   Associate Professor of Medicine, Director, Coronary Care Unit and Electrophysiology Laboratory, University Hospital, State University of New York Health Science Center, Brooklyn, NY

Gan-Xin Yan, MD, PhD   Research Scientist, Masonic Medical Research Laboratory, Utica, NY; Senior Research Scientist, Lankenau Institute for Medical Research, Lankenau Hospital, Winnewood, PA

Yee Guan Yap, BMedSci, MBBS, MRCP   British Heart Foundation Research Fellow in Cardiology, Department of Cardiological Sciences, St. George's Hospital Medical School, London, United Kingdom

Shiwen Yuan, MD, PhD   Cardiologist, Department of Cardiology, University Hospital, Lund, Sweden

Markus Zabel, MD   Fellow in Electrophysiology, Department of Medicine, Division of Cardiology, Klinikum Benjamin Franklin, Free University, Berlin, Germany

Wojciech Zareba, MD, PhD   Associate Professor of Medicine, Cardiology Unit, University of Rochester Medical Center, Rochester, NY

Contents

Preface iii

Basic Studies

1. Electrical Heterogeneity and the Development of
   Arrhythmias 3
   Charles Antzelevitch, Wataru Shimizu, and Gan-Xin Yan

2. Repolarization Inhomogeneities in Ventricular
   Myocardium: Studies Using the Optical Mapping
   Technique 23
   *Fadi G. Akar, Joseph M. Pastore, Kenneth R. Laurita, and
   David S. Rosenbaum*

Methodological Aspects

3. QT Dispersion: Methodology and Clinical Significance 41
   *Pierre Maison-Blanche, Fabio Badilini, Jocelyne Fayn, and
   Philippe Coumel*

4. QT Dispersion on 12-Lead Electrocardiogram in Normal
   Subjects: Reproducibility and Relation to T Wave 59
   Yee Guan Yap and A. John Camm

5. Correlations Between Monophasic Action Potential
   Recordings and Surface Electrocardiograms with Regard
   to the Evaluation of Dispersion of Ventricular
   Repolarization 75
   Markus Zabel and Michael R. Franz

6. Automatic Detection of Spatial and Temporal
   Heterogeneity of Repolarization 85
   Wojciech Zareba, Jean Philippe Couderc, and Arthur J. Moss

7. Evaluation of Ventricular Activation-Recovery Coupling
   Using an Electroanatomical Mapping Technique.................. 109
   Lior Gepstein, Gal Hayam, and Shlomo A. Ben-Haim

8. Global Dispersion of Ventricular Repolarization: Findings
   from Monophasic Action Potential Mapping Using the
   CARTO System 121
   *Shiwen Yuan, Ole Kongstad, Eva Hertervig, Magnus Holm,
   and S. Bertil Olsson*

Dispersion of Ventricular Repolarization and Ventricular Arrhythmias

9. Increased Dispersion of Repolarization: A Major Mechanism Behind the Genesis of Malignant Ventricular Arrhythmias in Cardiac Diseases................................ 143
   Jan P. Amlie

10. Dispersion of "Refractoriness" and Ventricular Tachycardia or Fibrillation After Myocardial Infarction...... 165
    Michiel J. Janse

11. The Electrophysiological Mechanism of Torsade de Pointes in the Long QT Syndrome...................................... 175
    Nabil El-Sherif, Gioia Turitto, Dmitry O. Kozhevnikov, and Mark Restivo

12. Spatial Dispersion of Ventricular Repolarization in the Long QT Syndrome... 199
    Carlo Napolitano, Silvia G. Priori, and Peter J. Schwartz

Dispersion of Ventricular Repolarization and Cardiac Disorders

13. Role of Ischemia on Dispersion of Repolarization................. 211
    Peter Taggart and Peter Sutton

14. Dispersion of Repolarization in Patients with Dilated Cardiomyopathy.. 229
    Wolfram Grimm, Katrin Leuchtenberger, and Bernhard Maisch

15. Dispersion of Repolarization in Patients with Hypertension 239
    Juha S. Perkiömäki

16. QT Dispersion in Patients with Congestive Heart Failure and Ventricular Arrhythmias 253
    Michel Galinier, Atul Pathak, Bruno Dongay, Daniel Curnier, Joelle Fourcade, Serge Boveda, and Jean-Paul Bounhoure

Dispersion of Ventricular Repolarization and Antiarrhythmic Treatment

17. Modulation of Dispersion of Ventricular Repolarization by Antiarrhythmic Drugs 267
    Stefan H. Hohnloser

18. Effect of Class I Drugs on Dispersion of Repolarization....... 279
    Lennart Bergfeldt

19. Effect of Class III Drugs on Dispersion of Repolarization in Patients with Myocardial Infarction 289
C.P. Day

20. Effect of Defibrillation on Dispersion of Repolarization 297
Paulus Kirchhof, C. Larissa Fabritz, Lars Eckardt, Günter Breithardt, Wilhelm Haverkamp, and Michael R. Franz

Index 319

Basic Studies

1

Electrical Heterogeneity and the Development of Arrhythmias

Charles Antzelevitch,
Wataru Shimizu, and
Gan-Xin Yan

Summary

Recent studies from a number of laboratories point to the presence of at least three electrophysiologically distinct cell types in ventricular myocardium: epicardial cells, endocardial cells, and M cells. Epicardial and M cells, but not endocardium, display action potentials with a notched or spike and dome morphology, the result of a prominent transient outward current (I_{to})-mediated phase 1. M cells are distinguished from endocardial and epicardial cells by the ability of their action potential to prolong disproportionately in response to a slowing of rate and/or to agents with Class III actions. This intrinsic electrical heterogeneity contributes to the inscription of the electrocardiogram (ECG) as well as to the development of a variety of cardiac arrhythmias. The transmural dispersion of early and late repolarization is in large part responsible for the inscription of the J wave and T wave of the ECG. Full repolarization of epicardium defines the peak of the T wave, and full repolarization of the M cells defines the end of the T wave. Thus the interval between the peak and the end of the T wave provides a valuable index of transmural dispersion of repolarization (TDR). Heterogeneous response of the three cell types to pharmacological agents and/or pathophysiological states often results

Supported by grants from the National Institutes of Health (HL 47678), the American Heart Association, New York State Affiliate, and the Masons of New York State and Florida.

From Olsson SB, Amlie JP, Yuan S (eds): *Dispersion of Ventricular Repolarization: State of the Art.* ©Futura Publishing Company, Inc., Armonk, NY, 2000.

in amplification of intrinsic electrical heterogeneities, thus providing a substrate as well as a trigger for the development of reentrant arrhythmias, including torsade de pointes (TdP), commonly associated with the long QT syndrome (LQTS), and the polymorphic ventricular tachycardia/ventricular fibrillation (VT/VF) encountered in the Brugada syndrome. In a model of the latter, early repolarization of the epicardial action potential results in abnormal *abbreviation* of action potential duration (APD) due to an all-or-none repolarization at the end of phase 1 of the epicardial action potential. Loss of the action potential dome in epicardium but not endocardium creates a large dispersion of repolarization across the ventricular wall, resulting in a transmural voltage gradient that manifests in the ECG as an ST segment elevation (or idiopathic J wave) and a vulnerable window during which reentry may be initiated by an extrasystole. Under these conditions, heterogeneous repolarization of the epicardial action potential gives rise to phase 2 reentry, which provides an extrasystole capable of precipitating VT/VF (or rapid TdP). Experimental models displaying these phenomena show ECG characteristics similar to those of the Brugada syndrome as well as those encountered during acute ischemia. TDR is also importantly amplified in LQTS. A much greater *prolongation* of the M cell action potential contributes to the development of long QT intervals, wide-based or notched T waves, and a large TDR, which provides the substrate for the development of a polymorphic VT closely resembling TdP. An early–afterdepolarization-induced triggered beat is thought to provide the extrasystole that precipitates TdP. Pharmacological models of the LQT1, LQT2, and LQT3 forms of LQTS mimic the distinctive electrocardiographic, electrophysiological, and pharmacological responses observed in patients with these three different genetic syndromes. In LQTS as in the Brugada syndrome, a mutation in an ion channel gene is responsible for the development of a large TDR, which creates an arrhythmogenic substrate capable of causing life-threatening cardiac arrhythmias.

Electrical Heterogeneity in the Heart

A growing number of studies report regional differences in the electrical properties of cells that comprise the ventricular myocardium (for reviews see Reference 1). Electrical and pharmacological distinctions between endocardium and epicardium of the canine, feline, rabbit, rat, and human heart have been described.[1,2] Distinctions in the electrophysiological characteristics and pharmacological responsiveness of M cells located in the deep structures of the canine, guinea pig, rabbit, and human ventricles have also been well documented in studies of enzymatically dissociated myocytes and tissues from the M region as well as of arterially perfused wedge preparations and in vivo models.[3-26]

Epicardial, endocardial, and M cells differ with respect to repolarization characteristics. Ventricular epicardium and M cells commonly display action potentials with a prominent notch, due to a prominent phase 1, which is largely due to a prominent 4-aminopyridine-sensitive I_{to}. The absence of a prominent notch in the endocardium is a consequence of a much smaller I_{to}. Regional differences in I_{to}, first suggested on the basis of action potential data,[27] have now been demonstrated using whole cell patch clamp techniques in canine,[4] feline,[28] rabbit,[29] rat,[30] and human[31,32] ventricular myocytes. Not only is I_{to} much larger in epicardium than in endocardium, it is also much larger in the right than the left ventricular epicardium. As a consequence, right ventricular epicardium displays a much more prominent action potential notch than left ventricular epicardium.[33] The transmural gradient in the amplitude of the I_{to}-mediated action potential notch underlies the normal J wave or Osborne wave of the ECG.[34,35] Exaggeration of this gradient has been linked to the appearance of pathophysiological J waves, ST segment elevation, and the development of VT/VF in the Brugada syndrome as well as in experimental models of acute ischemia.[36-39]

The M cell is distinguished by the ability of its action potential to prolong more than that of epicardium or endocardium in response to a slowing of rate and/or in response to APD-prolonging agents.[5,14,40] The ionic bases for these features of the M cell include the presence of a smaller slowly activating delayed rectifier current (I_{Ks})[10] but a larger late sodium current (late I_{Na}).[41] No transmural differences were observed in the rapidly activating delayed rectifier (I_{Kr}) and inward rectifier (I_{K1}) currents. Of note, transmural and apicobasal differences in the density of I_{Kr} channels have been described in the 11-week-old ferret heart.[42] I_{Kr} message and channel protein was found to be larger in the epicardium.

Histologically, M cells are similar to epicardial and endocardial cells. Electrophysiologically and pharmacologically, they represent a hybrid between Purkinje and ventricular cells (Table 1).

I_{Kr} blockers, including d-sotalol, E-4031, almokalant, and erythromycin, produce a much greater prolongation of APD in M cells than in epicardium or endocardium (Table 2). Surface epicardial and endocardial tissues when isolated from the canine left ventricle show very little response. A similar preferential prolongation of the M cell APD is seen with agents that increase calcium current (I_{Ca}), such as Bay K 8644, as well as with agents that increase late I_{Na} such as ATX-II and anthopleurin-A. An exception to this rule applies to agents that block I_{Ks}, including azimilide, quinidine, pentobarbital, amiodarone, and chromanol 293B. Chromanol 293B is the more specific of the I_{Ks} blockers. In isolated tissues, chromanol 293B produces a similar percentage prolongation of APD in the three transmural cell types. The situation is a bit more complicated for drugs affecting two or more ion channels, such as quinidine, pentobarbital,

Table 1
Electrophysiological Distinctions among Epicardial, Endocardial, M Cells, and Purkinje Fibers Isolated from the Canine Heart

	Purkinje	M Cells	Epicardial	Endocardial
Long APD, steep APD-rate	Yes	Yes	No	No
Develop EADs in response to agents with Class III actions	Yes	Yes	No	No
Develop DADs in response to digitalis, high Ca^{2+}, catecholamines	Yes	Yes	No	No
Display marked increase in APD in response to I_{Kr} blockers	Yes	Yes	No	No
Display marked increase in APD in response to I_{Ks} blockers	No	Yes	Yes	Yes
α1-Agonist-induced change in APD	↑	↓	↔	↔
V_{max}	High	Intermediate	Low in surface tissues	
Phase 4 depolarization	Yes	No	No	No
Depolarize in $[K^+]_o$ < 2.5 mmol/L	Yes	No	No	No
Acceleration-induced EADs and APD prolongation in presence of I_{Kr} block	No	Yes	No	No
EADs sensitive to $[Ca^{2+}]_i$	No	Yes	–	–
Develop DADs with Bay K 8644	No	Yes	No	No
Found in bundles	Yes	No	No	No

APD = action potential duration; DAD = delayed afterdepolarization; EAD = early afterdepolarization. Modified from Reference 1 with permission.

amiodarone, and azimilide. In the case of quinidine, relatively low therapeutic levels of the drug (3 to 5 μmol/L; 1.14 to 1.89 μg/mL) produce a marked prolongation of the M cell APD but not of epicardium and endocardium, consistent with a predominant effect of quinidine to block I_{Kr} at this concentration.[43-46] At higher concentrations (10 to 30 μmol/L; 3.78 to 11.37 μg/mL), quinidine produces a further prolongation of the epicardial and endocardial action potential, consistent with an effect of the drug to block I_{Ks}, but *abbreviates* the APD of the M cell, due to its action to block late I_{Na}.

Although transitional cells are found throughout the wall in the canine left ventricle, M cells displaying the longest action potentials (at basic cycle lengths ≥2000 ms) are often localized in the deep subendocardium to mid-myocardium in the anterior wall,[23] in the deep subepicardium to mid-myocardium in the lateral wall,[5] and throughout the wall in the

Table 2
Early Afterdepolarization-Induced Triggered Activity and/or
Prominent Action Potential Prolongation Recorded in
Isolated Epicardial, M, and Endocardial Tissue Slices

	Epicardium	Endocardium	M Cells
Quinidine (3-5 μmol/L)	–	–	+++
4-Aminopyridine (2.5-5 mmol/L)	–	–	+++
Amiloride (1-10 μmol/L)	–	–	++
Clofilium (1 μmol/L)	–	–	+++
Bay K 8644 (1 μmol/L)	–	–	++
Cesium (5-10 mmol/L)	–	–	++
Sotalol (100 μmol/L)	–	–	+++
Erythromycin (10-100 ug/mL)	–	–	+++
E-4031 (1-5 μmol/L)	–	–	+++
ATX-II (10-20 nmol/L)	+++	++	++++
Quinidine (>10 μmol/L)	+	++	++
Azimilide (5-10 μmol/L)	+	++	+++
Chromanol 293B (10-100 μmol/L)	+++	+++	+++

+/– = Little to no response; ++++ = Largest response. Modified from Reference 1 with permission.

region of the right ventricular outflow tracts.[1] M cells are also present in the deep layers of endocardial structures, including papillary muscles, trabeculae, and the interventricular septum.[8] Unlike Purkinje fibers, they are not found in discrete bundles. The first description of cells with an unusually long APD and rapid $\dot{V}_{max}$ was made in a papillary muscle preparation.[47]

In the canine left ventricle, M cells with the longest action potentials are found in the deep subendocardium, and transitions in APD_{90} are fairly gradual across the ventricular wall, except in the region between epicardium and deep subepicardium.[23] A sharp rise in tissue resistivity is measured in this region and is likely responsible for the sharp increase in APD_{90}. The increased tissue resistivity reduces electrotonic interaction, which allows cells in this region to exhibit more of their intrinsic properties. Thus, the degree of electrical heterogeneity across the intact ventricular wall depends on: 1) intrinsic action potential characteristics of neighboring cells; and 2) the extent to which they are electrically coupled in the syncytium.[48]

The shift in the position of the M cells from the deep subepicardium to the deep subendocardium appears to follow the transmural shift in the muscular layers that envelop the heart, as described by Streeter et al,[49,50] and more recently by Lunkenheimer and coworkers.[51]

Cells with the characteristics of M cells have been described in the canine, guinea pig, rabbit, and human ventricles.[3-25] Three studies have failed to discern M cells in the ventricles of the pig, guinea pig, and rat,[15,52,53] due largely to methodological problems.[1] Another study, while clearly demonstrating the presence of M cells in the ventricles of the canine heart in vitro, failed to delineate the unique cell type in vivo.[14,54] The combination of pentobarbital anesthesia, bipolar recording techniques, and use of high doses of quinidine, all of which strongly suppress TDR, may underlie the disparity.[1]

Because of the preferential response of M cells, agents with Class III actions and some ion channel mutations serve to amplify TDR, thus creating the substrate for the development of TdP.

Our principal focus in the remainder of this chapter is to examine how amplification of the transmural heterogeneities normally present in the early and late phases of the action potential can lead to the Brugada and LQTSs, respectively.

Brugada Syndrome

The Brugada syndrome is characterized by an ST segment elevation in the right precordial leads V_1 to V_3 (unrelated to ischemia, electrolyte abnormalities, or structural heart disease) and a high risk of sudden cardiac death[55-64] (for reviews see References 37, 39, and 65).

The incidence of the Brugada syndrome is greatest in males of Asian origin. The age at which the arrhythmic event occurs ranges between 2 and 77 years, with a mean age of 35 to 41 years.[57,64,65] A familial occurrence has long been recognized and an autosomal dominant mode of inheritance with variable expression has been described.[66] The Brugada syndrome appears unrelated to any chromosomal loci thus far described for arrhythmogenic right ventricular dysplasia (ARVD).[67] The only gene thus far linked to the Brugada syndrome is the cardiac sodium channel gene *SCN5A*.[68] Chen et al[68] described several mutations in *SCN5A* at sites other than those known to contribute to the LQT3 form of LQTS.

The cellular mechanism underlying this syndrome is thought to involve an outward shift of the current active at the end of phase 1 of the right ventricular epicardial action potential (where I_{to} is largest). Such a shift can cause all-or-none repolarization at the end of phase 1 and, thus, loss of the epicardial action potential dome, leading to marked abbreviation of the action potential. Some pathophysiological conditions (e.g., ischemia, metabolic inhibition, hypothermia) and some pharmacological interventions (e.g., I_{Na} or I_{Ca} blockers or I_{K-ATP} activators) have been shown to cause loss of the dome and abbreviation of the action potential in canine and feline ventricular cells in which I_{to} is prominent.

Under ischemic conditions and in response to a number of drugs, canine ventricular epicardium exhibits an all-or-none repolarization as a result of the rebalancing of currents flowing at the end of phase 1 of the action potential. Failure of the dome to develop occurs when outward currents (principally I_{to}) overwhelm the inward currents (chiefly I_{Ca}), resulting in a marked abbreviation of the action potential. The loss of the action potential dome in epicardium but not in endocardium creates a voltage gradient during phases 2 and 3 of the action potentials that manifests as an ST segment elevation. Studies involving the arterially perfused ventricular wedge preparation provide direct evidence in support of the hypothesis that loss or depression of the action potential dome in epicardium but not in endocardium underlies the development of a prominent ST segment elevation in the Brugada syndrome and in other syndromes associated with an ST segment elevation.[36,38]

Loss of the action potential dome at some epicardial sites but not others also leads to the development of a marked dispersion of repolarization within ventricular epicardium. Propagation of the action potential dome from sites at which it is maintained to sites at which it is lost causes local reexcitation by a mechanism termed "phase 2 reentry," leading to the development of a very closely coupled extrasystole, capable of initiating circus movement reentry.[69] Phase 2 reentry has been observed in canine epicardium exposed to: 1) K^+ channel openers such as pinacidil[70]; 2) sodium channel blockers such as flecainide[71]; 3) increased $[Ca^{2+}]_o$[72]; 4) metabolic inhibition[73]; and 5) simulated ischemia.[69] I_{to} block with 4-aminopyridine restores electrical homogeneity and abolishes reentrant activity in all cases.

Phase 2 reentry induces circus movement reentry in isolated sheets of right ventricular epicardium.[69] More recent studies have demonstrated these phenomena in the intact wall of the canine right ventricle (Fig. 1).[2,74] The arrhythmia often takes the form of a polymorphic VT, resembling a rapid TdP, which in some cases cannot be readily distinguished from VF. Investigators in the field have long appreciated the fact that circus movement reentry is more often than not precipitated by an extrasystole. The mechanism described here provides not only the substrate for the development of circus movement reentry in the form of epicardial and TDR, but also the phase 2 reentrant extrasystole that triggers the VT/VF episode.

A prominent I_{to} is a prerequisite for phase 2 reentry. Agents that inhibit I_{to}, including 4-aminopyridine and quinidine, are effective in restoring the action potential dome, and thus electrical homogeneity, and in aborting all arrhythmic activity in experimental models of this syndrome.[2,38] Class Ia and Ic antiarrhythmic agents that block I_{Na} but little to

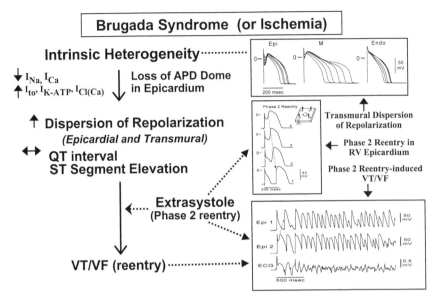

Figure 1. Proposed cellular and ionic mechanisms for the Brugada syndrome. The middle inset is modified from Reference 69, with permission.

no I_{to} (flecainide, ajmaline, and procainamide) exacerbate or unmask the Brugada syndrome, whereas those with actions to block both I_{Na} and I_{to} (quinidine and disopyramide) can exert an ameliorative effect.[38] The anticholinergic effects of quinidine and disopyramide may also contribute to their effectiveness. In the clinic, amiodarone and β-blockers have been shown to be without effect.[57] The only therapeutic measure with proven effectiveness is the implantable cardioverter-defibrillator. These findings highlight the need for a cardioselective I_{to} blocker, which may prove to be effective in the Brugada syndrome as well as other syndromes associated with an ST segment elevation.

Long QT Syndrome

The congenital and acquired (drug-induced) LQTSs are characterized by the development of long QT intervals in the ECG, abnormal T waves, and the atypical polymorphic tachycardia known as TdP.[75-79] Genetic linkage studies have identified four forms of the congenital LQTS caused by mutations in ion channel genes located on chromosomes 3, 7, 11, and 21. Mutations in *KvLQT1* and *minK (KCNE1)* are responsible for defects in I_{Ks}, which underlies the LQT1 and LQT5 forms of LQTS, whereas mutations in *HERG* and *SCN5A* are responsible for defects in the rapidly activating component of I_{Kr} and I_{Na}, which underlie the LQT2 and LQT3 syndromes.

Mutations in a *minK*-related protein MiRP1, which associates with *HERG* to form the I_{Kr} channel, appear responsible for the LQT6 form of LQTS.[80]

Recent studies have examined the electrophysiological, electrocardiographic, and pharmacological characteristics of the LQT1, LQT2, and LQT3 syndromes using arterially perfused canine left ventricular wedge preparations that permit simultaneous recording of transmembrane activity from epicardial, M, and endocardial or Purkinje sites and a pseudo-ECG along the same axis. This methodology makes possible correlation of transmembrane and electrocardiographic activity.[16,21-24,81] The wedge preparation is capable of developing and sustaining a variety of arrhythmias, including TdP. The pharmacological models mimic the clinical congenital syndromes with respect to prolongation of the QT interval, T wave morphology, rate dependence of repolarization, and response to antiarrhythmic drugs.[16,21-24]

Preferential prolongation of APD in cells in the M region underlie LQTS, contributing to the development of long QT intervals, abnormal T waves, and TdP (Figs. 2 and 3). Support for this hypothesis derives from a number of studies involving the arterially perfused wedge preparation.[16,21,23,24,81,82]

The I_{Ks} blocker chromanol 293B was used to mimic LQT1, and the β-adrenergic agonist isoproterenol was used to assess β-adrenergic influence. I_{Ks} block alone produced a homogeneous prolongation of repolarization and refractoriness across the ventricular wall and never induced arrhythmias. The addition of isoproterenol caused abbreviation of epicardial and endocardial APD with little or no change in the APD of the M cell, resulting in a marked augmentation of TDR and the development of spontaneous and stimulation-induced TdP.[21] These cellular changes give rise to a broad-based T wave and the long QT interval characteristics of LQT1. The development of TdP in the model is sensitive to β-adrenergic stimulation, consistent with a sensitivity of congenital LQTS, LQT1 in particular, to sympathetic stimulation.[78,83-88]

d-Sotalol, an I_{Kr} blocker, was used to mimic LQT2 and the most common acquired (drug-induced) form of LQTS. In this experimental model, a greater prolongation of the M cell action potential and slowing of phase 3 of the action potential of all three cell types results in a low-amplitude T wave, a long QT interval, a large TDR, and the development of spontaneous as well as stimulation-induced TdP (Figs. 2 and 3). The addition of hypokalemia gives rise to low-amplitude T waves with a deeply notched or bifurcated appearance, similar to those commonly seen in patients with the LQT2 syndrome.[16,24] Isoproterenol further exaggerates TDR, thus increasing the incidence of TdP.[89]

ATX-II was used to mimic LQT3. This agent increases late I_{Na} which helps to sustain the action potential plateau.[16] ATX-II markedly prolongs the QT interval, delays the onset of the T wave—in some cases also

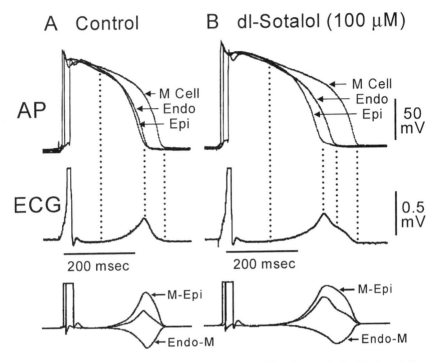

Figure 2. Voltage gradients on either side of the M region underlie the inscription of the electrocardiographic T wave. **Top:** Action potentials simultaneously recorded from endocardial, epicardial, and M region sites of an arterially perfused canine left ventricular wedge preparation. **Middle:** Electrocardiogram (ECG) recorded across the wedge. **Bottom:** Computed voltage differences between the epicardium and M region action potentials ($\Delta V_{M\text{-}Epi}$) and between the M region and endocardium responses ($\Delta V_{Endo\text{-}M}$). If these traces are representative of the opposing voltage gradients on either side of the M region, responsible for inscription of the T wave, then the weighted sum of the two traces should yield a trace (**middle trace in bottom grouping**) resembling the ECG, which it does. The voltage gradients are weighted to account for differences in tissue resistivity between M and Epi and Endo and M regions, thus yielding the opposing currents flowing on either side of the M region. **A.** Under control conditions the T wave begins when the plateau of epicardial action potential separates from that of the M cell. As epicardium repolarizes, the voltage gradient between epicardium and the M region continues to grow, giving rise to the ascending limb of the T wave. The voltage gradient between the M region and epicardium ($\Delta V_{M\text{-}Epi}$) reaches a peak when the epicardium is fully repolarized; this marks the peak of the T wave. On the other end of the ventricular wall, the endocardial plateau deviates from that of the M cell, generating an opposing voltage gradient ($\Delta V_{Endo\text{-}M}$) and corresponding current that limits the amplitude of the T wave and contributes to the initial part of the descending limb of the T wave. The voltage gradient between the endocardium and the M region reaches a peak when the endocardium is fully repolarized. The gradient continues to decline as the M cells repolarize. All gradients are extinguished when the longest M cells are fully repolarized. **B.** d-Sotalol (100 μmol/L) prolongs the action potential of the M cell more than those of the epicardial and endocardial cells, giving rise to a

widening it—and produces a sharp rise in TDR as a result of a greater prolongation of the APD of the M cell. The differential effect of ATX-II to prolong the M cell action potential is likely due to the presence of a larger late sodium current in the M cell.[41] ATX-II produces a marked delay in onset of the T wave because of a relatively large effect of the drug on epicardial and endocardial APD. This feature is consistent with the late-appearing T wave (long isoelectric ST segment) observed in patients with the LQT3 syndrome. Also in agreement with the clinical presentation of LQT3, the model displays a steep rate dependence of the QT interval and develops TdP at slow rates. Surprisingly, in the ATX-II model of LQT3, β-adrenergic influence in the form of isoproterenol, *reduces* TDR by abbreviating the APD of the M cell more than that of epicardium or endocardium, and thus reducing the incidence of TdP. While the β-adrenergic blocker propranolol is protective in LQT1 and LQT2 wedge models, it has the opposite effects in LQT3, acting to amplify transmural dispersion and promoting TdP.[89]

Torsade de Pointes

The LQTS can be life-threatening because it is accompanied by the development of TdP, an atypical polymorphic VT that can degenerate to VF. TdP has been reported in patients receiving potassium channel blockers such as d-sotalol and quinidine, usually at slow rates or after long pauses. These conditions are similar to those under which these agents induce early afterdepolarizations (EADs) and triggered activity in isolated Purkinje fibers and M cells, suggesting a role for EAD-induced triggered activity in the genesis of TdP. While EADs may underlie the premature beat that initiates TdP, recent studies provide evidence in support of circus movement reentry as the mechanism responsible for the maintenance of the arrhythmia.[1,3,16,17,21,24,78,81,90,91] In the wedge, TdP develops spontaneously in all three models and can be readily induced by introduction of a single premature beat to the epicardial surface (the site of earliest repolarization).

The available data provide support for the hypothesis presented in Figure 4. The hypothesis presumes the presence of electrical heterogeneity, principally in the form of TDR, under baseline conditions. This intrinsic

---

Figure 2 *(continued).* widening of the T wave and a prolongation of the QT interval. The greater separation of epicardial and endocardial repolarization times also gives rise to a notch in the descending limb of the T wave. Once again, the T wave begins when the plateau of epicardial action potential diverges from that of the M cell. The same relationships as described for **A** are observed during the remainder of the T wave. The d-sotalol-induced increase in dispersion of repolarization across the wall is accompanied by a corresponding increase in the T_{peak}-T_{end} interval in the pseudo-ECG. Modified from Reference 24 with permission.

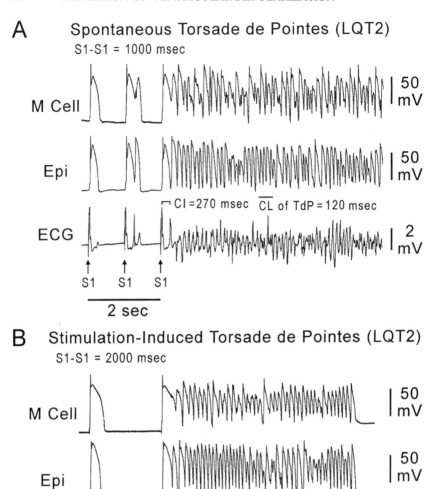

Figure 3. Spontaneous and stimulation-induced torsade de pointes developing in an arterially perfused canine left ventricular wedge pretreated with d-sotalol.

heterogeneity is amplified by agents that decrease net repolarizing current by reducing I_{Kr} or I_{Ks} or augmenting late I_{Ca} or late I_{Na} or by ion channel mutations that affect these currents and are responsible for the various forms of LQTS. I_{Kr} blockers and LQT2 mutations or late I_{Na} promoters and LQT3 mutations produce a preferential prolongation of the M cell action potential. As a consequence, the QT interval prolongs and is accompanied by a dramatic increase in TDR, which creates a vulnerable window for the development of reentry. The decrease in net repolarizing current can also give rise to EAD-induced triggered activity in M and Purkinje cells, which are responsible for the extrasystole that triggers TdP. β-Adrenergic agonists serve to further amplify transmural heterogeneity (transiently) in the case of I_{Kr} and LQT2, but to reduce it in the case of late I_{Na} enhancers or LQT3.[89] I_{Ks} blockers or LQT1 mutations cause a homogeneous prolongation of APD throughout the ventricular wall, leading to a prolongation of the QT interval but with no increase in TDR. Under these conditions, TdP does not occur spontaneously nor can it be induced by programmed stimulation until a β-adrenergic agonist is introduced. Isoproterenol dramatically increases transmural dispersion under these conditions by abbreviating the APD of epicardium and endocardium thus creating a vulnerable window that an EAD-induced trig-

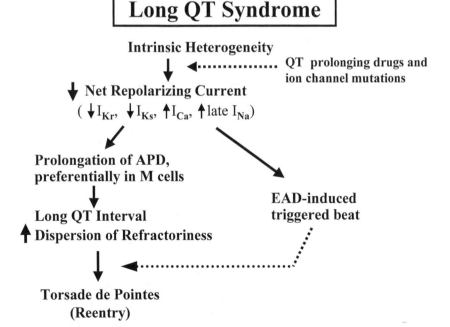

Figure 4. Proposed cellular and ionic mechanisms for the long QT syndrome.

gered response can capture to generate TdP, a circus movement arrhythmia.

We have highlighted two primary electrical diseases of the heart, displaying very different clinical phenotypes but sharing a final common pathway in the precipitation of VT/VF. The two syndromes share the ability to amplify the intrinsic heterogeneity that exists across the ventricular wall, in some cases by modifying the same gene (*SCN5A*) (Fig. 5).

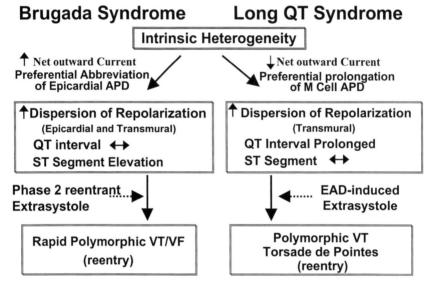

Figure 5. Similarities and differences in the mechanisms responsible for the development of arrhythmias in the Brugada and long QT syndromes.

References

1. Antzelevitch C, Shimizu W, Yan GX, et al. The M cell. Its contribution to the ECG and to normal and abnormal electrical function of the heart. *J Cardiovasc Electrophysiol* 1999;10:1124-1152.
2. Antzelevitch C, Yan GX, Shimizu W, Burashnikov A. Electrical heterogeneity, the ECG, and cardiac arrhythmias. In Zipes DP, Jalife J (eds): *Cardiac Electrophysiology: From Cell to Bedside.* 3rd ed. New York: W.B. Saunders Co.; 1999:222-238.
3. Antzelevitch C, Sicouri S. Clinical relevance of cardiac arrhythmias generated by afterdepolarizations: The role of M cells in the generation of U waves, triggered activity and torsade de pointes. *J Am Coll Cardiol* 1994;23:259-277.
4. Liu DW, Gintant GA, Antzelevitch C. Ionic bases for electrophysiological distinctions among epicardial, midmyocardial, and endocardial myocytes from the free wall of the canine left ventricle. *Circ Res* 1993;72:671-687.

5. Sicouri S, Antzelevitch C. A subpopulation of cells with unique electrophysiological properties in the deep subepicardium of the canine ventricle: The M cell. *Circ Res* 1991;68:1729-1741.

6. Sicouri S, Antzelevitch C. Drug-induced afterdepolarizations and triggered activity occur in a discrete subpopulation of ventricular muscle cell (M cells) in the canine heart: Quinidine and Digitalis. *J Cardiovasc Electrophysiol* 1993;4:48-58.

7. Sicouri S, Fish J, Antzelevitch C. Distribution of M cells in the canine ventricle. *J Cardiovasc Electrophysiol* 1994;5:824-837.

8. Sicouri S, Antzelevitch C. Electrophysiologic characteristics of M cells in the canine left ventricular free wall. *J Cardiovasc Electrophysiol* 1995;6:591-603.

9. Drouin E, Charpentier F, Gauthier C, et al. Electrophysiological characteristics of cells spanning the left ventricular wall of human heart: Evidence for the presence of M cells. *J Am Coll Cardiol* 1995;26:185-192.

10. Liu DW, Antzelevitch C. Characteristics of the delayed rectifier current (I_{Kr} and I_{Ks}) in canine ventricular epicardial, midmyocardial and endocardial myocytes: A weaker I_{Ks} contributes to the longer action potential of the M cell. *Circ Res* 1995;76:351-365.

11. Weissenburger J, Nesterenko VV, Antzelevitch C. Intramural monophasic action potentials (MAP) display steeper APD-rate relations and higher sensitivity to Class III agents than epicardial and endocardial MAPs: Characteristics of the M cell in vivo. *Circulation* 1995;92:I300. Abstract.

12. Sicouri S, Quist M, Antzelevitch C. Evidence for the presence of M cells in the guinea pig ventricle. *J Cardiovasc Electrophysiol* 1996;7:503-511.

13. Li GR, Feng J, Carrier M, Nattel S. Transmural electrophysiologic heterogeneity in the human ventricle. *Circulation* 1995;92:I158. Abstract.

14. Anyukhovsky EP, Sosunov EA, Rosen MR. Regional differences in electrophysiologic properties of epicardium, midmyocardium and endocardium: In vitro and in vivo correlations. *Circulation* 1996;94:1981-1988.

15. Rodriguez-Sinovas A, Cinca J, Tapias A, et al. Lack of evidence of M-cells in porcine left ventricular myocardium. *Cardiovasc Res* 1997;33:307-313.

16. Shimizu W, Antzelevitch C. Sodium channel block with mexiletine is effective in reducing dispersion of repolarization and preventing torsade de pointes in LQT2 and LQT3 models of the long-QT syndrome. *Circulation* 1997;96:2038-2047.

17. El-Sherif N, Caref EB, Yin H, Restivo M. The electrophysiological mechanism of ventricular arrhythmias in the long QT syndrome: Tridimensional mapping of activation and recovery patterns. *Circ Res* 1996;79:474-492.

18. Weirich J, Bernhardt R, Loewen N, et al. Regional- and species-dependent effects of K$^+$-channel blocking agents on subendocardium and mid-wall slices of human, rabbit, and guinea pig myocardium. *Pflugers Arch* 1996;431:R130. Abstract.

19. Burashnikov A, Antzelevitch C. Acceleration-induced action potential prolongation and early afterdepolarizations. *J Cardiovasc Electrophysiol* 1998;9:934-948.

20. Shimizu W, McMahon B, Antzelevitch C. Sodium pentobarbital reduces transmural dispersion of repolarization and prevents torsade de pointes in models of acquired and congenital long QT syndromes. *J Cardiovasc Electrophysiol* 1999;10:156-164.

21. Shimizu W, Antzelevitch C. Cellular basis for the electrocardiographic features of the LQT1 form of the long QT syndrome: Effects of ß-adrenergic agonists, antagonists and sodium channel blockers on transmural dispersion of repolarization and torsade de pointes. *Circulation* 1998;98:2314-2322.
22. Shimizu W, Antzelevitch C. Cellular and ionic basis for T wave alternans under long QT conditions. *Circulation* 1999;99:1499-1507.
23. Yan GX, Shimizu W, Antzelevitch C. Characteristics and distribution of M cells in arterially-perfused canine left ventricular wedge preparations. *Circulation* 1998;98:1921-1927.
24. Yan GX, Antzelevitch C. Cellular basis for the normal T wave and the electrocardiographic manifestations of the long QT syndrome. *Circulation* 1998; 98:1928-1936.
25. Balati B, Varro A, Papp JG. Comparison of the cellular electrophysiological characteristics of canine left ventricular epicardium, M cells, endocardium and Purkinje fibres [In Process Citation]. *Acta Physiol Scand* 1998;164:181-190.
26. Sicouri S, Moro S, Elizari MV. d-Sotalol induces marked action potential prolongation and early afterdepolarizations in M but not epicardial or endocardial cells of the canine ventricle. *J Cardiovasc Pharmacol Ther* 1997;2:27-38.
27. Litovsky SH, Antzelevitch C. Transient outward current prominent in canine ventricular epicardium but not endocardium. *Circ Res* 1988;62:116-126.
28. Furukawa T, Myerburg RJ, Furukawa N, et al. Differences in transient outward currents of feline endocardial and epicardial myocytes. *Circ Res* 1990; 67:1287-1291.
29. Fedida D, Giles WR. Regional variations in action potentials and transient outward current in myocytes isolated from rabbit left ventricle. *J Physiol (Lond)* 1991;442:191-209.
30. Clark RB, Bouchard RA, Salinas-Stefanon E, et al. Heterogeneity of action potential waveforms and potassium currents in rat ventricle. *Cardiovasc Res* 1993;27:1795-1799.
31. Wettwer E, Amos GJ, Posival H, Ravens U. Transient outward current in human ventricular myocytes of subepicardial and subendocardial origin. *Circ Res* 1994;75:473-482.
32. Nabauer M, Beuckelmann DJ, Uberfuhr P, Steinbeck G. Regional differences in current density and rate-dependent properties of the transient outward current in subepicardial and subendocardial myocytes of human left ventricle. *Circulation* 1996;93:168-177.
33. Di Diego JM, Sun ZQ, Antzelevitch C. I_{to} and action potential notch are smaller in left vs. right canine ventricular epicardium. *Am J Physiol* 1996;271:H548-H561.
34. Yan GX, Antzelevitch C. Cellular basis for the electrocardiographic J wave. *Circulation* 1996;93:372-379.
35. Antzelevitch C, Sicouri S, Lukas A, et al. Regional differences in the electrophysiology of ventricular cells: Physiological and clinical implications. In Zipes DP, Jalife J (eds): *Cardiac Electrophysiology: From Cell to Bedside.* Philadelphia: W.B. Saunders Co.; 1995:228-245.
36. Antzelevitch C. The Brugada syndrome. *J Cardiovasc Electrophysiol* 1998; 9:513-516.
37. Gussak I, Antzelevitch C, Bjerregaard P, et al. The Brugada syndrome: Clinical, electrophysiological and genetic aspects. *J Am Coll Cardiol* 1999;33:5-15.
38. Yan GX, Antzelevitch C. Cellular basis for the Brugada syndrome and other mechanisms of arrhythmogenesis associated with ST segment elevation. *Circulation* 1999;100:1660-1666.

39. Antzelevitch C, Brugada P, Brugada J, et al. *The Brugada Syndrome*. Armonk: Futura Publishing Co., Inc.; 1999:1-99.
40. Antzelevitch C, Sicouri S, Litovsky SH, et al. Heterogeneity within the ventricular wall: Electrophysiology and pharmacology of epicardial, endocardial and M cells. *Circ Res* 1991;69:1427-1449.
41. Eddlestone GT, Zygmunt AC, Antzelevitch C. Larger late sodium current contributes to the longer action potential of the M cell in canine ventricular myocardium. *PACE* 1996;19:II569. Abstract.
42. Brahmajothi MV, Morales MJ, Reimer KA, Strauss HC. Regional localization of ERG, the channel protein responsible for the rapid component of the delayed rectifier, K^+ current in the ferret heart. *Circ Res* 1997;81:128-135.
43. Sicouri S, Moro S, Litovsky SH, et al. Chronic amiodarone reduces transmural dispersion of repolarization in the canine heart. *J Cardiovasc Electrophysiol* 1997;8:1269-1279.
44. Sun ZQ, Eddlestone GT, Antzelevitch C. Ionic mechanisms underlying the effects of sodium pentobarbital to diminish transmural dispersion of repolarization. *PACE* 1997;20:1116. Abstract.
45. Conder ML, Smith MA, Atwal KS, McCullough JR. Effects of NE-10064 on K^+ currents in cardiac cells. *Biophys J* 1994;66:A326. Abstract.
46. Condor MD, Hess TA, Smith MA, et al. The effects of NE-10064 on cardiac sodium channels. *FASEB J* 1994;8(5 pt. 2):A609. Abstract.
47. Solberg LE, Singer DH, Ten Eick RE, Duffin EG. Glass microelectrode studies on intramural papillary muscle cells. *Circ Res* 1974;34:783-797.
48. Viswanathan PC, Shaw RM, Rudy Y. Effects of I_{Kr} and I_{Ks} heterogeneity on action potential duration and its rate-dependence: A simulation study. *Circulation* 1999;99:2466-2474.
49. Streeter DD, Spotnitz HM, Patel DP, et al. Fiber orientation in the canine left ventricle during diastole and systole. *Circ Res* 1969;24:339-347.
50. Streeter DD. Gross morphology and fiber geometry of the heart. In Berne RM (ed): *Handbook of Physiology. Section 2: The Cardiovascular System*. Baltimore: Waverly Press, Inc.; 1979:61-112.
51. Lunkenheimer PP, Redmann K, Scheld H, et al. The heart muscle's putative secondary structure. Functional implications of a band-like anisotropy. *Technol Health Care* 1997;5:53-64.
52. Bryant SM, Wan X, Shipsey SJ, Hart G. Regional differences in the delayed rectifier current (I_{Kr} and I_{Ks}) contribute to the differences in action potential duration in basal left ventricular myocytes in guinea-pig. *Cardiovasc Res* 1998;40:322-331.
53. Shipsey SJ, Bryant SM, Hart G. Effects of hypertrophy on regional action potential characteristics in the rat left ventricle: A cellular basis for T-wave inversion? *Circulation* 1997;96:2061-2068.
54. Anyukhovsky EP, Sosunov EA, Gainullin RZ, Rosen MR: The controversial M cell. *J Cardiovasc Electrophysiol* 1999;10:244-260.
55. Brugada P, Brugada J. Right bundle branch block, persistent ST segment elevation and sudden cardiac death: A distinct clinical and electrocardiographic syndrome: A multicenter report. *J Am Coll Cardiol* 1992;20:1391-1396.
56. Brugada J, Brugada P. Further characterization of the syndrome of right bundle branch block, ST segment elevation, and sudden cardiac death. *J Cardiovasc Electrophysiol* 1997;8:325-331.
57. Brugada J, Brugada R, Brugada P. Right bundle-branch block and ST-segment elevation in leads V_1 through V_3. A marker for sudden death in patients without demonstrable structural heart disease. *Circulation* 1998;97:457-460.

58. Aizawa Y, Tamura M, Chinushi M, et al. Idiopathic ventricular fibrillation and bradycardia-dependent intraventricular block. *Am Heart J* 1993;126:1473-1474.
59. Aizawa Y, Tamura M, Chinushi M, et al. An attempt at electrical catheter ablation of the arrhythmogenic area in idiopathic ventricular fibrillation. *Am Heart J* 1992;123:257-260.
60. Bjerregaard P, Gussak I, Kotar SL, Gessler JE. Recurrent syncope in a patient with prominent J-wave. *Am Heart J* 1994;127:1426-1430.
61. Martini B, Nava A, Thiene G, et al. Ventricular fibrillation without apparent heart disease: Description of six cases. *Am Heart J* 1989;118:1203-1209.
62. Miyazaki T, Mitamura H, Miyoshi S, et al. Autonomic and antiarrhythmic drug modulation of ST segment elevation in patients with Brugada syndrome. *J Am Coll Cardiol* 1996;27:1061-1070.
63. Kasanuki H, Ohnishi S, Ohtuka M, et al. Idiopathic ventricular fibrillation induced with vagal activity in patients without obvious heart disease. *Circulation* 1997;95:2277-2285.
64. Nademanee K. Sudden unexplained death syndrome in southeast Asia. *Am J Cardiol* 1997;79(6A):10-11.
65. Marcus FI. Idiopathic ventricular fibrillation. *J Cardiovasc Electrophysiol* 1997;8:1075-1083.
66. Corrado D, Nava A, Buja G, et al. Familial cardiomyopathy underlies syndrome of right bundle branch block, ST segment elevation and sudden death [see comments]. *J Am Coll Cardiol* 1996;27:443-448.
67. Ahmed F, Li D, Karibe A, et al. Localization of a gene responsible for arrhythmogenic right ventricular dysplasia to chromosome 3p23. *Circulation* 1998;98:2791-2795.
68. Chen Q, Kirsch GE, Zhang D, et al. Genetic basis and molecular mechanisms for idiopathic ventricular fibrillation. *Nature* 1997;392:293-296.
69. Lukas A, Antzelevitch C. Phase 2 reentry as a mechanism of initiation of circus movement reentry in canine epicardium exposed to simulated ischemia. The antiarrhythmic effects of 4-aminopyridine. *Cardiovasc Res* 1996;32:593-603.
70. Di Diego JM, Antzelevitch C. Pinacidil-induced electrical heterogeneity and extrasystolic activity in canine ventricular tissues: Does activation of ATP-regulated potassium current promote phase 2 reentry? *Circulation* 1993;88:1177-1189.
71. Krishnan SC, Antzelevitch C. Flecainide-induced arrhythmia in canine ventricular epicardium: Phase 2 reentry? *Circulation* 1993;87:562-572.
72. Di Diego JM, Antzelevitch C. High [Ca^{2+}]-induced electrical heterogeneity and extrasystolic activity in isolated canine ventricular epicardium: Phase 2 reentry. *Circulation* 1994;89:1839-1850.
73. Antzelevitch C, Sicouri S, Lukas A, et al. Clinical implications of electrical heterogeneity in the heart: The electrophysiology and pharmacology of epicardial, M and endocardial cells. In Podrid PJ, Kowey PR (eds): *Cardiac Arrhythmia: Mechanism, Diagnosis and Management.* Baltimore: Williams & Wilkins; 1995:88-107.
74. Antzelevitch C, Shimizu W, Yan GX, Sicouri S. Cellular basis for QT dispersion. *J Electrocardiol* 1998;30(suppl):168-175.
75. Schwartz PJ, Periti M, Malliani A. The long QT syndrome. *Am Heart J* 1975;89:378-390.
76. Moss AJ, Schwartz PJ, Crampton RS, et al. The long QT syndrome: A prospective international study. *Circulation* 1985;71:17-21.

77. Zipes DP. The long QT interval syndrome: A Rosetta stone for sympathetic related ventricular tachyarrhythmias. *Circulation* 1991;84:1414-1419.
78. Shimizu W, Ohe T, Kurita T, et al. Effects of verapamil and propranolol on early afterdepolarizations and ventricular arrhythmias induced by epinephrine in congenital long QT syndrome. *J Am Coll Cardiol* 1995;26:1299-1309.
79. Roden DM, Lazzara R, Rosen MR, et al. Multiple mechanisms in the long-QT syndrome: Current knowledge, gaps, and future directions. *Circulation* 1996;94:1996-2012.
80. Abbott GW, Sesti F, Splawski I, et al. MiRP1 forms I_{Kr} potassium channels with HERG and is associated with cardiac arrhythmia. *Cell* 1999;97:175-187.
81. Antzelevitch C, Sun ZQ, Zhang ZQ, Yan GX. Cellular and ionic mechanisms underlying erythromycin-induced long QT and torsade de pointes. *J Am Coll Cardiol* 1996;28:1836-1848.
82. Shimizu W, Antzelevitch C. Characteristics of spontaneous as well as stimulation-induced torsade de pointes in LQT2 and LQT3 models of the long QT syndrome. *Circulation* 1997;96:I554. Abstract.
83. Schwartz PJ. The idiopathic long QT syndrome: Progress and questions. *Am Heart J* 1985;109:399-411.
84. Moss AJ, Schwartz PJ, Crampton RS, et al. The long QT syndrome: Prospective longitudinal study of 328 families. *Circulation* 1991;84:1136-1144.
85. Crampton RS. Preeminence of the left stellate ganglion in the long Q-T syndrome. *Circulation* 1979;59:769-778.
86. Timothy KW, Zhang L, Meyer KJ, Vincent GM. Differences in precipitators of cardiac arrest and sudden death in chromosome 11 versus 7 genotype long QT syndrome patients. *Circulation* 1996;94:I204. Abstract.
87. Ali RH, Zareba W, Rosero SZ, et al. Adrenergic triggers and non-adrenergic factors associated with cardiac events in long QT syndrome patients. *PACE* 1997;20:1072. Abstract.
88. Schwartz PJ, Malteo PS, Moss AJ, et al. Gene-specific influence on the triggers for cardiac arrest in the long QT syndrome. *Circulation* 1997;96:I212. Abstract.
89. Shimizu W, Antzelevitch C. Differential effects of ß-adrenergic agonists and antagonists on transmural dispersion of repolarization and torsade de pointes in LQT1, LQT2 and LQT3 models of the long QT syndrome. *Circulation* 1998;98:I10. Abstract.
90. El-Sherif N, Chinushi M, Caref EB, Restivo M. Electrophysiological mechanism of the characteristic electrocardiographic morphology of torsade de pointes tachyarrhythmias in the long-QT syndrome. Detailed analysis of ventricular tridimensional activation patterns. *Circulation* 1997;96:4392-4399.
91. Akar FG, Yan GX, Antzelevitch C, Rosenbaum DS. Optical maps reveal reentrant mechanism of torsade de pointes based on topography and electrophysiology of mid-myocardial cells. *Circulation* 1997;96(8):I355. Abstract.

2

Repolarization Inhomogeneities in Ventricular Myocardium:
Studies Using the Optical Mapping Technique

Fadi G. Akar, Joseph M. Pastore,
Kenneth R. Laurita, and David S. Rosenbaum

Ventricular dispersion of repolarization (DOR) has long been associated with susceptibility to reentrant arrhythmias.[1,2] Theoretically, the manifestation of DOR depends on two factors: 1) the intrinsic variation of action potential characteristics of cells, and 2) the extent of intercellular electrical coupling between adjacent cells.[3] Previously, it was assumed that partial uncoupling, such as in ischemia or infarction, is required for the formation of an arrhythmogenic substrate. In this chapter, we focus on heterogeneities of repolarization present in well-coupled (i.e., normal) myocardium, and their role in promoting arrhythmias.

Although heterogeneity of ionic properties of cells isolated from various regions of the heart is well documented,[4] the extent to which ionic current heterogeneities are functionally expressed in the normal heart is not known. Due to limitations of conventional electrophysiological recording techniques, quantitative assessment of spatial gradients of cellular repolarization has been difficult. In recent years the technique of high-resolution optical action potential mapping has been used increasingly to investigate the extent to which spatial diversity of cellular repolarization properties influence the formation of DOR in the normal heart.[5-7]

From Olsson SB, Amlie JP, Yuan S (eds): *Dispersion of Ventricular Repolarization: State of the Art.* ©Futura Publishing Company, Inc., Armonk, NY, 2000.

Cellular repolarization is closely associated with susceptibility to arrhythmias, and hence, a detailed study of its dynamics across the heart is of considerable interest. Moreover, the expression of outward ionic currents responsible for both early and late phases of repolarization has been shown to vary considerably across the heart. For example, a relatively strong expression of the transient outward potassium current, I_{to}, in epicardial cells is responsible for their distinct "spike and dome" morphology. Also due to their strong I_{to} content, epicardial cells have shorter action potential durations (APDs) at normal heart rates than do endocardial cells, which are essentially devoid of I_{to}.[8-10] On the other hand, M cells, located in midmyocardial layers, exhibit a relatively low density of the slowly activating delayed rectifier potassium current, I_{ks}. Due to their unique ionic composition (i.e., weak late repolarizing currents), M cells display an enhanced sensitivity to interventions that prolong APD such as bradycardia and Class III antiarrhythmic drugs.[11-16]

In addition to differences in the electrophysiological properties of cells isolated from various layers of myocardium, we have recently shown that cellular kinetics of repolarization vary across even a single layer of myocardium.[17,18] Specifically, we found that the cellular kinetics of repolarization across the guinea pig ventricular epicardium are heterogeneous, varying systematically from apex to base.[17]

With these recent findings, it is becoming abundantly apparent that heterogeneities of cellular repolarization properties exist not only between cells of different chambers of the heart (i.e., atria, ventricles, nodal tissue), but also in cells of different muscle layers of individual chambers (i.e., epicardial, midmyocardial, endocardial), and even within a single muscle layer (apical ventricle versus basal ventricle). As is discussed, such diversity in electrophysiological characteristics of cellular ionic properties can strongly influence the formation of arrhythmogenic substrates, even in the normal heart.

Transepicardial Gradients of Repolarization

It had been assumed for some time that cells forming a certain layer of myocardium are identical in terms of their ionic compositions, and hence generate identical action potentials. With the advent of optical mapping, which allows for the high-resolution recording of action potentials from hundreds of sites simultaneously in the intact heart,[19] it has become apparent that heterogeneities of cellular electrical behavior are in fact present across a single layer of myocardium, the epicardial surface.

We and others have shown that the APDs of cells located in the basal region of the anterior surface of the guinea pig left ventricle are longer than those of cells located near the apex.[6,7] The gradual increase in APD from apex to base (i.e., transepicardial APD gradient) is present during normoxic perfusion of the heart and under steady state pacing and, hence, is an intrinsic property of normal myocardium.

Intrinsic APD gradients present in the normal heart during both baseline pacing and sinus rhythm can result in further heterogeneities of repolarization when an abrupt change in the basic cycle length (BCL) occurs, such as the case during a premature ventricular beat. For example, as BCL is shortened, APD is altered heterogeneously due to the intrinsic gradient of baseline APD present at the time of the BCL change. We have shown that apical and basal myocardium manifest inherently different responses to BCL shortening, suggesting a difference in their restitution kinetics.[20]

Restitution Kinetics in the Normal Heart are Heterogeneous

APD restitution refers to the process by which a cell's action potential responds to a premature beat.[21-23] Although APD usually shortens exponentially with a decreasing diastolic interval (DI), this relationship is not always maintained. In some species, such as the rabbit, APD paradoxically lengthens with decreasing DI over certain portions of the restitution curve.[21] Since cellular restitution is thought to reflect the time-dependent kinetics of membrane ionic currents governing repolarization, heterogeneity in the spatial distribution or expression of ion channel function could manifest itself as a heterogeneity of restitution between cells. During premature stimulation of the heart, intercellular heterogeneity of restitution kinetics may significantly influence the ensuing pattern of repolarization, thereby profoundly affecting DOR.

Conventional electrophysiological recording techniques are limited to measuring action potentials at only a few sites, and thus determining the role of cellular heterogeneities of restitution on repolarization at the whole heart or tissue levels has been difficult. Optical mapping with voltage-sensitive dyes, on the other hand, enables the measurement of action potentials with high voltage and spatial resolutions from hundreds of recording sites. Also, optical action potentials represent an average of local transmembrane activity and are not sensitive to biological variability between individual myocytes.[19] This makes optical mapping well suited for measuring intrinsic (i.e., cellular) properties of intact preparations.

Heterogeneities of cellular restitution along the epicardial surface and their role in the formation of an arrhythmogenic substrate were investigated. APD restitution was measured simultaneously from 128 recording sites using the protocol described in Figure 1 (panel A). The relationship between APD following a premature stimulus (APD_p) and the preceding

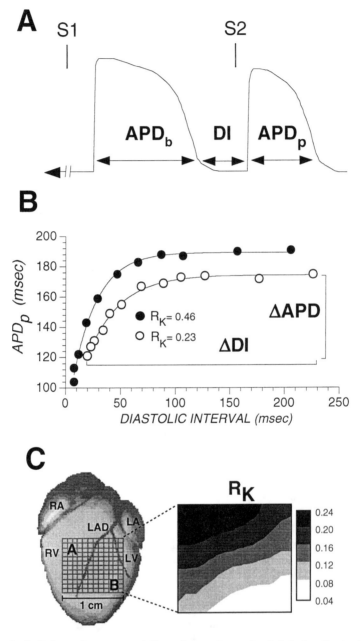

Figure 1. A. Schematic representation of an action potential during the last beat of a 50-beat baseline drive train (S1) and a single premature beat (S2). Superimposed are: APD_b = action potential duration (APD) of the baseline beat; DI = diastolic interval; APD_p = APD of the premature beat. **B.** Two restitution curves

DI is illustrated in Figure 1. Although for the majority of recording sites restitution followed a single exponential curve, nonexponential behavior was not uncommon.[6] Due to variations in the characteristics of restitution curves measured from hundreds of sites across the epicardial surface, we avoided defining a mathematical relationship between APD and DI a priori. Instead, we defined an empirical restitution rate constant, R_K, which did not assume a preset mathematical relation between APD and DI.[6] Greater values of R_K indicated a faster time course of restitution and a greater degree of APD adaptation for a given change in DI.

Shown in panel B of Figure 1 are restitution curves measured from two ventricular sites, one where APD varied relatively slowly with DI ($R_K = 0.23$) and the other where APD varied rapidly ($R_K = 0.46$). The spatial variation of restitution across the epicardial surface is shown in panel C of Figure 1. R_K normally ranged between 0.04 and 0.24, varying by as much as 500% within an area of $1\ cm^2$. Moreover, spatial heterogeneity of R_K was not random; rather, an organized gradient of R_K across the epicardial surface was observed. In particular, the gradient of R_K was oriented parallel to cardiac fibers, despite the high degree of electrotonic coupling between cells in this direction. These findings suggest the presence of considerable heterogeneity of membrane ionic processes in the apicobasal direction, enough to overcome the homogenizing effects of electrotonic interactions.

Epicardial Restitution Heterogeneity Promotes DOR

Heterogeneity of restitution kinetics between cells across the epicardial surface is expected to appreciably influence the sequence and pattern

---

Figure 1 *(continued)*. calculated from action potentials recorded in guinea pig, one at a site where APD_b was longest (closed circles) and the other where APD_b was shortest (open circles). Shown are the parameters used to estimate the rate constant of restitution (R_K) at the site where R_K was smallest, where ΔAPD is the extent of APD_p shortening over the range of diastolic intervals tested (ΔDI). R_K was also calculated (parameters not shown) at the site where R_K was greatest for comparison. We found that R_K is a robust measure of the kinetics of the rapid phase of the restitution response since its relative magnitude is insensitive to the specific range of diastolic intervals used to define it, provided this range is consistently defined for each site and that the maximum diastolic interval is taken from the flat portion of the restitution curve. **C.** Diagram of the mapping field ($1\ cm^2$ grid) and its position relative to the intact guinea pig heart preparation. Spatial dispersion of restitution kinetics (R_K) calculated from a representative experiment (not the same as in **B**) is shown in the contour map. The distribution of R_K was essentially identical when pacing was performed from site A and B, indicating that R_K was independent of propagation direction and was a suitable measure of restitution properties intrinsic to each cell. RA = right atrium; LA = left atrium; RV = right ventricle; LV = left ventricle; LAD = left anterior descending coronary artery.

of repolarization following a premature beat. Shown in Figure 2 is the pattern of depolarization (panels A, C, and E) and repolarization (panels B, D, and F) during baseline ventricular pacing (left), premature stimulation at an intermediate coupling interval (center), and at a coupling interval just beyond (<2 ms) the effective refractory period of the baseline beat (right). During baseline pacing, the impulse propagated uniformly from the site of stimulation (panel A), and a significant gradient of repolarization was present, with latest repolarization occurring near the base of the heart and earliest repolarization occurring near the apex (panel B). The repolarization gradient (solid arrow) during baseline pacing was generally

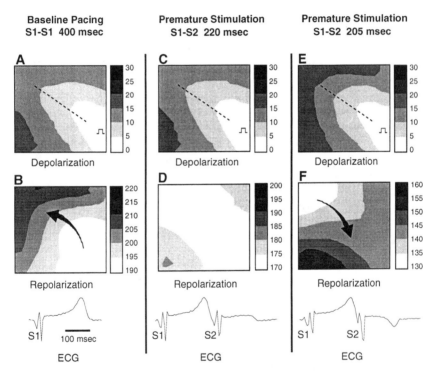

Figure 2. Contour maps of depolarization (**A, C,** and **E**) and repolarization (**B, D,** and **F**) during baseline pacing (**A, B**), a premature stimulus at an intermediate coupling interval (**C, D**), and a premature stimulus at a coupling interval near the refractory period (**E, F**), measured from the epicardial surface of a guinea pig. The electrocardiogram (ECG) recorded during the last baseline beat (S1) and the premature stimulus (S2) is shown across the bottom. Depolarization and repolarization times are in milliseconds. The site of pacing (⊓ symbol) was identical for all recordings. The dashed lines (**A, C,** and **E**) indicate epicardial fiber direction. In contrast to depolarization, the gradient of repolarization (solid arrow) was markedly influenced by a premature stimulus. Reduced heterogeneity (**D**) and inversion of repolarization gradients (**F**) are reflected in the ECG by T wave flattening (bottom middle) and inversion (bottom right), respectively.

oriented in an apex-to-base direction, parallel to cardiac muscle fibers (dashed line).

A premature stimulus introduced at an intermediate coupling interval produced no significant change in the pattern of depolarization (panel C); however, it essentially eradicated the repolarization gradient present during baseline pacing (panel D). In contrast, a premature stimulus introduced at a very short coupling interval resulted in a slight slowing of conduction velocity as evidenced by the crowding of isochrone lines (panel E). The overall pattern of depolarization, however, remained unchanged. Importantly, repolarization following the tightly coupled premature stimulus changed substantially as the gradient of repolarization was reestablished. However, the orientation of the repolarization gradient was completely reversed compared to that during baseline pacing. We have termed such profound coupling interval "dependent alteration of dispersion gradients modulated dispersion."[17] Interestingly, the eradication and subsequent reversal of the repolarization gradient by intermediate and short premature coupling intervals, respectively, were paralleled by the flattening and subsequent inversion of the electrocardiographic T wave. This suggested that dispersion gradients were modulated throughout the myocardium and not only in the mapping region shown in Figure 2.

Modulated dispersion can be explained by heterogeneity of cellular restitution kinetics across the epicardial surface. In general, where APD during baseline pacing (APD_b) is longest, R_K is fastest and vice versa. Since R_K is faster at sites having longer APD_b, APD_p shortened more rapidly at these sites compared with sites with shorter APD_b (i.e., smaller R_K), effectively eliminating repolarization heterogeneity across the epicardial surface. With further shortening of S1S2 coupling interval, cells initially having the longest APD now displayed the shortest APD because of their relatively fast R_K. Thus, the APD gradient was restored but was oriented in the opposite direction.

The timing of repolarization of a cardiac myocyte is determined by the sum of the time required for the impulse to propagate to and depolarize that myocyte, and the myocyte{{quotesingle}}s intrinsic APD. Therefore, spatial heterogeneity of repolarization between cells is determined by the combined effect of conduction gradients (i.e., conduction velocity) and spatial gradients of APD. Our data indicate that the magnitude and orientation of repolarization gradients are primarily determined by changes in spatial distribution of APD. There is also evidence suggesting that this may be the case under conditions of abnormal repolarization. For example, in experimental models of congenital long QT syndrome, DOR is predominantly caused by regional heterogeneity of APD.[5] On the other hand, in the case of chronic myocardial infarction when conduction is markedly slowed, propagation delays may play a more significant role in promoting heterogeneity of ventricular repolarization. Thus, the factors contributing to DOR in the heart are dependent on the specific pathophysiological substrate involved.

Modulated Dispersion Affects Susceptibility to Ventricular Fibrillation

Premature impulses are traditionally viewed as "triggers," which, in the presence of a suitable arrhythmogenic "substrate," can promote reentrant excitation. Our data, however, demonstrate a dynamic interrelationship between the trigger and the substrate. In addition to acting as an arrhythmogenic trigger, a premature stimulus actively modulates the underlying electrophysiological properties of the heart. Classically, it is known that premature stimuli delivered at progressively shorter coupling intervals shorten refractoriness at the stimulus site, allowing capture of subsequent stimuli at increasing degrees of prematurity. By shortening the cardiac wavelength via their effect on APD, premature stimuli may increase the likelihood of inducing reentry (a concept similar to "peeling back" refractoriness). Modulated dispersion, by taking into account the delicate interaction between the premature impulse and the underlying electrophysiological substrate, offers an alternative hypothesis. In addition to shortening refractoriness, the premature stimulus is believed to alter the arrhythmogenic substrate by modulating spatial DOR in a coupling-interval–dependent manner. The modulated dispersion hypothesis was tested using high-resolution action potential mapping with voltage-sensitive dye as a tool for assessing the formation of DOR in the wake of premature stimuli. Vulnerability to ventricular fibrillation (VF) following a premature beat was quantified using a modified VF threshold (VFT) protocol, where a train (100 Hz) of S3 pulses were applied during the T wave of the premature beat (S2). The minimum current strength that successfully initiated VF was defined as the VFT (i.e., S3-VFT). S3-VFT was measured as DOR was modulated over a broad range of S1S2 coupling intervals.

To quantitatively determine the relationship between S1S2 coupling interval and ventricular repolarization properties, mean repolarization time (S2-RT) and DOR time (S2-DISP) were calculated for each S1S2 coupling interval. Shown in Figure 3 (panel A) are S2-RT (open circles) and S2-DISP (closed circles) generated during each prematurely stimulated beat. In a representative experiment, S2-RT decreased monotonically from 221 ms to 145 ms as S1S2 coupling interval was shortened from 300 ms to 230 ms. These changes were attributed to coupling-interval–dependent changes in APD, which were largest at short S1S2 coupling intervals, as predicted from restitution properties of cardiac myocytes. In contrast, as coupling interval was shortened, DOR was modulated in a biphasic fashion. For S1S2 coupling intervals near the baseline pacing

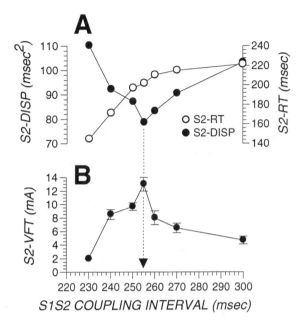

Figure 3. A. Mean repolarization (S2-RT; open circles) and dispersion of repolarization (S2-DISP; filled circles) of an S2 premature beat as a function of S1S2 coupling interval. These values were calculated from 128 optical action potentials recorded from the epicardial surface of guinea pig ventricle. Dispersion of repolarization was calculated by the variance of repolarization times measured over the entire mapping field. **B.** Changes in vulnerability to ventricular fibrillation induced by an S3 pulse train (S3-VFT) in the wake of repolarization patterns induced by various S1S2 coupling intervals. Dispersion of repolarization (**A**, filled circles) and vulnerability to fibrillation (**B**) were modulated in a similar biphasic fashion, with minimum vulnerability (i.e., maximum S3-VFT) and minimum dispersion occurring at the same S1S2 coupling interval (255 ms, dashed arrow). Reproduced from Reference 6.

rate, DOR was relatively high, decreasing as S1S2 coupling interval was shortened to a critical value (255 ms; Fig. 3, dashed arrow). With further shortening of S1S2 coupling interval, DOR rose sharply to a level slightly higher than that measured during baseline pacing.

Illustrated in Figure 3 (panel B) is the effect of cycle-length–dependent modulation of repolarization on susceptibility to VF. Clearly, vulnerability of the heart to VF, as measured by the S3-VFT protocol, was modulated in a biphasic fashion in parallel to DOR (filled circles, panel A). As S1S2 coupling interval was shortened to a critical value (Fig. 3, dashed arrow), S3-VFT increased (i.e., vulnerability decreased). With further shortening of S1S2, however, S3-VFT decreased (i.e., vulnerability increased) to levels below those present at baseline pacing. These data indicate that the electrophysiological substrate for VF is not static but can potentially form, disappear, and reform in a predictable fashion during a perturbation of stimulus cycle length.

It is generally assumed that the shortening of a premature stimulus coupling interval increases the likelihood of inducing reentry. However, Figure 3 illustrates a paradoxical decrease in arrhythmia vulnerability as premature stimulus coupling interval was initially shortened over a broad range of coupling intervals. The attenuation of repolarization gradients by a premature stimulus may serve as a protective mechanism in electrophysiologically normal myocardium. These findings further illustrate the importance of accounting for global changes in DOR throughout the heart, and not just the refractory period at one site, for the development of a more comprehensive understanding of arrhythmia-prone electrophysiological substrates.

Role of Repolarization Alternans in the Formation of Arrhythmogenic Substrates

We have seen thus far that gradients of APD are present across the epicardial surface of the guinea pig left ventricle, with APD being longest toward the base and shortest at the apex. This variation in electrical behavior present in normal myocardium is uniquely expressed upon the introduction of a premature beat. While these heterogeneities are present in the normal heart under baseline pacing, factors exist during which such heterogeneities are magnified. For example, repolarization alternans, which is manifest as a periodic change in the time course of repolarization, repeating once every other beat, has been described.[24,25] Repolarization alternans is of particular interest because T wave alternans is a marker of vulnerability to ventricular arrhythmias[24,25] and often immediately precedes arrhythmias in various pathologic conditions including Prinzmetal's angina,[26] acute myocardial infarction,[27,28] catecholamine excess, electrolyte imbalances,[29] and the long QT syndrome.[30,31] It is now evident that microvolt-level T wave alternans, which is visually undetectable on clinical electrocardiographic tracings, is common in patients at risk for sudden cardiac death.[24,32] We recently found that repolarization alternans occurring between cells having different restitution properties is a novel mechanism by which arrhythmogenic substrates can form.[18]

T wave alternans of the surface electrocardiogram (ECG) arises from alternans of repolarization occurring at the level of the single cell. Once again, the technique of high-resolution optical mapping was applied to the endocardial cryoablated, Langendorff-perfused guinea pig heart model to investigate the cellular basis for electrocardiographic T wave alternans.[18] Optical action potentials were recorded from 128 sites simultaneously at a time when T wave alternans was induced by rapid steady state ventricular pacing.

A tracing of the ECG and an optical action potential recorded simultaneously during two sequential beats of T wave alternans are compared in Figure 4. The tracings recorded during each beat are superimposed, and the difference between them indicates the magnitude of alternation. T wave alternans of the surface ECG coincided with and was explained by alternation of phases 2 and 3 of the action potential; i.e., T wave alternans arises from alternation of repolarization occurring at the level of the cell. In this experimental model, the magnitude of T wave alternans peaked near the crest of the T wave, with relatively little alternation involving the ST segment (Fig. 4). Interestingly, the distribution of T wave alternans in the endocardial cryoablated guinea pig model is similar to the distribution of T wave alternans typically observed in high-risk arrhythmia patients.[24] Note also that the magnitude of cellular alternans (i.e., 20 mV) is nearly two orders of magnitude greater than the magnitude of T wave alternans recorded simultaneously from the ECG (i.e., 400 μV).

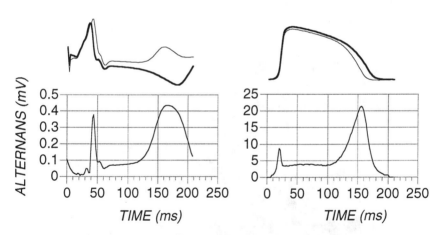

Figure 4. Changes in transmembrane potential of guinea pig ventricular myocytes that underlie T wave alternans on the surface ECG. **Top:** An electrocardiogram (ECG) **(left)** and representative action potential **(right)** recorded from one of 128 mapping sites. Tracings recorded from two consecutive beats are superimposed for the purposes of illustrating electrical alternans. The magnitude of electrical alternans during each time point of the cardiac cycle is represented by the difference between the amplitudes of the signals recorded on consecutive beats. T wave alternans in the range of 100 to 430 μV was distributed symmetrically around the T wave **(bottom left)**. Electrocardiographic T wave alternans was explained by beat-to-beat alternation in the onset of phase 3 of the action potential. The magnitude of alternation of transmembrane potential amplitude (21 mV, **bottom right**) was more than an order of magnitude larger than the magnitude of T wave alternans on the surface ECG (0.43 mV, **bottom left**).

Spatial Heterogeneity of Action Potential Alternans Parallels Heterogeneity of Restitution

Electrocardiographic T wave alternans has been shown to occur above a critical heart rate in patients whose heart rate was modulated by exercise.[33,34] Similarly, alternans in APDs recorded from isolated ventricular myocytes are induced above a critical threshold heart rate. Consequently, it is not surprising that an alternans heart rate threshold is present in action potentials recorded from cells in the intact heart.[18] Using multisite optical action potential recordings, we found that the heart rate threshold for repolarization alternans varied between cells across the epicardial surface of the guinea pig heart.[18] Moreover, the magnitude and phase of cellular alternans were also heterogeneously distributed in a systematic pattern (Fig. 5) that closely followed the known distribution of cellular restitution. Repolarization time alternans, which was calculated from the difference in cellular repolarization time measured during sequential beats

LOCAL REPOLARIZATION ALTERNANS (ms)

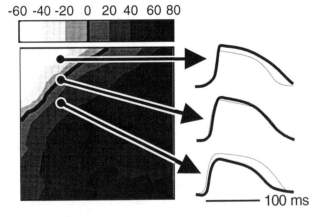

Figure 5. Distribution of action potential alternans in the intact ventricle. Shown is a plot of local repolarization alternans measured as the difference in repolarization time between consecutive beats at each ventricular recording site. Local repolarization alternans varies from apex to base according to known distribution of cellular restitution properties across the epicardial surface of guinea pig (Fig. 1, **C**). Notice the change in phase of repolarization alternans denoted by the thick black line and demonstrated by action potential recordings shown for selected sites. These action potentials were recorded from two sequential beats (depicted by bold and thin traces) to illustrate the relative phase of repolarization alternans between cells. The alternation of action potentials with opposite phase is termed "discordant alternans."

for all 128 sites, is plotted in Figure 5. Positive and negative values indicate relative prolongation and shortening of local repolarization on a particular beat, respectively. Note that during a given beat, repolarization is prolonged near the base of the heart and shortened near the apex, indicating regional differences in the phase of alternation across the epicardial surface. Such disruption in the phase of the APD variation has been termed "discordant alternans." In our preparations, discordant alternans occurred despite the presence of normal intercellular coupling and was most likely explained by regional heterogeneities in membrane restitution kinetics. Such inhomogeneous alternations of repolarization occurring between neighboring regions of cells suggest that the ionic currents determining repolarization differ substantially between these regions so as to overcome the synchronizing effect of electrotonic interactions. The sharp increase in DOR due to discordant alternation of repolarization may provide a mechanism by which electrical alternans could lead to VF and sudden death.[18]

Summary

It is evident that cellular repolarization properties vary extensively between cardiac cells. However, the influence such heterogeneities of repolarization have on arrhythmia vulnerability in the intact heart is not well appreciated. Using high-resolution optical action potential mapping with voltage-sensitive dyes, we have demonstrated the influence of spatial heterogeneity of cellular restitution kinetics on the spatiotemporal dynamics of ventricular repolarization. During premature stimulation of the heart, repolarization gradients are modulated in a systematic and predictable manner that is highly dependent on the timing of the premature impulse. We have termed this "coupling interval dependence modulated dispersion." Modulated dispersion may strongly influence the heart's vulnerability to fibrillation and the electrophysiological requirements for reentry via its dynamic effects on DOR.

Spatial heterogeneities of repolarization properties appear to also play a critical role in the development of arrhythmogenic substrates during T wave alternans. Heterogeneous ion channel function and expression, as manifest by regional variation in cellular restitution properties, create a situation where cellular repolarization within adjacent regions of myocardium alternate with differing amplitude and phase. Regional differences in the phase of alternans (i.e., discordant alternans) produce critical gradients of repolarization which may form a suitable substrate for unidirectional block and reentrant ventricular arrhythmias. These findings demonstrate the complexity of arrhythmogenic substrates that are dependent on dynamic and heterogeneous processes such as repolarization. Obviously, the factors that determine DOR in the heart are dependent on the specific pathophysiological substrate involved. Further studies are required to enhance our understanding of mechanisms by which heterogeneities of restitution, repolarization, and alternans influence the electrophysiological substrate for reentry in the presence and absence of cardiac pathology.

References

1. Kuo C, Munakata K, Reddy CP, Surawicz B. Characteristics and possible mechanisms of ventricular arrhythmia dependent on the dispersion of action potential durations. *Circulation* 1983;67:1356-1357.
2. Surawicz B. Ventricular fibrillation and dispersion of repolarization. *J Cardiovasc Electrophysiol* 1997;8:1009-1012.
3. Lesh MD, Pring M, Spear JF. Cellular uncoupling can unmask dispersion of action potential duration in ventricular myocardium: A computer modeling study. *Circ Res* 1989;65:1426-1440.
4. Hume JR, Uehara A. Ionic basis of the different action potential configurations of single guinea pig atrial and ventricular myocytes. *J Physiol (Lond)* 1984; 368:525-544.
5. Akar FG, Yan G, Antzelevitch C, Rosenbaum DS. Optical maps reveal reentrant mechanism of torsade de pointes based on topography and electrophysiology of mid-myocardial cells. *Circulation* 1997;96(8):I555. Abstract.
6. Laurita KR, Girouard SD, Akar FG, Rosenbaum DS. Modulated dispersion explains changes in arrhythmia vulnerability during premature stimulation of the heart. *Circulation* 1998;98:2774-2780.
7. Efimov IR, Huang DT, Rendt JM, Salama G. Optical mapping of repolarization and refractoriness from intact hearts. *Circulation* 1994;90:1469-1480.
8. Litovsky SH, Antzelevitch C. Transient outward current prominent in canine ventricular epicardium but not endocardium. *Circ Res* 1988;62:116-126.
9. Furukawa T, Myerburg RJ, Furukawa N, et al. Differences in transient outward currents of feline endocardial and epicardial myocytes. *Circ Res* 1990; 67:1287-1291.
10. Fedida D, Giles WR. Regional variations in action potentials and transient outward current in myocytes isolated from rabbit left ventricle. *J Physiol (Lond)* 1991;442:191-209.
11. Sicouri S, Antzelevitch C. A subpopulation of cells with unique electrophysiological properties in the deep subepicardium of the canine ventricle: The M cell. *Circ Res* 1991;68:1729-1741.
12. Drouin E, Charpentier F, Gauthier C, et al. Electrophysiologic characteristics of cells spanning the left ventricular wall of human heart: Evidence for presence of M cells. *J Am Coll Cardiol* 1995;26:185-192.
13. Sicouri S, Quist M, Antzelevitch C. Evidence for the presence of M cells in the guinea pig ventricle. *J Cardiovasc Electrophysiol* 1996;7:503-511.
14. Liu D-W, Antzelevitch C. Characteristics of the delayed rectifier current (I_{Kr} and I_{Ks}) in canine ventricular epicardial, midmyocardial, and endocardial myocytes: A weaker I_{Ks} contributes to the longer action potential of the M cell. *Circ Res* 1995;76:351-365.
15. Gintant GA. Two components of delayed rectifier current in canine atrium and ventricle: Does I_{Ks} play a role in the reverse rate dependence of class III agents? *Circ Res* 1996;78:26-37.

16. Sanguinetti MC, Jurkiewicz NK. Two components of cardiac delayed rectifier K+ current: Differential sensitivity to block by class III antiarrhythmic agents. *J Gen Physiol* 1990;96:195-215.
17. Laurita KR, Girouard SD, Rosenbaum DS. Modulation of ventricular repolarization by a premature stimulus: Role of epicardial dispersion of repolarization kinetics demonstrated by optical mapping of the intact guinea pig heart. *Circ Res* 1996;79:493-503.
18. Pastore JM, Girouard SD, Laurita KR, et al. Mechanism linking T wave alternans to the genesis of cardiac fibrillation. *Circulation* 1999;99:1385-1394.
19. Girouard SD, Laurita KR, Rosenbaum DS. Unique properties of cardiac action potentials recorded with voltage-sensitive dyes. *J Cardiovasc Electrophysiol* 1996;7:1024-1038.
20. Rosenbaum DS, Kaplan DT, Kanai A, et al. Repolarization inhomogeneities in ventricular myocardium change dynamically with abrupt cycle length shortening. *Circulation* 1991;84:1333-1345.
21. Hiraoka M, Kawano S. Mechanism of increased amplitude and duration of the plateau with sudden shortening of diastolic intervals in rabbit ventricular cells. *Circulation* 1987;60:14-26.
22. Kobayashi Y, Peters W, Khan SS, et al. Cellular mechanisms of differential action potential duration restitution in canine ventricular muscle cells during single versus double premature stimuli. *Circulation* 1992;86:955-967.
23. Watanabe M, Otani NF, Gilmour RF Jr. Biphasic restitution of action potential duration and complex dynamics in ventricular myocardium. *Circ Res* 1995;76:915-921.
24. Rosenbaum DS, Jackson LE, Smith JM, et al. Electrical alternans and vulnerability to ventricular arrhythmias. *N Engl J Med* 1994;330:235-241.
25. Sutton PMI, Taggart P, Lab M, et al. Alternans of epicardial repolarization as a localized phenomenon in man. *Eur Heart J* 1991;12:70-78.
26. Kleinfeld MJ, Rozanski JJ. Alternans of the ST-segment in Prinzmetal's angina. *Circulation* 1977;55:574-577.
27. Puletti M, Curione M, Righetti G, Jacobellis G. Alternans of the ST-segment and T-wave in acute myocardial infarction. *J Electrocardiol* 1980;13:297-300.
28. Dilly SG, Lab MJ. Electrophysiological alternans and restitution during acute regional ischemia in myocardium of anesthetized pig. *J Physiol (Lond)* 1988;402:315-333.
29. Reddy CVR, Kiok JP, Khan RG, El-Sherif N. Repolarization alternans associated with alcoholism and hypomagnesemia. *Am J Cardiol* 1984;53:390-391.
30. Shimizu W, Yamada K, Arakaki Y, et al. Monophasic action potential recordings during T-wave alternans in congenital long QT syndrome. *Am Heart J* 1996;132:699-701.
31. Platt SB, Vijgen JM, Albrecht P, et al. Occult T wave alternans in long QT syndrome. *J Cardiovasc Electrophysiol* 1996;7:144-148.
32. Rosenbaum DS, Albrecht P, Cohen RJ. Predicting sudden cardiac death from T wave alternans of the surface electrocardiogram: Promise and pitfalls. *J Cardiovasc Electrophysiol* 1996;7:1095-1111.
33. Wayne VS, Bishop RL, Spodick DH. Exercise-induced ST segment alternans. *Chest* 1983;83:824-825.
34. Hohnloser SH, Klingenheben T, Zabel M, et al. T wave alternans during exercise and atrial pacing in humans. *J Cardiovasc Electrophysiol* 1997;8:987-993.

Methodological Aspects

3

QT Dispersion:
Methodology and Clinical Significance

Pierre Maison-Blanche, Fabio Badilini,
Jocelyne Fayn, and Philippe Coumel

Introduction

The QT interval on the surface electrocardiogram (ECG) is considered a surrogate of cellular action potential duration. However, it only yields a limited view of the complex electrogenesis of ventricular repolarization. Evidence of T wave end inequality between leads on the surface ECG traces back to a report by Wilson et al,[1] and was revived by the concept of QT dispersion. Because of its apparent simplicity, the concept of QT dispersion rapidly became popular, and a growing literature is now devoted to its potential prognostic interest. A principal reason for the success of the concept in the cardiologist community is the term coined for its designation. For clinicians, "dispersion" immediately calls to mind "inhomogeneity" in the distribution of both action potential duration and conduction wavefronts. All of these electrophysiological parameters are known to be highly arrhythmogenic. Now, the problem is in the realization that we may be somewhat abused by our semantics.

All of the information about ventricular electrical activity is contained in a *single* image—the spatial QRS and T loops that can be characterized by their morphology, planarity, speed, etc. When projected on the orthogonal axes XYZ, or on the frontal, sagittal, and horizontal planes, they form the QRS-T complexes. A single structure such as a three-dimensional loop cannot generate any "dispersion." However, any projection on a two-dimensional plane implies the loss of a part of the information, and

From Olsson SB, Amlie JP, Yuan S (eds): *Dispersion of Ventricular Repolarization: State of the Art.* ©Futura Publishing Company, Inc., Armonk, NY, 2000.

identifying "dispersion" from various projections may just be a way to characterize the lost information. In particular, every time the tip of the electrical vector progresses perpendicular to the plane or the axis of projection, the resulting activity becomes transiently nil, as if the original source had disappeared.

Whether QT dispersion is a reality or an illusion, the practical problem remains that even an illusion should be evaluated as exactly as possible, in order to assess its clinical implications.

Methodological Aspects

Current Status of Scalar 12-Lead QT Dispersion

Problems of Definitions

Potential drawbacks of using interlead difference in QT interval as a surrogate of repolarization inhomogeneity were reviewed extensively by Statters et al[2] in 1994. First, the definition itself of QT dispersion is not clearly established; most studies have used the range of QT intervals for all available leads, but the standard deviation of the QT interval may be preferable as it is less dependent on extreme values. Other studies have proposed the use of the variation coefficient (QT standard deviation/ mean QT). In the attempt to take into account the inability to measure all leads, some authors have corrected the QT duration range by applying the square root of the number of measured leads.[3] A second unsolved issue remains the exact definition of the T wave offset. While most studies consider it the return to the isoelectric line or the nadir between the T wave and the U wave, others claim that the method of Lepeschkin and Surawicz[4] (intersection between the isoelectric line and the tangent to descending limb of the T wave) is more reliable. Another critical point raised by Statters et al[2] is the possible use of a subset of leads, as it could be inappropriate to merge the information from the limb leads with that of precordial chest leads. Another matter of dispute is whether QT dispersion should be corrected for heart rate, although this specific issue had been related mainly to the nonsimultaneous acquisition of leads typical of some poor commercial systems.

Inconsistency of Manual Measurements of QT Intervals on Paper Printouts

Murray et al[5] used a database of 512 digitized ECGs to compare QT interval measures from different paper ECG formats. In this study, measurements were performed by four independent cardiologists. They showed significant changes in QT outputs with different paper speeds (the QT interval lengthened by 16 ms between 50 and 25 mm/s). There were also significant changes with amplifier gain (5 ms between 10 and 15 mm/mV). Interestingly, they also found a relation between QT interval and the amplitude of the T wave: QT intervals increased by 10 ms for a doubled T wave height. Finally, there were consistent differences between cardiologists, the greatest mean difference reaching 20 ms. The authors concluded that, regarding manual measurement of ventricular repolarization, it would be preferable that a single cardiologist be in charge of the database, and different paper speed and different gain should not be used. In addition, small differences in QT dispersion should be taken with caution, particularly in presence of large T wave amplitude variations.

In the same year, Kautzner and colleagues[6] published a similar study focusing on interobserver reproducibility of both QT duration and dispersion in normal subjects. Of note, standard 12-lead ECGs were printed at 25 mm/s but measures of each lead were achieved using a digitizing pad with a resolution of 0.1 mm (i.e., 4 ms for that paper speed). Each recording was analyzed by two observers. In accordance with Murray and colleagues, they reported that the longest QT interval is often seen in leads with highest amplitude (precordial leads V_2 and V_3) whereas the shortest QT interval is most frequently seen in leads with a flattened T wave (Fig. 1). The main results from this study are well known in the cardiologist community, now well aware of the striking difference between the reproducibility of QT duration and that of QT dispersion. Interobserver differences of various QT duration parameters were negligible (2% to 4%) when compared with QT interval dispersion (27% to 33%). Logically, Kautzner and coworkers concluded that their findings jeopardized the application of manual QT dispersion assessment for risk stratification studies.

Current Implications

After a long series of many encouraging articles showing the strong discriminant and prognostic power of QT dispersion,[7-16] more recent literature is less enthusiastic. There is accumulated evidence that manual measures of QT dispersion, but not QT duration, on paper printouts are irrelevant. The first implication is that all previously published material based on manual measurement should be taken with extreme caution.

In contrast to these positive studies that are based mainly on a retrospective analysis of an ECG database, Zabel et al[17] prospectively collected 12-lead resting ECGs in 280 consecutive patients referred for acute myocardial infarction (MI). In this study the 12-lead ECGs were optically scanned and digitized before automatic analysis of QT dispersion and other repolarization variables. After a mean follow-up of 32 months, QT dispersion was not predictive for global mortality or arrhythmic death. The study by Zabel et al emphasizes the need for a deep reevaluation of

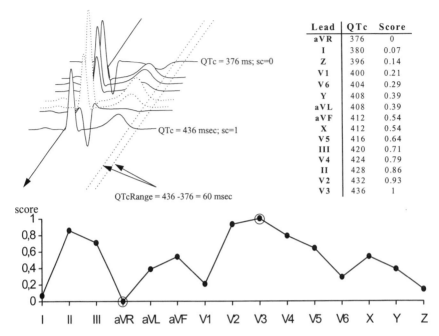

Figure 1. Descriptive example of weighted score distribution in one subject. **Top left:** The electrocardiographic leads are sorted according to increasing rate-corrected QT (QTc) duration (only a subset of 15 leads has been depicted). In this example, QTcRange is 60 ms. To evaluate the relative importance of each lead with respect to repolarization dispersion, a weighted score distribution was introduced (see Reference 12 for further details). The two extreme leads (aVR: shortest QTc, and V_3 longest QTc) are given scores of 0 and 1, respectively. **Top right:** Table displays all 15 leads with corresponding QTc interval (ms) and score value. Leads with intermediate QTc intervals are assigned intermediate score values. Leads with the same QTc (for instance V_6 and Y) are given the same score. In this specific example, all 15 leads have a measured QTc. **Bottom:** Graphic representation of score distribution. On the horizontal axis, leads are organized from left to right as frontal, precordial, and orthogonal. Open circles identify the two extreme leads.

the concept of scalar QT dispersion from both technical and pathophysiological standpoints.

Scalar QT Dispersion in the Era of Digital Computerized Electrocardiology

Computerized ECG has been available for more than 15 years, and there is extensive medical literature on this digitized technology. It is interesting to note how such progress had not reached the cardiologist community when the concept of scalar QT dispersion started to gain popularity. However, we will hereafter discuss the invaluable advantages of modern electrocardiology when applied to ventricular repolarization.

Technical Aspects of ECG Recordings and Storage

Today computer processing of the ECG is a routine procedure, with easy waveform calculation in microvolts and milliseconds. Most commercially available 12-lead resting ECG recorders acquire digitally the surface analog ECG signals with sampling rates from 250 to 1000 sample^{s-1} (Hz), with excellent amplitude resolution (≤ 5 μV). The size of an electronic file containing 10 seconds of ECG data is only a few kilobytes. As discussed in the section of this chapter entitled "ECG Fundamentals and Projection Effect," modern systems only store two of the six limb leads (the remainder being calculated whenever necessary), thus permitting a savings of one third of the data. Although memory size is becoming less and less important, a 30% storage capacity increase is still practical.

In the era of digital imaging and quality control, it is thus amazing and unacceptable that the most commonly used method of storage and documentation is still on paper. Thanks to the efforts of the Common Standards for Quantitative Electrocardiography (CSE) working party, there is now a widely accepted ECG format, and clinicians and researchers can freely exchange digital data through diskettes or simply modem transmission.[18]

If from one side we should all be partisans of digitized ECG, from the other it is fair to admit that the majority of ECGs, even those obtained in large-scale trials, are stored as hard copy paper records. Today this limitation has been overcome. Initially, digitizing pads were used, and certainly provided an improvement, although they do not allow further analysis of the ECG waveforms.[17,19] Techniques have been developed to convert paper records, through scanners, into digital images. At this step, direct digital acquisition or scanning procedures provide comparable data quality.

Computerized Analysis of Ventricular Repolarization

A substantial number of research groups have worked on automatic repolarization waveform analysis.[12,20-24] More recently, a commercial system proposed an option for such algorithm.[25,26] In the context of QT dispersion, the rationale of this research is to ensure 100% reproducibility. From a practical point of view, automatic analysis takes only few seconds to process an ECG and, together with a well-designed graphic viewer, it allows multiple display modes. Figures 1 and 2 are two examples from our personal system.

In general, the dispersion of a time interval can derive from the variability of both its beginning and its end points. However, in the

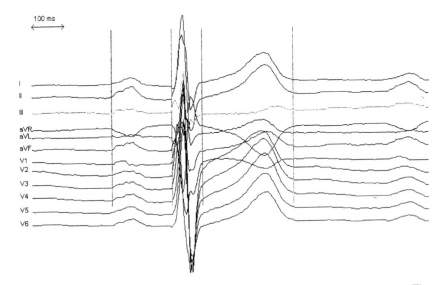

Figure 2. Graphic representation of a digitized 12-lead electrocardiogram. The 12 leads are vertically aligned. In each lead the cardiac complex displayed is the median template obtained from 10 seconds of continuous data. In this example, lead III was automatically excluded by the computer program for QT measurement (reduced amplitude). The four vertical cursors represent, respectively, the position of P wave onset, QRS onset and offset, and T wave offset. The T wave end was actually obtained as the median position from 11 individual leads.

context of QT dispersion, the clinical interest resides entirely in the terminating point (either the apex or end of the T wave) and variations due to QRS onset may be troublesome. Unfortunately, the literature is not particularly clear with respect to this feature. This was highlighted by the CSE Working Party, under the direction of Jos Willems. Five experts defined QRS wave onset and offset in a database, including normal ECGs and a set of pathologies such as ventricular hypertrophy and MI.[23] QRS onset dispersion was in the order of 5 ms, as later confirmed by Kors and van Herpen,[26] who compared QT dispersion using both lead-independent and lead-dependent QRS onsets.

This value is considered negligible when compared with T offset dispersion and the QRS onset of all leads is generally fixed to a single global value (median of 12, earliest of 12…), with only the apex and end of T waves allowed to change. In this way, computerized QT dispersion reflects the dispersion of a point within the repolarization phase.

T Offset Detection: None of the published methods has proven powerful. Indeed, any measurement method that relies on a single point is susceptible to noise and to the changes of T wave morphology. As a brief description, in our laboratory T wave is first low-pass filtered by a recursive birectional Butterworth filter (other methods use alternative filtering techniques). Then the first derivative signal is calculated and its zero crossings (i.e., changes of signs) are detected. One of these zero crossings is chosen to be the T peak location based on additional heuristic criteria. The first derivative waveform is also used to detect the T offset based on comparison with an adaptive threshold.[27] Alternatively, in other systems the T offset can be detected with a computer "translation" of the Surawicz approach,[4] i.e., as the intersection between the tangent line on the maximum slope after the T apex and the isoelectric line identified in the TP segment.[24] Another classic program simply defines the end of T as the return to baseline of the ECG incremented by a threshold.[21]

Computerized methods work fine in the presence of high-quality ECG and monophasic T waves, since most algorithms have been validated using normal ECGs. Unfortunately, this is not true for abnormal ECGs with the T wave not clearly defined morphologically or characterized by irregular shapes. McLaughlin et al[28] showed that below 0.25 mV of T wave amplitude, automatic QT interval measurement was inaccurate. Savelieva et al, from St. George Hospital,[25] compared QT dispersion measurements obtained by both manual reading and the QT Guard analysis software package by Marquette Medical Systems (Milwaukee, WI).[24] They found a lack of agreement between manual and automatic measurements and concluded that computerized analysis cannot be performed blindly. We share the concerns of Malik's group, and it is now widely accepted as a strong recommendation that visual expert reviewing of automatic measurement be mandatory.

Automatic and Manual Exclusion of Leads: Most algorithms are tuned to automatically exclude "difficult" T wave leads. This exclusion is reasonably based on noise content and/or T wave amplitude. Although many systems allow the possibility for the insertion of calipers on these excluded leads, it is unlikely that a manual reliable measure could be meaningful (Fig. 2). Another alternative, regardless of the ECG characteristics, is to impose beforehand a specific lead for exclusion. The default set-up of the QT Guard system, for example, eliminates lead V_1 because of the frequent occurrence of a flat T wave in this lead. Of note, these automatic interventions, if they may introduce a clinical bias, still maintain 100% reproducibility.

In contrast, user interactive modification of ECG calipers can have a major impact on reproducibility of QT dispersion. To a certain degree, it could produce worse results than manual measurements from good quality paper printouts, particularly if performed under poor screen size and resolution modes.

Delete-Only Strategy: A good compromise between the need for correction and that for preserving reproducibility is the choice of a delete-only strategy. This approach was evaluated in our laboratory using a set of 50 recordings randomly selected from a database of Marquette MacView ECG files of young healthy male subjects. For the purpose of this study, the ECGs were analyzed by a blinded single expert three different times. Reading 2 was 15 days after reading 1, whereas reading 3 was 15 days after reading 2 (1 month after reading 1).

The program used is a Windows-based application that permits analysis of MacView ECG files (250-Hz sampling) stored on PC floppy diskettes. Among many variables (see below), the program provides QT intervals. QT dispersion is based on the n measured QT intervals and is assessed by either its range (i.e., longest minus shortest QT of the sequence) or its standard deviation (Table 1).

User intervention consists of the eventual modification of single-lead cursor. For this specific study, we have limited this last intervention to a *delete-only* operation, i.e., we deliberately avoided the modification of single-lead measurements, only allowing the possibility to exclude a suspicious or noisy beat from the automatic analysis. Then, QT dispersion parameters are recalculated taking into account the manually excluded leads. The parameters tested for reproducibility were QT duration (either absolute or rate-corrected by Fridericia's formula) and QT dispersion (both QT range and standard deviation). Reproducibility was assessed using Bland-Altman method[29] by comparing readings 1 and 2 (15 days apart), readings 2 and 3 (15 days apart), and readings 2 and 3 (30 days apart). Reproducibility was quantified by the concentration of the differences around the mean value of all the differences, which represents the statistical bias. The coefficient of reproducibility (CR) is defined as the 95% confidence interval of the differences (i.e., CR=3.92 SD by assuming a normal distribution). Table 2 gives mean ± standard deviations for QT and QT dispersion. Table 3 displays reproducibility parameters among readings.

Our findings in healthy subjects support the concept that interlead variation of QT duration can be quantified with good confidence provided that ECG acquisition, analysis, and review are performed with adequate technology by experienced cardiologists who are well trained for the algorithm they use. Our experience with our program may not be valid with another. In addition, whether similar results can be obtained in populations with more complex T wave morphologies still must be confirmed.

Other Repolarization Variables

Due to the technical problems and pitfalls related to a measurement method that relies on a single point, alternative approaches that do not require the localization of the T wave offset were recently introduced.

Table 1
12-Lead QT Measurement Output

	I	II	V_1	V_2	V_3	V_4	V_5	V_6	III	aVR	aVL	aVF
QTm	276	284	284	272	280	280	284	284	-9	284	272	288
QTo	360	368	364	364	372	376	372	364	-9	368	340	364
RTm	241	246	268	251	219	240	244	244	-9	248	223	249
RTo	325	330	348	343	311	336	332	324	-9	332	291	325
SoTm	184	192	192	180	188	188	192	192	-9	192	180	196
SoTo	268	276	272	272	280	284	280	272	-9	276	248	272
SoUm	-9	-9	-9	-9	-9	-9	-9	-9	-9	-9	-9	-9
SoUo	-9	-9	-9	-9	-9	-9	-9	-9	-9	-9	-9	-9
t50	172	184	184	160	172	176	180	180	-9	176	164	196
t25-75	72	68	176	96	88	80	72	68	-9	68	76	72
t20-80	88	92	220	124	116	100	92	88	-9	84	100	104
AmpT	380	400	-92	551	605	580	483	400	-9	-390	190	209
Area	9.67	10.21	2.89	19.20	19.00	16.10	12.37	9.99	-9	9.82	5.18	5.58
Ether	1.65	1.62	2.53	2.05	1.95	1.66	1.75	1.67	-9	1.86	2.06	1.48

Table 2
Mean ± Standard Deviation for QT and QT Dispersion

	QT	QTc	QT Range	QT SD
Reading 1	389±24	390±17	27±8	8.7±2.3
Reading 2	391±25	391±17	21±7	7.2±2.0
Reading 3	391±25	392±17	26±7	8.4±2.2

Mean ± SD of parameters analyzed. Data are expressed in ms.

Table 3
Reproducibility Parameters among Readings

	QT	QTc	QT Range	QT SD
Bias (ms)	−1.18	−1.14	5.36	1.48
Mean absolute difference (ms)	2.98	2.98	5.68	1.52
Mean relative error (%)	0.3	0.3	22.4	18.5
Coefficient of reproducibility (ms)	16	16	30.45	8

Test of reproducibility between first and second reading.

	QT	QTc	QT Range	QT SD
Bias (ms)	−1.76	−1.70	1.04	0.28
Mean absolute difference (ms)	3.12	3.10	4.40	1.08
Mean relative error (%)	0.4	0.5	4	3
Coefficient of reproducibility (ms)	16	16	31.36	8

Test of reproducibility between first and third reading.

	QT	QTc	QT Range	QT SD
Bias (ms)	−0.58	−0.56	−4.32	−1.2
Mean absolute difference (ms)	1.62	1.6	5.12	1.40
Mean relative error (%)	0.1	0.1	18.2	15.3
Coefficient of reproducibility (ms)	11	10	28.4	7.9

Test of reproducibility between second and third reading.

Years ago Merri et al[22] introduced new parameters of ventricular repolarization such as T wave area (absolute repolarization area), symmetry (ratio between early and late repolarization area), and tA50 (time interval to accumulate the first 50% of the total area). These parameters are not strictly independent of T wave offset but are much less affected by its misplacement. These variables appear to be very discriminant between men and women but an interlead variation associated with them has yet to be demonstrated.

Recently Couderc et al[30] suggested that a fixed ECG segment could be used to perform ventricular repolarization analysis. In this study, the so-called "T window" started 100 ms after the preceding R peak and ended 220 ms before the one that followed. The first derivative of the signal in this window was the retained repolarization variable. The practical implication of using a repolarization segment based on the location of QRS peaks remains to be established.

ECG Fundamentals and Projection Effect

The standard 12-lead ECG includes bipolar limb leads (I, II, III), "unipolar" limb leads (aVR, aVL, aVF), and "unipolar" precordial leads (V_1 through V_6). It is important to remember that the so-called unipolar leads are in reality bipolar leads in the sense that they measure voltage differences between two points. Simply, one of the two points is the Wilson central terminal, which only influences the baseline level of the other point—what is referred to as the exploring electrode.[31] Thus, the widely accepted assumption that precordial leads reflect local information must be taken with caution.

Limb leads are closely related. Actually, only two are independent and the other four can be derived with simple mathematical equations. In fact, 12-lead ECG systems only record two limb leads and six precordials. For example, if we record leads I and II, the other four limb leads can be calculated as follows:

$$III = II - I \qquad \text{(Einthoven's law)}$$
$$aVR = -\tfrac{1}{2}\,(I + II)$$
$$aVL = I - \tfrac{1}{2}II$$
$$aVF = II - \tfrac{1}{2}I$$

Of course, if any other two leads are recorded, the above equations can be rearranged to have on their right hand sides the two known leads. Macfarlane[31] clearly stated that the above equations do not take into account body size and internal thoracic structure.

The early literature on QT dispersion completely ignored the implication of limb lead dependencies. The reason is difficult to understand. More recent literature actually focused on this particular issue, which has dramatic consequences on the concept of QT dispersion as discussed below. In a remarkable paper Kors and van Herpen[26] demonstrated how using the above equations when one of the limb leads terminates (i.e., reaches the 0 value) then the five other must end at the same time (when a second lead reaches the 0 value). In other words, a 0 level reached for any two leads will imply a 0 level for all of the other four. Thus, QT dispersion of limb leads should mathematically be constrained to only two durations.[26] This mathematical observation implies that extraction of more than two different QT durations in this set of leads is either a manual or a computer error. Accordingly, Kors suggested that QT dispersion be derived from 8 measurements, 6 from precordial leads and 2 from limb leads. Regarding limb leads, a possible solution would be to use the shortest QT and the median of the other five QT values measured.

Another milestone in the understanding of the electrophysiological background of QT dispersion was recently reported by Macfarlane et al[32] and Lee et al[33] in two separate studies. Based on the Dower mathematical transformation,[34] both studies derived the 12-lead ECG from the XYZ orthogonal representation and compared several ECG parameters as measured on the two different sets of leads (generic expression: derived lead = aX + bY + cZ). In the study by Macfarlane et al, 1220 derived 12-lead ECGs from the CSE database were compared with original orthogonal ECGs. Computer analysis was performed by the Glasgow program,[20] which provides QT interval for the 12 leads plus the XYZ leads individually. QT dispersion was calculated for all sets of leads. The 12-lead derived ECG gave a significantly longer QT dispersion than the orthogonal XYZ themselves (27.47 ± 10.8 ms versus 17.1 ± 10.0 ms). Macfarlane and colleagues concluded that projecting the electrical activity on 12 separate lead axes produces a larger QT dispersion only related to arithmetic, and therefore suggested that part of 12-lead QT dispersion is due to projection effect. The study by Lee and colleagues concentrated on the comparison between originally acquired and derived precordial leads in a data set of 129 normal subjects. Precordial QT dispersion for the derived ECG was nearly identical to that obtained from original ECG (40 ± 20 versus 41 ± 18). Since by definition derived ECGs do not contain any local effect, Lee's group concluded that QT dispersion of precordial leads should only reflect projection phenomenon or measurement error.

Clinical Significance

Finally, after years of misinterpretation of thousands of ECG recordings, the fundamentals of electrocardiology have been rediscovered, thanks to the involvement of distinguished experts in the field. The bipolar nature of all surface ECG leads has been restored, limb lead redundancy cannot now be ignored, and the existence of a projection effect has been demonstrated.

Should we now abandon the concept of interlead variation of QT duration? We believe the answer to this question is critical and that the most recent results may help. Our group[12] and that of Brohet in Brussels[35] reported on the discriminant power of XYZ QT dispersion. We compared the ECG recordings among 92 normal subjects and 71 patients following MI and we found that, although reduced when compared with 12 leads, dispersion in XYZ leads could discriminate (Table 4). Zaidi and coworkers even stated that the discriminant power of XYZ leads (in this case repre-

Table 4
ECG Variables in Controls and in Post-MI Patients

ECG Variables	XYZ Lead		12 Lead	
	Controls (n=92)	Post-MI (n=71)	Controls (n=92)	Post-MI (n=71)
RR (ms)	–	–	884±150	1036±166
QRS (ms)	–	–	90±9*	94±11
QTc (ms)	397±19[†]	407±29	398±19[†]	412±27
QTc range (ms)	9±7[‡]	21±13	34±11[‡]	51±19

MI = myocardial infarction. *P<0.01; [†]P<0.001; [‡]P<0.0001, controls versus MI.

sented by the percentage of inferior and anterior MI patients whose rate-corrected QT [QTc] dispersion values exceeds the 97.5 percentile value obtained from their normal population) was much greater than that of 12 leads. Thus, reduced magnitude of QTc dispersion may not necessarily imply a lesser discriminant power. On the contrary, as stated above, larger 12-lead QTc dispersion may be affected by nonphysiological components of ventricular repolarization dispersion. It remains to be demonstrated whether this lead configuration may provide a prognostic index of ventricular repolarization inhomogeneity.

Using the MEANS program, de Bruyne et al[36] recently compared QT dispersion from 8 leads (the 6 precordial plus the shortest limb lead and the median of the other 5) and from all 12 leads in the prospective Rotterdam study. The rationale for the use of two QTc dispersion definitions was that the pure 12-lead QT dispersion reflects error of the computer program. The results of this study showed that increased QTc dispersion is a strong and independent risk marker for cardiac mortality. Interestingly, QTc dispersion in 12 leads was larger than that in 8 leads, but with little effect on the associated risk.

These data suggest that the discriminant or predictive value of QT dispersion probably reflects T wave intrinsic properties. Findings from our group[37] showed that the presence of an electrophysiological substrate for repolarization inhomogeneity is associated with alterations in the morphology of spatial T wave loop structure. T loop analysis was performed by using an algorithm that has been previously described.[38] A main feature of this method is to evaluate a three-dimensional structure in a space defined by its three principal axes of inertia.[39] In this space, the morphology of the loop is determined by the three eigenvalues relative to the principal axes: λ_1, λ_2, and λ_3. In general, the energy of the loop is concentrated in a plane defined by λ_1 and λ_2 (called the preferential plane) so that the value of the third dimension (λ_3) is small with respect to that of λ_1 and λ_2. Furthermore, in the preferential plane, the T loop is usually narrow (ellipsoidal shape), thus leading to a value of λ_2 that is smaller than the value of λ_1. The T loop shape in the preferential plane was quantified by a roundness parameter (RP) defined as RP = $(\lambda_2/\lambda_1)^{1/2}$. This parameter provides an estimation of the loop narrowness in the preferential plane: the smaller the RP, the thinner the loop (theoretically, a perfectly round loop will have RP = 1). The planarity of the loop was directly assessed by the value of λ_3. For a globally planar loop (i.e., a loop fully contained in the preferential plane), $\lambda_3 = 0$; the larger the loss of planarity, the larger the λ_3. A schematic representation of the T loop parameters is shown in Figure 3.

In this study we explored conventional 12-lead resting ECG QT dispersion and the corresponding morphology of the spatial T wave loop in 25 normal subjects, in 30 post-MI patients, and in 17 individuals with congenital long QT syndrome (LQTS). Standard and XYZ ECG leads were simultaneously digitized (250 Hz) and automatically analyzed. All scalar measurements of QT dispersion were significantly larger in the two patho-

CAVIAR Fundamentals

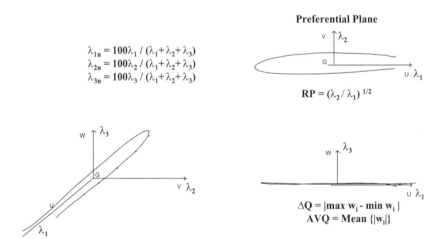

Figure 3. Schematic representation of T loop parameters. **Bottom left:** A T wave loop is drawn with respect to its axes of inertia u, v, and w. A digitized sample (P_i) on the loop is then characterized by three coordinate values relative to these axes: u_i, v_i, and w_i. The three eigenvalues λ_1, λ_2, and λ_3 (indicated in parenthesis) provide information on the amount of inertia in each of the directions u, v, and w. The normalized eigenvalues λ_{1n}, λ_{2n}, and λ_{3n} express the percent of explained inertia for each of the directions. The **top right** panel shows the projection of the loop on the preferential plane (plane formed by u and v axes), and provides a view of loop roundness, whereas the **bottom right** panel is the projection on the plane formed by first and third principal axes (u and w) and gives an idea of loop planarity. See Reference 37 for definition of all parameters.

logic populations; however none of them could discriminate post-MI groups from LQTS groups (QT dispersion = 33.3, 61.4, and 62.7 ms, respectively, for the three populations). Conversely, a loss of planarity and an increased roundness of the T wave loop were observed in the two pathologic groups, with the former effect more pronounced in the LQTS (P=0.04 compared with post-MI) and the latter in the post-MI group (P= 0.02 compared with LQTS). Figures 4 and 5 show representative examples of a normal subject and a post-MI patient. The exaggerated roundness of the post-MI loop is noteworthy. We concluded that changes in the morphology of the spatial T wave loop are associated with QT dispersion and can discriminate between different substrates of repolarization inhomogeneity.

More recently, another elegant study confirmed our initial report.[40] From the CSE database, the authors compared scalar QT dispersion and T loop parameters after reconstruction of XYZ leads from the standard ECG leads. T loop morphology was characterized by its initial and termi-

Control

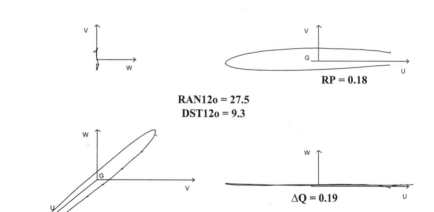

Figure 4. Normal subject. Example of a T wave loop relative to a normal subject together with overlapped 12-lead electrocardiographic scalar leads (**top left**). The T loop is displayed in the **bottom left** panel whereas its projections on the preferential plane and on the vertical plane are respectively shown in the **top right** and **bottom right** panels. The typical elongated and planar shape of the normal T wave loop (quantified by a small value of RP and ΔQ) can be appreciated. RAN12o and DSTo (in ms) correspond to the QT dispersion values calculated from scalar leads (range and standard deviation).

post MI

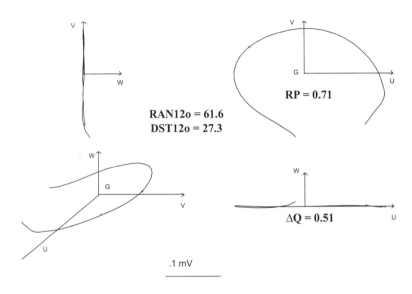

RAN12o = 61.6
DST12o = 27.3

RP = 0.71

ΔQ = 0.51

.1 mV

Figure 5. Post myocardial infarction (MI) patient. Example of a T wave loop relative to a post-MI patient together with overlapped 12-lead electrocardiographic scalar leads. The increased roundness of the loop (RP = 0.71) can be noticed. For more details, see legend of Figure 3.

nal axes, width, and maximal amplitude. In contrast to our study, each T loop parameter was determined using the original XYZ set of coordinates. Kors and coauthors[40] found that QT dispersion was smallest for large, narrow T loops (54.2 ms) and largest for small, wide loops (69.5 ms).

Finally, when applied to the Rotterdam database, these T loop parameters were found to be independent indicators of cardiac events.[41] Subjects with abnormal T loop had a more than fourfold risk for cardiac death and sudden cardiac death.

It is difficult to foresee whether the many obvious advantages of using vectorcardiography will overcome the reluctance of cardiologists to return to this technology.

References

1. Wilson, Macleod AG, Barker PS, et al. The interpretation of the initial deflections of the ventricular complex of the electrocardiogram. *Am Heart J* 1931;6:637-664.
2. Statters DJ, Malik M, Ward DE, et al. QT dispersion: Problems of methodology and clinical significance. *J Cardiovasc Electrophysiol* 1994;5:672-685.

3. Day CP, McComb JM, Matthews J, et al. Reduction in QT dispersion by sotalol following myocardial infarction. *Eur Heart J* 1991;12:423-427.
4. Lepeschkin E, Surawicz B. The measurement of the Q-T interval of the electrocardiogram. *Circulation* 1952;51:378-388.
5. Murray A, McLaughlin NB, Bourke JP, et al. Errors in manual measurement of QT intervals. *Br Heart J* 1994;71:386-390.
6. Kautzner J, Yi G, Camm J, et al. Short- and long-term reproducibility of QT, QTc, and QT dispersion measurement in healthy subjects. *PACE* 1994;17:928-937.
7. Moreno FL, Villanueva T, Karagounis LA, et al. Reduction in QT interval dispersion by successful thrombolytic therapy in acute myocardial infarction. *Circulation* 1994;90:94-100.
8. Manttari M, Oikarinen L, Manninen V, et al. QT dispersion as a risk factor for sudden cardiac death and fatal myocardial infarction in a coronary risk population. *Heart* 1997;78:268-272.
9. Zaidi M, Robert A, Fesler R, et al. Dispersion of ventricular repolarization in hypertrophic cardiomyopathy. *J Electrocardiol* 1996;26(suppl):89-94.
10. Hii JT, Wyse DG, Gillis AM, et al. Precordial QT interval dispersion as a marker of torsade de pointes. *Circulation* 1992;6:1376-1382.
11. Buja G, Miorelli M, Turrini P, et al. Comparison of QT dispersion in hypertrophic cardiomyopathy between patients with and without ventricular arrhythmias and sudden death. *Am J Cardiol* 1993;72:973-976.
12. Sainte Beuve C, Badilini F, Maison-Blanche P, et al. QT dispersion. Comparison of orthogonal, quasi-orthogonal and 12-lead configurations. *Ann Noninvas Electrocardiol* 1999;4(2):167-175.
13. Glancy JM, Weston PJ, Bhullar HK, et al. Reproducibility and automatic measurement of QT dispersion. *Eur Heart J* 1996;17:1035-1039.
14. Zareba W, Moss AJ, le Cessie S. Dispersion of ventricular repolarization and arrhythmic cardiac death in coronary artery disease. *Am J Cardiol* 1994;74:550-553.
15. Priori SG, Napolitano C, Diehl L, et al. Dispersion of the QT interval: A marker of therapeutic efficacy in the idiopathic long QT syndrome. *Circulation* 1994;89:1681-1689.
16. Karagounis L, Anderson J, Moreno F, et al. Multivariate associates of QT dispersion in patients with acute myocardial infarction: Primacy of patency status of the infarct-related artery. *Am Heart J* 1998;135:1027-1035.
17. Zabel M, Kligenheben T, Franz M, et al. Assessment of QT dispersion for prediction of mortality or arrhythmic events after myocardial infarction. Results of a prospective, long-term follow-up study. *Circulation* 1998;97:2543-2550.
18. Willems J, Arnaud P, Van Bemmel JH, et al. Assessment of the performance of electrocardiographic computer programs with the use of a reference data base. *Circulation* 1985;71:526-534.
19. Bhullar HK, Fothergill JC, Goddard WP, et al. Automated measurement of QT interval dispersion from hard-copy ECGs. *J Electrocardiol* 1993;26(suppl):321-331.
20. Macfarlane PW, Devine B, Latif S, et al. Methodology of ECG interpretation in the Glasgow program. *Methods Inf Med* 1990;29:354-361.
21. van Bemmel JH, Kors JA, van Herpen G. Methodology of the modular ECG analysis system MEANS. *Methods Inf Med* 1990;29:346-353.

22. Merri M, Benhorin J, Alberti M, et al. Electrocardiographic quantitation of ventricular repolarization. *Circulation* 1989;80:1301-1308.
23. Willems JL, Abreu-Lima C, Arnaud P, et al. The diagnostic performance of computer programs for the interpretation of electrocardiograms. *N Engl J Med* 1991;325:1767-1773.
24. Xue Q, Reddy S. New algorithms for QT dispersion analysis. *Comput Cardiol* 1996;23:293-296.
25. Savelieva I, Gang Y, Guo X, et al. Agreement and reproducibility of automatic versus manual measurement of QT interval and QT dispersion. *Am J Cardiol* 1998;81:471-477.
26. Kors JA, van Herpen G. Measurement error as a source of QT dispersion: A computerized analysis. *Heart* 1998;80:453-458.
27. Badilini F, Maison Blanche P, Childers R, et al. QT interval analysis on ambulatory electrocardiogram recordings: A selective beat averaging approach. *Med Biol Eng Comput* 1999;37:71-79.
28. McLaughlin NB, Campbell RWF, Murray A. Comparison of automatic QT measurement techniques in the normal 12 lead electrocardiogram. *Br Heart J* 1995;74:84-89.
29. Bland JM, Altman DG. Statistical methods for assessing agreement between two methods of clinical measurement. *Lancet* 1986;1:307-310.
30. Couderc JP, Zareba W, Konecki J, et al. New technique for quantifying spatial dispersion of ventricular repolarization morphology in digitized ECGs. *J Am Coll Cardiol* 1999;33(suppl):351A. Abstract.
31. Macfarlane PW. Lead systems. In Macfarlane PW, Veitch Lawrie TD (eds): *Comprehensive Electrocardiology*. New York: Pergamon Press; 1989:315-352.
32. Macfarlane PW, McLaughlin SC, Rodger JC. Influence of lead selection and population on automated measurement of QT dispersion. *Circulation* 1998;98:2160-2167.
33. Lee KW, Kligfield P, Okin PM, et al. Determinants of precordial QT dispersion in normal subjects. *J Electrocardiol* 1998;31(suppl):128-133.
34. Dower GE, Bastos Machado H, Osborne JA. On deriving electrocardiogram from vectorcardiographic leads. *Clin Cardiol* 1980;3:87-95.
35. Zaidi M, Robert A, Fesler R, et al. Computer-assisted study of the ECG indices of the dispersion of ventricular repolarization. *J Electrocardiol* 1996;29:199-211.
36. de Bruyne MC, Hoes AW, Kors JA, et al. QTc dispersion predicts cardiac mortality in the elderly. The Rotterdam study. *Circulation* 1998;97:467-472.
37. Badilini F, Fayn J, Maison-Blanche P, et al. Quantitative aspects of ventricular repolarization: Relationship between three dimensional T-wave loop morphology and scalar QT dispersion. *Ann Noninvas Electrocardiol* 1997;2(2):146-157.
38. Fayn J, Rubel P, Mohsen N. An improved method for the precise measurement of serial ECG changes in QRS duration and QT interval. Performance assessment on the CSE noise-testing database and on healthy 720 case-set population. *J Electrocardiol* 1991;24(suppl):123-127.
39. Rubel P, Fayn J, Mohsen N. Stability of surface T wave and corrected QT interval in a normal male population. In Butrous GS, Schwartz PJ (eds): *Clinical Aspects of Ventricular Repolarization*. London: Farrand Press; 1989:57.
40. Kors JA, van Herpen G, van Bemmel JH. QT dispersion in an attribute of T-loop morphology. *Circulation* 1999;99:1458-1463.
41. Kors JA, de Bruyne MC, Hoes AW, et al. T-loop morphology as a marker of cardiac events in the elderly. *J Electrocardiol* 1998;31(suppl):54-59.

4

QT Dispersion on 12-Lead Electrocardiogram in Normal Subjects:
Reproducibility and Relation to T Wave

Yee Guan Yap and A. John Camm

Introduction

QT dispersion (QTd) is usually defined empirically as the maximum QT interval minus the minimum QT interval as measured from the 12 leads of the electrocardiogram (ECG)[1] (Fig. 1). It is a representation of the spatial variability of the QT interval using simultaneously or nearly simultaneously recorded surface ECG leads. QTd has been proposed as an indirect measure of spatial heterogeneity of ventricular repolarization,[1,2] reflecting spatial differences in myocardial recovery time. This concept is supported by studies performed on patients with the long QT syndrome that have shown large spatial differences in myocardial recovery time as demonstrated by both the duration of monophasic action potentials in different parts of the ventricle[3] and the QT interval from body surface ECG mapping.[4] The presence of dispersion of recovery time may be arrhythmogenic by initiating ventricular arrhythmia via reentry or triggered automaticity mechanisms.[1,5,6] In spite of the electrophysiological implications of QTd, many controversies still exist about its significance and measurement. It is unclear whether the interlead variability in the QT interval duration is a result of technical factors such as variable projection of a single repolarization vector onto different ECG leads (a projection

From Olsson SB, Amlie JP, Yuan S (eds): *Dispersion of Ventricular Repolarization: State of the Art.* ©Futura Publishing Company, Inc., Armonk, NY, 2000.

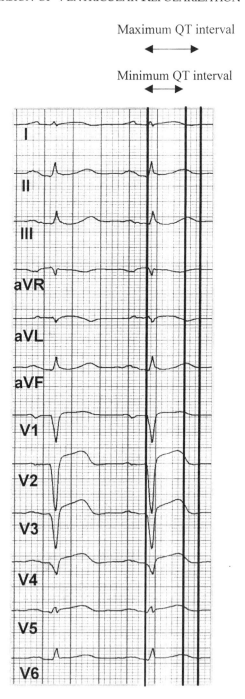

Maximum QT interval

Minimum QT interval

Figure 1. Measurement of QT dispersion. QT dispersion = maximum QT − minimum QT intervals.

phenomenon) and differences in unipolar versus bipolar leads, or a result of natural dispersion of repolarization (a local effect). Indeed, QTd may simply be a result of inaccuracy in QT interval measurement when the T wave amplitude is low and the T wave offset is difficult to define or complicated by an abnormal morphology or superimposed U wave.

The concept of measuring QTd for the prediction of ventricular arrhythmia is an attractive one, as it is simple to understand, inexpensive, and noninvasive, and it can be readily applied clinically. However, the measurement of QTd depends critically on the techniques used which have not been standardized.[1,6-8] Inconsistent methods employed in measuring QTd partly explain the disparity in the reproducibility and clinical value of QTd from various studies. Previous reports used digitizers, photocopy enlargement, and user interactive digital computing systems[9-11]; but recent technical advances now allow direct ECG acquisition for electronic analysis and automatic QT interval and QTd measurements, although the reproducibility of such methods will require validation. Uncertainties over the minimal number of leads required for QTd measurement, lead selection (i.e., 12-lead versus six precordial leads only), the need for adjustment for missing leads and heart rate may all influence the result of QTd measurement. For QTd to be useful as a predictor, it must be reproducible. Therefore, when measuring QTd, the methodology must be scrutinized vigorously before the results can be accepted.

Lead Adjustment and Number of Valid Leads

One of the confounding factors in QTd measurement is the number of leads available for measurement. This is normally because the end of T wave is not clearly distinguishable in one or more leads as a result of a flat T wave across several leads or of interruption of the T wave by a U wave. Less often, recording noise or the presence of ventricular ectopics excludes certain leads from measurement of the QT interval. As a result, adjustment formulas for missing leads have been suggested by some workers.[7,12] Hnatkova and coworkers[7] assessed the effects of lead adjustment formulas on QTd in a group of 27 healthy subjects. They found that QTd performed poorly when one or more leads were missing, but was appropriately adjusted with a factor of $1/\sqrt{n}$ where n is the number of measured leads. They suggested that such an adjustment removed the systematic bias introduced by the missing leads and significantly reduced the mean relative error caused by the omission. However, when such a lead-adjustment formula was applied to patients after myocardial infarction (MI), a different trend emerged. Glancy and colleagues[12] analyzed QTd retrospectively on 461 ECGs from 226 post-MI patients. They found that lead-adjusted QTc dispersion (QTd adjusted for heart rate using Bazett's formula) using the above factor produced a large, significant increase of the QTd when the number of measurable leads decreased from 12 to 8 (28.9±10.3 versus 38.7±16.1; P<0.001). Others found that QTc dispersion increased in proportion to the square root of the number of leads in post-MI patients treated with sotalol.[13] It is important to realize that rate correction for QTd is no longer necessary or appropriate (see below). Nevertheless, even allowing for such difference in the measurement techniques between studies, the fact that lead adjustment formulas produce different trends in different populations suggests that the formulas themselves are probably inappropriate or influenced by various factors such as the population studied or drugs. Thus, it seems that lead adjustment should not be applied for QTd measurement.

Although no lead adjustment formula seems appropriate, the number of measurable leads (so-called valid leads) on an ECG for QTd measurement is important. Most investigators have not specified the actual number of leads that were measured in their studies, although some had a minimum number of leads required (e.g., six or eight leads) before the ECGs were included for QTd measurement. The greater the number of valid leads that are measured, the more accurately QTd may reflect the dispersion of repolarization across the myocardium and the less likely for the result to be spurious. Hnatkova et al[7] showed that when the number of missing leads for QTd measurement was increased from one to four leads, the mean relative error of QTd measurement increased from 6.1% to 18.5%. In MI patients, when the number of measurable leads decreased from 12 to eight leads, there was a small, nonsignificant increase in rate-corrected QTd (QTcd) measurement from 100±35.5 to 109.5±47.9 ms.[12] Gang et al[13] reported that in healthy subjects the mean number of valid leads available for QTd measurement was between 10.14 and 10.23 for global QTd and 4.96 and 4.97 for precordial QTd when measured in the supine position using an automated method. There have yet been no data on the number of valid leads measurable and required in at-risk populations, particularly in patients after MI, for QTd to truly reflect the underlying dispersion of repolarization. This is because the T wave is commonly abnormal (biphasic or inverted) in MI patients; this can seriously affect the number of valid leads available for measurement. Thus, the minimum number of leads required in order to have a reproducible and clinically valid QTd measurement is still unknown.

In addition to number of valid leads available for QTd measurement, the specific lead that is missing is also likely to influence the measurement of QTd. In healthy subjects, the shortest QT interval was most often found in leads aVL and V_1, whereas the longest QT interval was most often recorded in leads V_2 and V_3.[7] Therefore, the omission of one or more of these leads will have a larger impact on the assessment of QTd than omission of other leads. In patients with MI, the longest QT interval measured was most usually found in lead V_4 and the shortest was lead

V_1, although the most common lead omitted for QT interval measurement was aVR and the least common was lead V_3.[12]

Lead Selection

There was an uncertainty in earlier studies regarding the lead selection for QTd measurement in order to obtain maximum information on ventricular recovery time. Some investigators used 12-lead measurement (global)[1,14] whereas others used the precordial leads only.[10,15] Van de Loo et al[16] showed that in healthy subjects, QTd measured from six precordial chest leads correlated weakly with that obtained from the 12-lead ECGs in the same population (r=0.32). In contrast, Priori and colleagues[15] showed that in patients with congenital long QT syndrome, assessment of QTd in the six precordial leads correlated well with results obtained from analysis of 12-lead ECGs. In patients with anterior wall MI, while there was a good correlation in QTd assessed with six precordial and 12 leads, it was not as good in patients with inferior MI.[16] Therefore, it is apparent in certain populations including healthy subjects and long QT syndrome patients that six precordial leads may be sufficient for the measurement of QTd, but this may not be true in others. With respect to the reproducibility of both techniques, 12-lead QTd was more reproducible than the precordial QTd (see below). This is important especially when QTd is being used as a clinical tool. In general, therefore, it is preferable to use 12 leads for the determination of QTd.

Recently, Macfarlane et al[17] argued that QTd should be measured using eight leads only (six precordial leads and any two limb leads) because all six limb leads can be derived from any two using Einthoven's law. Therefore, if the T wave has ended in two limb leads, e.g., I and II, then the QT interval in the remaining four limb leads cannot be greater except because of a projection effect, allowing for small measurement error, and the fact that the QRS onset may vary slightly from lead to lead. In their study, Macfarlane et al showed that in a normal population, QTd measured from all 12 leads was 4 ms longer than QTd measured from leads I, II, and V_1 through V_6 (20.76±7.8 ms). Unfortunately, this concept has not yet been widely adopted and investigated and its clinical value cannot be ascertained.

Heart Rate Correction

Unlike QT interval measurement, there has been some uncertainty about the need to correct QTd for heart rate. In animal studies, epicardial mapping with direct measurement of repolarization at multiple sites has shown that although the repolarization time (action potential duration [APD]) should be corrected for heart rate, the dispersion of repolarization (maximum APD – minimum APD) does not change with heart rate and need not be corrected for it.[18] Subsequent studies have confirmed this view.[19,20]

Subramanian and colleagues[19] performed a study to assess the effect of heart rate on QTd using fixed atrial pacing at various cycle lengths on patients undergoing electrophysiological study in a drug-free state. They showed that QTd remained relatively constant and did not change as a function of the atrial paced rate while QTc dispersion significantly increased at shorter cycle lengths. Furthermore, heart-rate–induced changes in QT interval and APD at 90% repolarization (APD_{90}) were not associated with alteration in QTd. Thus, QTd is not altered by isolated changes in heart rate, and "correction" of the QTd is misleading since the changes in this parameter at different heart rates may largely reflect the changes in cycle length and not alterations in cardiac repolarization. Other workers also showed that QTd measured automatically remained relatively unchanged and did not correlate with R-R interval changes following exercise.[20] QTd should therefore not be corrected for heart rate.

Effects of T Wave

The most crucial and difficult aspect of the methodology of measuring the QT interval and QTd is the identification of the offset of T wave, which in turn is influenced by the presence of U wave, T wave amplitude, and baseline noise. Hence, not all ECG leads had measurable QT intervals. In healthy subjects, the most frequently measured leads for QT interval measurement are II, V_3, and V_4 (99.1%), and the least measurable lead was aVL (30.4%).[8] Many conditions can produce U waves, including congenital and drug-induced long QT syndromes, which can obscure the T wave offset. This is particularly difficult if a U wave is present that merges with the T wave. In this situation, the end of T wave is defined by some as the nadir between the T and U wave for QT interval and QTd measurement.[6] Others, however, have chosen to exclude these leads completely[21] whereas some include the lead and measure to the end of the U wave. It is important to note that QTd is a function of T wave duration.[22] Therefore, the presence of a merged T/U wave complex signifies an abnormal ventricular repolarization, and the exclusion of a U wave from T/U complex for QTd measurement will decrease the power of the QTd measurement to reflect any abnormality of repolarization and may be misleading. Indeed, if the leads with T/U phenomena were excluded from analysis, a falsely low value of QTd would be obtained.[21] Therefore, U waves should be included for QT interval and QTd measurement if it is part of the T/U complex but excluded if it is distinct from the T wave.

The amplitude of T wave is equally important and can influence the definition of the T wave offset for QTd measurement. Small T waves introduce greater variability in measurement.[23] In leads where the T wave amplitude is low, the terminal portion can be indistinguishable from spontaneous fluctuation of the baseline. Accurate QT measurement requires a T wave amplitude of at least 250 μV. However, the exclusion of small T waves may also affect the accuracy and reliability of QTd analysis. The selection of such a threshold level is therefore a compromise between excluding too many small T waves and maximizing the number of leads available for analysis. In a population consisting of patients with MI and arrhythmias (supraventricular and ventricular) and healthy controls, there was an average fall of 30% in QTd values when T waves with an amplitude of less than 100 μV were excluded and a 51% fall when those of less than 250 μV were excluded.[24] Murray et al[24] suggested that 100 μV is a reasonable compromise for QTd analysis.

The end of the T wave can sometimes be very difficult to define despite a perfectly formed T wave. During the offset of the T wave, the slow moving deflection of the T wave can be contaminated with noise. Furthermore, the shape of the T wave itself can be very variable (Fig. 2), from small and flat to biphasic. Various attempts have been made to determine the end of the T wave for QT interval measurement. Several algorithms that have been proposed for determining the end of the T wave include: the threshold method (TH), the differential threshold method (DTH), the slope method (SL), and the peak slope method (PSI) (Fig. 3). For the TH method, the T wave offset is determined as the interception of a threshold level with the T wave. In DTH method, the T wave offset is defined as the interception of a threshold level and the differential of the T wave. For both TH and DTH methods, the threshold levels are calculated as a fraction, in the range of 0.05 to 0.15, of the amplitude of the T wave or differential T wave, respectively. The final two algorithms are based on slope features. In SL method, the end of T wave is taken as the interception of an isoelectric level and a line tangential to the point of maximum T wave slope. Finally, the PSI method calculates the end of T wave as the interception point between an isoelectric level and the line that passes through the peak of the T wave and the point of maximum T wave slope. McLaughlin and colleagues[25] assessed the effects of various filtering bandwidths, isoelectric level, and threshold level settings on the above four algorithms in identifying the end of T wave using both manual and automatic methods. They found that the mean QT interval measurement was extremely variable with different filtering, isoelectric, and threshold levels: up to 62 ms for TH methods, 33 ms for DTH, 17 ms for SL, and 26 ms for PSI. Thus, various commonly used algorithms for T wave identification are influenced closely by the filtering and technique variables. Comparison of studies using different techniques must take into account such potential confounding factors; these authors

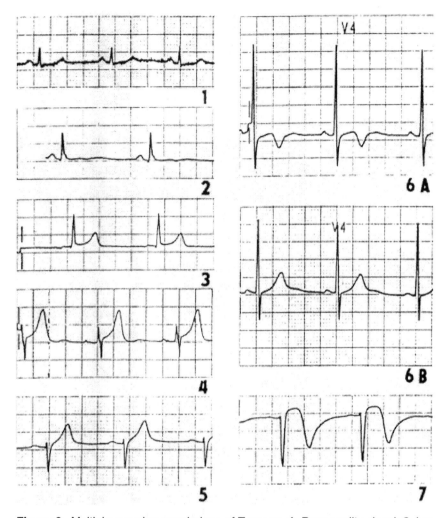

Figure 2. Multiple complex morphology of T waves. **1.** Poor quality signal; **2.** low amplitude; **3.** distinct T wave; **4.** distinct T and U waves; **5.** possible T/U fusion; **6A.** partial T/U wave fusion; **6B.** partial T/U wave fusion (sudden slope change); **7.** complete T/U wave fusion. Adapted from Kautzner J, Gang Y, Kishore AGR, et al. Interobserver reproducibility of QT interval measurement and QT dispersion in patients after acute myocardial infarction. *Ann Noninvas Electrocardiol* 1996;1(4):363-374.

recommended that generally, the TH method should not be used for clinical purposes for the reason mentioned.

Realizing the importance and difficulty of measuring T wave offset for QT interval and QTd measurement, Xue and Reddy[26] compared the reproducibility of QTd measurements using five different algorithms: two based on threshold method (TH and DTH), two based on maximum

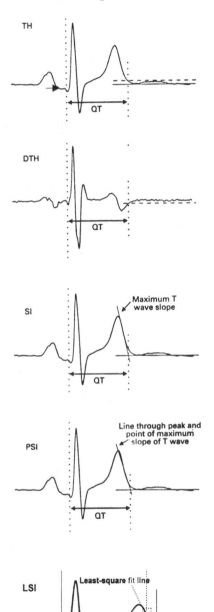

Figure 3. The main algorithms used for determining the end of the T wave include: **A.** the threshold method (TH), which is the interception of a threshold level and the T wave; **B.** the differential threshold method (DTH), which is the interception of a threshold level and the differential of the T wave; **C.** the slope method (SL), which is the interception of a line tangential to the point of maximum T wave slope and isoelectric level; **D.** the peak slope method (PSI), which is the interception of an isoelectric level and the line passing through the peak and point of maximum slope of the T wave; and **E.** the least-square fitting method, in which a least-square fitted line around the region of the maximum slope point is computed and the intersection of this line with the isoelectric line (the least-square index) is used for the T wave offset.

T wave slope (SL and the least-square fitting method), and finally, a T wave area method (TA). TA is a threshold method based on the integral of the T wave using the point at which the T wave area reaches 90% of the entire T wave area. In the least-square fitting method, a least-square fitted line around the region of the maximum slope point is computed, and the intersection of this line with the isoelectric line (the least-square index) is used for the T wave offset. In the threshold methods, three algorithms based on a percentage (10%, 15%, or 20%) of the maximum T peak (TH) or maximum differential T peak (DTH) were compared. In the T wave slope method, only one algorithm was possible that used the intersection of the maximum slope line with the isoelectric line of the TP segment as the T wave offset. In the least-square fitting method, three algorithms were compared using 2, 6, and 8n sample points for the fitting lines, where n is the number of samples above and below the inflex point for the computation of the downslope inflex tangent. For the TA method, the threshold was set at 90% of the total T wave area. They found that even in normal ECGs, the values of QTd performed on the same ECGs could vary from algorithm to algorithm by approximately 9 ms, ranging from 18 ms (TA) to 27 ms (DTH, 10%). For the threshold methods, a larger percentage of threshold (20%) had better reproducibility of QTd than a smaller percentage of threshold (10%), and in the least-square fitting method, the reproducibility was better with more points (i.e., eight better than two). More importantly, these investigators showed that the slope-based methods in general had better reproducibility than the threshold methods in determining T wave offset with least-square fitting algorithm achieved the best reproducibility in QTd measurement.

There are two reasons why slope-based algorithms had better reproducibility than threshold-based methods. First, the maximum slope point of the T wave is more stable, or more reproducible, than threshold methods, which are based on T wave amplitude. Second, the straight line corresponding to the maximum slope is better than the original curve for obtaining a stable point of intersection with a horizontal line, the same reason why a higher threshold can improve reproducibility, since the horizontal threshold line intersects with a more stable portion of the T wave. The least-square fit algorithm achieved better reproducibility than the simple slope method, mainly because of more stable fitting due to more sample points. The least-square fit algorithm is now being adopted as the standard algorithm used for detecting T wave offset for automated QT interval and QTd measurement in some commercial products. It is important to realize that compared with threshold method, the slope method may theoretically cut off the terminal portion of the T wave and reduce its accuracy for QT interval measurement.

Reproducibility of QTd

The clinical value of QTd critically depends on the reproducibility of the method employed for its measurement, whether it is manual or automated. For QTd to be useful as a stratification tool, it must be reproducible. It is important to realize that the identification of electrocardiographic waveforms also depends on subjective observations and that the individual approaches by different observers may constitute a significant bias.

Kautzner and colleagues[8] examined the short- and long-term reproducibility of QT interval and QTd measurement in healthy subjects using a digitizing board with a 0.1-mm resolution. With use of this method, the measurement of QT interval from standard ECG recordings was feasible and not operator-dependent, with an interobserver relative error of less than 4%. The duration of the QT interval in healthy volunteers was stable and its short-term (1 day) and long-term (1 week and 1 month) reproducibility was high with an intrasubject relative error of less than 6%. In contrast, QTd measurement (without any correction for heart rate or missing leads) was highly nonreproducible, between subsequent recordings (relative error 26% to 35%) and between observers (relative error 28%). Thus, the low reproducibility with the digitizing method reduced the applicability of such a method for QTd measurement. This is probably not surprising given the poor human precision of operating a digitizing board as shown in a study by Malik and Bradford.[27] They found that even with a high-precision digitizing board (with a technical accuracy of ±50 microns), a median mean error of 1.2 mm and a median maximum error of 1.0 mm were found for repeated distance measurement. When simulating QTd measurement (measuring the same distance 12 times), a median value of 20 ms was found for ECG recorded at 25 mm/s paper speed. Accurate QT interval measurement and hence QTd assessment requires considerable experience in using the tool as well as identification of the T wave offset. This is particularly true when measuring QT intervals in MI patients, where large errors have been reported between observers not specifically experienced in QT interval measurement.[28] Furthermore, a major source of interobserver error is lack of rules on QT and QTd measurements.

To counteract the imprecision of measurement using a digitizing board, Glancy et al used a user interactive method whereby the ECGs were scanned onto a computer that would then allow a manual measurement on-screen.[11] They compared the reproducibility of their method with that of an automatic measurement using a specially designed algorithm on patients after MI. They found that the reproducibility of the mean QT interval using this method was good with an intrasubject error of 6 ms (relative error 1.4%) and interobserver error of 7 ms (1.8%), and the observers' versus automatic measurement errors were approximately 10.5 ms (26.5%). However, QTd measurement using both methods yielded large errors for all methods with an intrasubject error of 12 ms (19.8%), interobserver error of 15 ms (24%), and observers' versus automatic measurement error of approximately 26 ms (32%). The study showed that a user interactive method for measuring QTd did not fare that much better than the digitizing method in its reproducibility, and the authors called for caution when studies reported differences of magnitude close to the measurement error. Furthermore, comparison of QTd measurement between either different observers or across studies or different populations requires even greater caution.

While the automated system of QTd measurement is theoretically more reproducible, it is limited by the ability of the algorithm to recognize common T wave morphologies. As discussed earlier, Xue and Reddy[26] demonstrated that a least-square fitting slope-based algorithm for determining T wave offset had the best reproducibility in QTd measurement. This algorithm is now being incorporated into commercial software that provides automated measurement of QTd. In 70 healthy subjects, Gang et al[13] assessed the reproducibility and stability of automated QTd measurement using a least-square fitting algorithm for determining the T wave offset. They found that the reproducibility of QTd measured in supine position at a mean interval of 8 days apart had a poor reproducibility with a relative error of 30.3% for global QTd and 31.0% for precordial QTd measurement. Global QTd measurement was generally more stable and not affected by posture (supine or standing) or the respiratory cycle, whereas the precordial QTd was reduced significantly when the posture was changed from supine to standing but not affected by the respiratory cycle. In the supine position, in which QTd is normally measured, the relative error/reproducibility of QTd measurement could be slightly improved when five serial ECG recordings were averaged compared with two ECGs (13.0% versus 16.4%), although it did not reach a significant level. The authors suggested that averaging of results from several serial measurements should be used whenever possible in order to improve the reproducibility of QTd measurement with this method.

Although it has been shown that automated QTd measurement has a poor reproducibility, it is unclear whether it is more reliable and reproducible than manual measurement. Indeed, it is not obvious whether QTd results obtained with manual measurement are comparable to those obtained with an automated method. In healthy controls, an automated method using a least-square fitting algorithm for determining T wave offset has an equally poor intrasubject reproducibility (approximately 40%) as the manual method in global QTd measurement.[29] However, for precordial QTd measurement, the manual method was shown to be significantly less reproducible than the automated method (P<0.005). For

QT interval measurement, the automatic method had significantly lower intrasubject variability and appeared to be more stable than with manual measurement (P<0.05).

The agreement between automatic and manual methods in both QT interval and QTd measurements was extremely poor (r^2=0.10 to 0.25 for QT interval measurement; r^2= 0.06 for global QTd; r^2=0.01 for precordial QTd). One possible explanation for the lack of correlation between automated and manual QT interval and QTd measurements in this study is that with the manual method, ECGs with U waves were excluded from measurement, whereas in the automated method, no such discrimination was possible with the algorithm. The fact that the automated method had a better reproducibility in the QT interval measurement also implies that the algorithm used for determining the T wave offset with the manual method was different from and more variable than that of the automated method. This would also have accounted for the lack of agreement between both methods. The lack of agreement between automated and manual methods suggests that QT interval and QTd results obtained with one method cannot be blindly applied and compared with those obtained with the other method. This finding was substantiated in a study performed by another group.[24] Murray et al[24] showed that automated QTd measurement gave different results than manual measurement and that they had no correlation with each other irrespective of the algorithms used for determining T wave offset (TH, DTH, SL or PSI). Different techniques for QTd measurement (automated or manual) will produce different QTd results and new reference ranges will need to be adopted.

Despite the above studies, it is still unclear whether the automated or the manual method is better for QTd measurement, as both methods have equally poor intrasubject reproducibility. However, the fact that the automated method has at least a better reproducibility in QT interval measurement renders this a preferred method for measuring the QT interval and probably the QTd.

Conclusion

The technique for measuring QTd is still evolving. It is hindered predominantly by the algorithm used to describe the T wave offset. It is important to realize that different methods used for QTd measurement will produce different results, particularly in diseased groups where the T wave morphology may be abnormal. Hence, when comparing the results from different studies, the methods used must be considered to ensure that they are comparable. It is clear that QTd should not be corrected for missing leads, or for heart rate. Global QTd should probably be used rather than precordial QTd, and the number of valid leads should be specified. While the reproducibility for both manual and automated QTd measurement is poor, at least for QT interval measurement, the automatic method has significantly lower intrasubject variability and is more stable than the manual measurement. The automated method is therefore preferable for QTd measurement and is the only realistic practical means of measuring QTd clinically. The reproducibility of automated QTd measurement can be improved by taking the mean of several serial measurements. While the data on healthy controls are crucial in validating the technique of QTd, considerably more data are still needed in at-risk groups to determine the usefulness of QTd as a risk stratification tool in these patients.

References

1. Day CP, McComb JM, Campbell RWF. QT dispersion: An indication of arrhythmia in risk patients with long QT intervals. *Br Heart J* 1990;63:342-344.
2. Zabel M, Portnoy S, Franz MR. Electrocardiographic indexes of dispersion of ventricular repolarization: An isolated heart validation study. *J Am Coll Cardiol* 1995;25:746-752.
3. Gavrilescu S, Luca C. Right ventricular monophasic action potentials in patients with long QT syndrome. *Br Heart J* 1978;40:1014-1018.
4. Abildskov JA, Vincent GM, Evans K, Burgess MJ. Distribution of body surface ECG potentials in familiar QT interval prolongation. *Am J Cardiol* 1981;47:480. Abstract.
5. Kuo CS, Munakata K, Reddy CP, Surawicz B. Characteristics and possible mechanism of ventricular arrhythmia dependent on the dispersion of action potential durations. *Circulation* 1983;67:1356-1367.
6. Higham PD, Campbell RWF. QT dispersion. *Br Heart J* 1994;71:508-510.
7. Hnatkova K, Malik M, Kautzner J, et al. Adjustment of QT dispersion assessed from 12 lead electrocardiograms for different numbers of analysed electrocardiographic leads: Comparison of stability of different methods. *Br Heart J* 1994;72:390-396.
8. Kautzner J, Gang Y, Camm AJ, Malik M. Short- and long-term reproducibility of QT, QTc and QT dispersion measurement in healthy subjects. *PACE* 1994;17:928-937.
9. Campbell RWF, Gardiner P, Amos PA, et al. Measurement of the QT interval. *Eur Heart J* 1985;6:D81-D85.
10. Hii JTY, Wyse DG, Gillis AM, et al. Precordial QT interval dispersion as a marker of torsades de pointes. Disparate effects of a class Ia antiarrhythmic drugs and amiodarone. *Circulation* 1992;86:1376-1382.
11. Glancy JM, Weston PJ, Bhullar HK, et al. Reproducibility and automatic measurement of QT dispersion. *Eur Heart J* 1996;17:1035-1039.
12. Glancy JM, Garratt CJ, Woods KL, de Bono DP. Use of lead adjustment formulas for QT dispersion after myocardial infarction. *Br Heart J* 1995;74:676-679.
13. Gang Y, Guo X-H, Crook R, et al. Computerised measurement of QT dispersion in healthy subjects. *Heart* 1998;80:459-466.
14. Day CP, McComb J, Matthews J, Campbell RWF. Reduction in QT dispersion by sotalol following myocardial infarction. *Eur Heart J* 1991;12:423-427.

15. Priori SG, Napolitano C, Diehl L, Schwartz PJ. Dispersion of the QT interval: A marker of therapeutic efficacy in the long QT syndrome. *Circulation* 1994;89:1681-1689.
16. Van de Loo A, Arendts W, Hohnloser SH. Variability of QT dispersion measurements in the surface electrocardiogram in patients with acute myocardial infarction and in normal subjects. *Am J Cardiol* 1994;74:1113-1118.
17. Macfarlane PW, McLaughlin SC, Rodger C. Influence of lead selection and population on automated measurement of QT dispersion. *Circulation* 1998;98:2160-2167.
18. Zabel M, Woosley RL, Franz MR. Is dispersion of ventricular repolarization rate dependent? *PACE* 1997;20:2405-2411.
19. Subramanian R, Shalaby A, Sager P. Is QT dispersion altered by changes in heart rate? *J Am Coll Cardiol* 1999;33:129A.
20. Maarouf N, Aytemir K, Gallagher MM, et al. Is QT dispersion heart rate dependent? What are the values of correction formulas for QT interval? *J Am Coll Cardiol* 1999;33:113A.
21. Sylven JC, Horacek BM, Spencer CA, et al. QT interval variability on the body surface. *J Electrocardiol* 1984;17:179-188.
22. Fei L, Statters D, Camm AJ. AT-interval dispersion on 12-lead electrocardiogram in normal subjects: Its reproducibility and relation to the T wave. *Am Heart J* 1994;127:1654-1655.
23. McLaughlin NB, Campbell RWF, Murray A. Accuracy of four automatic QT measurement techniques in cardiac patients and healthy subjects. *Heart* 1996;76:422-426.
24. Murray A, McLaughlin NB, Campbell RWF. Measuring QT dispersion: Man versus machine. *Heart* 1997;77:539-542.
25. McLaughlin NB, Campbell RWF, Murray A. Comparison of automatic QT measurement techniques in the normal 12 lead electrocardiogram. *Br Heart J* 1995;74:84-89.
26. Xue Q, Reddy S. Algorithms for computerized QT analysis. *J Electrocardiol* 1998;30:181-186.
27. Malik M, Bradford A. Human precision of operating a digitizing board: Implications for electrocardiogram measurements. *PACE* 1998;21:1656-1662.
28. Ahnve S. Errors in the visual determination of corrected QT (QTc) interval during acute myocardial infarction. *J Am Coll Cardiol* 1985;5:699-702.
29. Savelieva I, Yi G, Guo X-H, et al. Agreement and reproducibility of automatic versus manual measurement of QT interval and QT dispersion. *Am J Cardiol* 1998;81:471-477.

5

Correlations Between Monophasic Action Potential Recordings and Surface Electrocardiograms with Regard to the Evaluation of Dispersion of Ventricular Repolarization

Markus Zabel and Michael R. Franz

Methodological Need for Validation

In numerous experimental and clinical studies,[1-5] heterogeneity of the ventricular repolarization process has been established as a significant cofactor in the genesis of ventricular tachyarrhythmias. This heterogeneity is usually referred to as dispersion of ventricular repolarization, or even shorter, as dispersion. Clinically important, dispersion of ventricular repolarization is believed to represent a simple-to-measure condition of the heart that provides information on the likelihood of malignant ventricular arrhythmias, thus on the risk of a given patient to suffer from sudden cardiac death. True dispersion of repolarization can only be measured invasively and directly from the myocardium, e.g., using catheter recordings by means of the monophasic action potential (MAP) contact electrode method.[6-8] As a noninvasive means, body surface potential mapping using more than 100 precordial electrocardiogram (ECG) leads has been shown to be useful in quantitating dispersion.[9-12] Neither method,

From Olsson SB, Amlie JP, Yuan S (eds): *Dispersion of Ventricular Repolarization: State of the Art.* ©Futura Publishing Company, Inc., Armonk, NY, 2000.

however, was practical as a simple and widely accessible clinical tool for evaluation of dispersion of repolarization in patients. In 1990, Day and coworkers[13] proposed the measurement of the maximum difference of QT intervals from the 12-lead surface ECG as a simple estimate of dispersion of ventricular repolarization, subsequently called QT dispersion (QTD). This marker has been evaluated in a large number of studies[14-26] but it is currently uncertain whether the initial goal to provide an easy method of risk stratification can be met. QTD was proposed in patients post myocardial infarction[17-20,25] or with congestive heart failure.[21-24] It seems to be quite useful for the assessment of arrhythmia risk in long QT patients[11-13,15] or for evaluation of proarrhythmia during therapy with action-potential–prolonging drugs.[13,14] In addition to other methodological problems of the QTD method, which were reviewed by Statters et al,[27] Surawicz,[28] and Coumel et al,[29] a common criticism was that the method lacked a proper validation. This chapter therefore summarizes the two validation studies published[30,31] in which true dispersion measurements from the myocardium were correlated with standard QTD and numerous other ECG variables of dispersion of ventricular repolarization.

Experimental and Human Validation Methods

To accomplish the objective of validating potentially useful ECG variables using myocardial repolarization measurements, a novel isolated Langendorff heart preparation was developed by Zabel et al.[30] A total of 10 silver-silver chloride electrode pellets were positioned on the walls of the tissue bath around an isolated rabbit heart with a diameter similar to that of a rabbit thorax. With custom amplifier configurations a volume-conducted, simulated 12-lead ECG could be recorded. In addition to that, up to eight contact MAP electrodes were mounted with equal distances on the epicardium of the centrally placed Langendorff-perfused rabbit heart while additional catheters allowed the simultaneous recording of endocardial MAPs from both ventricles. In the human heart, Franz et al[6] and Zabel et al[31] recorded sequential endocardial MAPs during cardiac catheterization in 11 patients. In this mapping protocol, which followed the recording of a 12-lead surface ECG, contact electrode catheters were used to record an average of eight MAPs from six prespecified left ventricular endocardial regions. Similarly, MAPs were recorded by means of a contact electrode probe in six patients during cardiac surgery. That section of the protocol covered an average of six epicardial mapping sites from both ventricles.[6,31] The dispersion of MAP durations at 90% repolarization (APD$_{90}$) was defined as APD$_{90}$max - APD$_{90}$min, whereas dispersion of recovery time (recovery time = APD$_{90}$ + activation time) was also calculated as the difference of maximum and minimum. In summary, the presented methodology permitted the direct comparison of surface ECG and myocardial MAP recordings.

ECG Variables of Dispersion of Ventricular Repolarization

In the experimental study[30] volume-conducted ECGs were recorded digitally, whereas ECGs from the human study were later digitized from paper.[30,32] All recordings were submitted to interactive analysis by means of custom written software, allowing the calculation of most ECG dispersion variables proposed in the literature heretofore.

Conventional ECG Variables

The computer program used customized algorithms to detect important features of the ECG waveforms such as Q onset, J point, T_{peak}, and T_{end}, and then displayed vertical spikes superimposed on the signal, marking these points for confirmation or manual correction by the observer. After complete analysis, JT, rate-corrected JT (JTc), QT, and rate-corrected QT (QTc) intervals were calculated as an average among all analyzable leads with rate correction done by the Bazett's formula. Conventional QT, JT, QTc, and JTc dispersion were calculated as the maximum minus the minimum interval duration of all analyzable ECG leads. Adjusted QTD[33] and relative QTD involving the standard deviation of QT intervals[15] were also determined. Finally, all ECG variables were recalculated on the basis of the six precordial leads only.[14,15]

New ECG Variables

Because the T wave is presumably generated from inhomogeneous recovery throughout the heart,[6,34-36] our group[30] hypothesized that T wave width measured by the T peak to T end interval and T wave area, representing a summation of T wave vectors, reflects dispersion of ventricular repolarization. These variables were validated in the experimental study described above[30] and were subsequently evaluated clinically[22,25] as well as in the human validation study also presented here.[31] In support of the initial hypothesis, the T peak to T end interval has recently been proposed by Shimizu and Antzelevitch[37,38] as an ECG marker of transmural dispersion of ventricular repolarization. Their experiments provide evidence that delayed repolarization of M cells residing in the mid-myocardium contributes significantly to the transmural dispersion.[37,38] These findings, however, were derived from a single ECG lead in an arterially perfused canine wedge preparation and must be confirmed in whole heart models. Finally, the ratio of the Q-T_{peak} to Q-T_{end} interval was suggested by us as a measure of the late repolarization phase.[31] Conventional and new ECG variables are summarized in Table 1.

Results of Experimental and Human Validation Studies

Experimental Study

In the experimental study,[30] QTD and JT dispersion showed a significant correlation with the dispersion of APD_{90} (r=0.61, P<0.001 and r=0.64, P<0.001, respectively) as well as with the dispersion of recovery time (r= 0.59, P<0.001 and r=0.58, P<0.001, respectively; Fig. 1, panel A). Among the newly studied variables, T wave area exhibited an excellent correlation with dispersion of APD_{90} and recovery time (r=0.79, P<0.0001 and r=0.82, P<0.0001, respectively, Fig. 1, panel B), as did the T peak to T end interval (r=0.81, P<0.001 and r=0.82, P<0.001, respectively, Fig. 1, panel C). The T peak to T end interval and the area under the T wave therefore were expected to reflect true myocardial dispersion in patients better than QTD and JT dispersion.

Human Study

Similar to the experimental protocol, QTD showed a good correlation with dispersion of repolarization time (RT) (r=0.67, P<0.01, Fig. 2, panel A) in the human validation study,[31] which was remarkably similar to that observed in the experimental study. Data were available from a total of 17 patients. Among the other variables, the $Q-T_{peak}/Q-T_{end}$ ratio averaged over all analyzable leads (r=-0.59, P<0.01; Fig. 2, panel B), and in V_3 alone

Table 1
ECG Variables of Dispersion of Ventricular Repolarization

ECG Variable	First Description	Reference #
QT dispersion	1990	13
QT_c dispersion	1990	13
JT dispersion	1992	14
JT_c disprsion	1992	14
Adjusted QT dispersion	1992	33
Relative QT dispersion	1994	15
Precordial QT dispersion	1992	14
Area under T wave	1995	30
T peak to T end interval	1995	30
$Q-T_{peak}$ to $Q-T_{end}$ ratio	1998	31

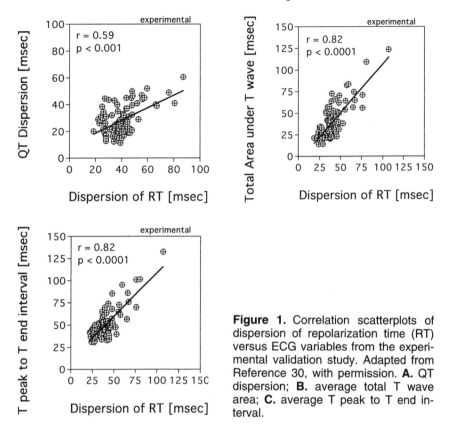

Figure 1. Correlation scatterplots of dispersion of repolarization time (RT) versus ECG variables from the experimental validation study. Adapted from Reference 30, with permission. **A.** QT dispersion; **B.** average total T wave area; **C.** average T peak to T end interval.

(r=-0.72, P<0.01; Fig. 2, panel C), exhibited one of the best correlations with dispersion of RT, which was further improved when only endocardial measurements were considered.[31] T area measures did not correlate with dispersion of RT but discriminated left ventricular hypertrophy. Beyond demonstrating a reasonable correlation between ECG variables of dispersion of repolarization and the direct myocardial MAP measurements, the study allowed a comparison among currently proposed ECG variables of dispersion of ventricular repolarization. Many of the studied ECG variables exhibit a similar and significant correlation with the invasive measurements. Importantly, this was true for the standard QTD (QT_{max} − QT_{min}), which had been widely used by many investigators. Adjusted and relative QTD did not show an improved association with the invasive measurements in the study. An identical association was found for precordial ECG variables, suggesting that most of the ventricular heterogeneity in repolarization is found within the six unipolar chest leads. Rate correction of QTD resulted in a decreased correlation with the myocardial measurements.

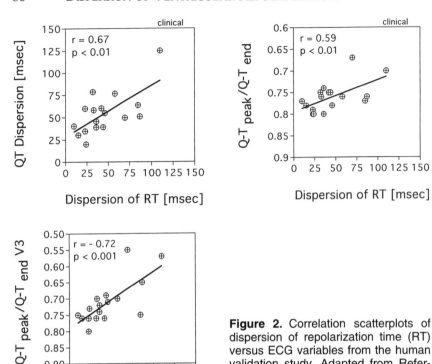

Figure 2. Correlation scatterplots of dispersion of repolarization time (RT) versus ECG variables from the human validation study. Adapted from Reference 31, with permission. **A.** QT dispersion; **B.** Q-T$_{peak}$/Q-T$_{end}$ ratio; **C.** Q-T$_{peak}$/Q-T$_{end}$ ratio in lead V$_3$.

Genesis of QTD—Local Differences of Repolarization or Different Projections of a Global T Wave Vector?

While the above validation studies establish a close correlation between dispersion at the myocardial level and variables that can be assessed from the 12-lead surface ECG, this does not prove a causal relationship between them, nor does it validate ECG dispersion variables as an index of arrhythmia risk. Due to the close correlation it can be assumed that the local variations in APD are mirrored by variations in the QT interval or by similar variables in the surface ECG. This so-called "local" hypothesis of QTD genesis is in contrast to a recently presented theory after which differences in QT duration—and thus QTD—can be explained by different projections of a common T wave vector.[39] While it may be very difficult beyond the straightforward correlations in the above two validation studies to explain the surface ECG on the basis of myocardial measurements (the "inverse" problem of electrocardiography), the hypothesis that all information is included in a single T wave vector may provide an oversimplification. The vectorcardiographic derivation of the common T wave vector from a sample number of surface ECG leads most likely averages out existing nondipolar contents within cardiac repolarization. Under certain arrhythmogenic clinical situations, it may be exactly this local deviation from dipolarity[11,40,41] that may reveal the arrhythmogenic substrate. The "local" repolarization hypothesis is furthermore supported by several body surface mapping studies. The study by Mirvis[10] in which 150 simultaneous precordial unipolar ECG leads were used was the first to reveal regional repolarization differences on the body surface. Subsequently, Cowan et al[42] first calculated interlead differences in the QT interval within the 12-lead surface ECG. In summary, it can be hypothesized that the T wave reflects a combination of local and global repolarization vector forces. Moreover, it can be expected that more local information from the vicinity of the unipolar electrodes is carried by the Wilson chest leads while more global repolarization vectors will be represented in the bipolar limb leads. It is therefore conceivable that the unipolar chest leads are most useful for QTD measurements. In addition, even the T wave of a single precordial lead seems to convey a large portion of the precordial or even 12-lead information content, as the $Q-T_{peak}/Q-T_{end}$ ratio measured from lead V_3 exhibited an excellent correlation with dispersion of ventricular repolarization as assessed by means of MAP recordings.

Conclusion

Dispersion of ventricular repolarization can be assessed from the 12-lead surface ECG, as has been validated in an experimental model and in the human heart. Several new ECG dispersion variables are available. A selection of several variables exhibits similar accuracy in their correlation with true myocardial dispersion. Variables involving the terminal part of repolarization such as the $Q-T_{peak}/Q-T_{end}$ ratio—even from a single lead—may add to the assessment of dispersion of ventricular repolarization from the human heart.

References

1. Han J, Moe GK. Nonuniform recovery of excitability in ventricular muscle. *Circ Res* 1964;14:44.
2. Merx W, Yoon MS, Han J. The role of local disparity in conduction and recovery time on ventricular vulnerability to fibrillation. *Am Heart J* 1977;94:603.
3. Kuo CS, Munakata K, Reddy CP, et al. Characteristics and possible mechanism of ventricular arrhythmia dependent on the dispersion of action potential durations. *Circulation* 1983;67:1356-1367.
4. Kuo CS, Reddy CP, Munakata K, et al. Mechanism of ventricular arrhythmias caused by increased dispersion of repolarization. *Eur Heart J* 1985;6(suppl D):63-70.

 5. Vassallo JA, Cassidy DM, Kindwall KE, et al. Nonuniform recovery of excitability in the left ventricle. *Circulation* 1988;78:1365-1372.
 6. Franz MR, Bargheer K, Rafflenbeul W, et al. Monophasic action potential mapping in human subjects with normal electrocardiograms: Direct evidence for the genesis of the T wave. *Circulation* 1987;75:379-386.
 7. Franz MR, Chin MC, Sharkey HR, et al. A new single catheter technique for simultaneous measurement of action potential duration and refractory period in vivo. *J Am Coll Cardiol* 1990;16:878-886.
 8. Franz MR. Method and theory of monophasic action potential recording. *Prog Cardiovasc Dis* 1991;33:347-368.
 9. Sylven JC, Horacek BM, Spencer CA, et al. QT interval variability on the body surface. *J Electrocardiol* 1984;17:179-188.
10. Mirvis DM. Spatial variation of QT intervals in normal persons and patients with acute myocardial infarction. *J Am Coll Cardiol* 1985;3:625-631.
11. De Ambroggi L, Bertoni T, Locati E, et al. Mapping of body surface potentials in patients with the idiopathic long QT syndrome. *Circulation* 1986;74:1334-1345.
12. De Ambroggi L, Negroni MS, Monza E, et al. Dispersion of ventricular repolarization in the long QT syndrome. *Am J Cardiol* 1991;68:614-620.
13. Day CP, McComb JM, Campbell RW. QT dispersion: An indication of arrhythmia risk in patients with long QT intervals. *Br Heart J* 1990;63:342-344.
14. Hii JTY, Wyse GD, Gillis AM, et al. Precordial QT interval dispersion as a marker of torsade de pointes. *Circulation* 1992;86:1376-1382.
15. Priori SG, Napolitano C, Diehl L, et al. Dispersion of the QT interval: A marker of therapeutic efficacy in the idiopathic long QT syndrome. *Circulation* 1994;89:1681-1689.
16. Barr CS, Naas A, Freeman M, et al. QT dispersion and sudden unexpected death in chronic heart failure. *Lancet* 1994;343:327-329.
17. Zareba W, Moss AJ, le Cessie S. Dispersion of ventricular repolarization and arrhythmic cardiac death in coronary artery disease. *Am J Cardiol* 1994; 74:550-553.
18. Moreno FL, Villanueva T, Karagounis LA, et al. Reduction in QT interval dispersion by successful thrombolytic therapy in acute myocardial infarction. TEAM-2 Study Investigators. *Circulation* 1994;90:94-100.
19. Perkiömäki JS, Koistinen MJ, Yli-Mayry S, et al. Dispersion of the QT interval in patients with and without susceptibility to ventricular tachyarrhythmias after previous myocardial infarction. *J Am Coll Cardiol* 1995;26:174-179.
20. Glancy JM, Garratt CJ, Woods KL, et al. QT dispersion and mortality after myocardial infarction. *Lancet* 1995;345:945-948.
21. Fei L, Goldman JH, Prasad K, et al. QT dispersion and RR variations on 12-lead ECGs in patients with congestive heart failure secondary to idiopathic dilated cardiomyopathy. *Eur Heart J* 1996;17:258-263.
22. Zabel M, Ney G, Fischer SR, et al. QRS width in the 12-lead surface ECG but not variables of QT dispersion predict mortality in the CHF-STAT trial. *PACE* 1996;19:589. Abstract.
23. Fu GS, Meissner A, Simon R. Repolarization dispersion and sudden cardiac death in patients with impaired left ventricular function. *Eur Heart J* 1997;18:281-289.
24. Pinsky DJ, Sciacca RR, Steinberg JS. QT dispersion as a marker of risk in patients awaiting heart transplantation. *J Am Coll Cardiol* 1997;29:1576-1584.
25. Zabel M, Klingenheben T, Franz MR, et al. Assessment of QT dispersion for prediction of mortality or arrhythmic events after myocardial infarction:

Results of a prospective long-term follow-up study. *Circulation* 1998; 97:2543-2550.
26. Zabel M, Franz MR, Klingenheben T, et al. QT dispersion as a marker of risk in patients awaiting heart transplantation? *J Am Coll Cardiol* 1998;31:1442-1443.
27. Statters DJ, Malik M, Ward DE, et al. QT dispersion: Problems of methodology and clinical significance. *J Cardiovasc Electrophysiol* 1994;5:672-685.
28. Surawicz B. Will QT dispersion play a role in clinical decision-making? *J Cardiovasc Electrophysiol* 1996;7:777-784.
29. Coumel P, Maison-Blanche P, Badilini F. Dispersion of ventricular repolarization: Reality? Illusion? Significance? *Circulation* 1998;97:2491-2493.
30. Zabel M, Portnoy S, Franz MR. Electrocardiographic indexes of dispersion of ventricular repolarization: An isolated heart validation study. *J Am Coll Cardiol* 1995;25:746-752.
31. Zabel M, Lichtlen PR, Haverich A, et al. Comparison of ECG variables of dispersion of ventricular repolarization with direct myocardial repolarization measurements in the human heart. *J Cardiovasc Electrophysiol* 1998;9:1279-1284.
32. Zabel M, Portnoy S, Fletcher RD, et al. A program for digitizing of ECG tracings on paper and accurate interactive measurement of QT intervals and ECG parameters of ventricular repolarization. *J Am Coll Cardiol* 1995;25:374A. Abstract.
33. Day CP, McComb JM, Campbell RWF. QT dispersion in sinus beats and ventricular extrasystoles in normal hearts. *Br Heart J* 1992;67:39-41.
34. Wilson FN, MacLeod AG, Barker PS, et al. The determination and the significance of the areas of the ventricular deflections of the electrocardiogram. *Am Heart J* 1934;10:46.
35. Harumi K, Burgess MJ, Abildskov JA. A theoretic model of the T wave. *Circulation* 1966;34:657-668.
36. Spach MS, Barr RC. Origin of epicardial ST-T wave potentials in the intact dog. *Circ Res* 1976;39:475-487.
37. Shimizu W, Antzelevitch C. Sodium channel block with mexiletine is effective in reducing dispersion of repolarization and preventing torsade de pointes in LQT2 and LQT3 models of the long-QT syndrome. *Circulation* 1997; 96:2038-2047.
38. Shimizu W, Antzelevitch C. Cellular basis for the ECG features of the LQT1 form of the long-QT syndrome: Effects of beta-adrenergic agonists and antagonists and sodium channel blockers on transmural dispersion of repolarization and torsade de pointes. *Circulation* 1998;98:2314-2322.
39. Kors JA, van Herpen G, van Bemmel JH. QT dispersion as an attribute of T-loop morphology. *Circulation* 1999;99:1458-1463.
40. Mitchell LB, Hubley-Kozey CL, Smith ER, et al. Electrocardiographic body surface mapping in patients with ventricular tachycardia. Assessment of utility in the identification of effective pharmacological therapy. *Circulation* 1992;86:383-393.
41. De Ambroggi L, Aime E, Ceriotti C, et al. Mapping of ventricular repolarization potentials in patients with arrhythmogenic right ventricular dysplasia: Principal component analysis of the ST-T waves. *Circulation* 1997;96:4314-4318.
42. Cowan JC, Yusoff K, Moore M, et al. Importance of lead selection in QT interval measurement. *Am J Cardiol* 1988;61:83-87.

6

Automatic Detection of Spatial and Temporal Heterogeneity of Repolarization

Wojciech Zareba, Jean Philippe Couderc, and Arthur J. Moss

The differences in morphology and duration of action potentials throughout ventricular myocardium contribute to a spatial heterogeneity of repolarization. There are substantial differences in repolarization morphology between anterior, inferior, and posterior walls of the left ventricle.[1] Similarly, action potential morphology recorded from left and right ventricles is different, contributing to the overall nonhomogeneity of repolarization in the myocardium.[2] In addition to these regional differences in repolarization, there are physiological transmural differences in the duration and shape of action potentials: the midmyocardial (M cell) zone is characterized by the longest duration of action potentials, the epicardial layer has the shortest duration of action potentials, and the duration of action potentials in endocardial layer is in the middle, between the epicardial and M cell zones.[3,4] Endocardial action potentials also differ in morphology, lacking the dome-shape phase present in action potentials recorded from epicardial and M cell layers.[3,4] The above two components, regional and transmural heterogeneity, indicate that the repolarization process has to be considered as at least a two-dimensional phenomenon. However, repolarization of a single cell, of a group of cells, and also of the entire myocardium is related to the electrical properties of the preceding beat. Both cycle length (heart rate) and repolarization duration of the preceding beat affect repolarization duration and morphology of the next beat.[5,6] Therefore, regional and transmural heterogeneity of repolarization

From Olsson SB, Amlie JP, Yuan S (eds): *Dispersion of Ventricular Repolarization: State of the Art.* ©Futura Publishing Company, Inc., Armonk, NY, 2000.

is influenced by the third (temporal) component, expressing changes in repolarization over time. For the above reasons, heterogeneity of repolarization should be considered a complex, three-dimensional electrophysiological phenomenon (Fig. 1).

Identifying optimal electrocardiographic (ECG) descriptors of this three-dimensional nature of heterogeneous repolarization is a major task of noninvasive electrocardiology. Numerous attempts have been made to evaluate the magnitude of spatial heterogeneity of repolarization in a standard 12-lead ECG. QT interval dispersion analysis (usually done manually) is the most popular method,[7-12] however, there are major technical and conceptual limitations of QT dispersion measurements. More recently, the automatic methods describing global repolarization morphology by analyzing T wave loop morphology,[13-15] T wave complexity,[16] or dispersion of T wave morphology[17] have been proposed and are described below. The direct relationship between these novel ECG parameters and heterogeneity of repolarization is not yet established.

Transmural heterogeneity of repolarization is even more difficult to assess in surface ECG recordings. In studies by Shimizu and Antzelevitch,[4] differential ECG recordings from perfused myocardial tissue wedge prep-

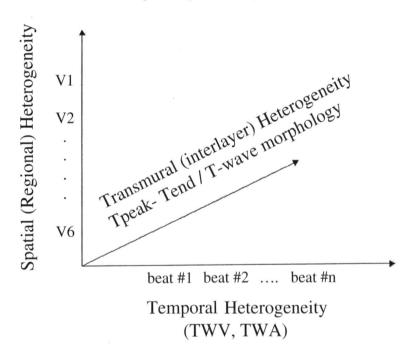

Figure 1. Schematic representation of three components (three-dimensional nature) of repolarization heterogeneity. TWV = T wave variability; TWA = T wave alternans.

arations showed that the T wave peak reflects the termination of repolarization in the epicardial layer, whereas T wave end reflects the termination of repolarization in M cell zone. The endocardial layer did not have a specific ECG manifestation, however notches and deflections on the descending arm of the T wave were suggested to reflect the end of endocardial repolarization.[4] The above observations indicate that measurements of the T peak-T end interval duration (or its ratio to the overall QT duration) would provide a noninvasive measure of transmural (epicardial-M cell) heterogeneity of repolarization. This very attractive concept is pertinent to ECG recordings derived from myocardial tissue but it cannot be adapted directly to standard 12-lead surface ECG recordings. Nevertheless, there are attempts to use the T peak-T end duration in electrocardiology.[18,19]

Temporal changes in repolarization duration, morphology, and spatial dispersion are being evaluated in surface ECG by quantifying the magnitude of QT variability,[20,21] T wave variability,[22,23] or T wave alternans (TWA).[24-26] These beat-to-beat variations are reflecting spatial heterogeneity of repolarization, since this phenomenon is believed to underlie beat-to-beat variability of repolarization.[27] There is a substantial progress in development of new methods (described below) quantifying beat-to-beat changes of repolarization.

All the above noninvasive ECG parameters attempting to describe the magnitude of spatial, transmural, or temporal heterogeneity of repolarization require automation. Measuring QT or QT peak intervals manually is not only erroneous but also insufficient in light of the recent understanding that abnormalities in repolarization morphology (not only duration) play a major role in arrhythmogenesis. In this chapter, we aim to provide an overview of automatic techniques used for quantifying three-dimensional features of repolarization heterogeneity and to share with you our own experience with these methods.

Automatic Analysis of
Spatial Dispersion of Repolarization

Interlead difference in the QT interval duration, called QT dispersion, was first proposed as a measure of repolarization heterogeneity in multilead body surface mapping.[7,28,29] In 1984, Sylven et al[7] recorded 120-lead body surface maps in 14 patients with mainly secondary QT prolongation, and demonstrated significantly increased interlead QT interval variability in comparison with the normal subjects. Similar observations were made in acute myocardial infarction patients studied by Mirvis[28] using 150-lead body surface mapping and in congenital long QT syndrome (LQTS) patients studied by De Ambroggi et al[29] using 117-lead maps. The body surface mapping, although providing detailed insight into the repolarization pattern, is not a practical approach to evaluating abnormalities of repolarization.

Instead, the analysis of repolarization in standard 12-lead ECG recordings has been considered the most applicable to clinical practice. The measurements of QT or JT interval duration in individual leads are usually done manually either on paper copy ECG or on digitizing boards. This latter approach, aiming to increase the precision of the QT measurements, may provide some improvement in quality of the analysis; however, it is still influenced by limitations of manual measurements (observer's inaccuracy and bias in determination of T wave endpoints). The reproducibility of manually measured QT dispersion remains low[30] and various automatic methods described below are being developed to overcome this limitation.

Repolarization-Duration–Based Methods

In 1989, Merri et al[8,31] proposed an automatic algorithm to quantify repolarization abnormalities and measure dispersion of repolarization from digitally acquired standard 12-lead and, subsequently, Holter ECGs. Several computer-derived parameters describing duration of the entire repolarization or its components have been designed: SoTm (S offset to T wave maximum), TmTo (T maximum to T offset), SoTo (S offset to T offset), RTm (R peak to T maximum), and RTo (R peak to T offset). T wave apex (maximum) in computer algorithms is usually detected by fitting a parabola to the signal in a 100-ms window centered on the maximum T wave amplitude and the vertex of the parabola defined T wave maximum (apex). The T wave offset is most frequently identified using the maximum slope from the final portion of the T wave. The crossing point between the baseline and this slope localizes the end of the T wave.[32] The standard deviation of the SoTm interval, measured automatically in precordial leads, has been proposed as a measure of repolarization dispersion.[8,33] This algorithm has been tested in digital 12-lead ECG recordings of more than 400 healthy subjects and subsequently applied to digital ECGs of LQTS patients, who showed significantly higher values of SoTm sd than healthy subjects (35±24 versus 17±15 ms, respectively; P<0.001).[8,10,33] Subsequently, we used the RTo interval, automatically computed in X, Y, and Z leads of digital Holter recordings, to determine the maximal dispersion of repolarization (RTd) in three-lead Holter ECG recordings.[34] A similar approach, based on the interlead comparison of automatically computed QT interval, was recently proposed by Caminal et al.[35]

To avoid the problem of accurate identification of T wave maximum and offset, Merri et al[8] proposed the area-based parameters describing duration of repolarization as a function of the shape of TU complex: time to accumulate 97%, first 50%, and middle 50% (between 25% and 75%) of the area under the curve of total repolarization time (Fig. 2). The ECG repolarization segment was determined by S wave offset (J point) and the onset of the following P wave, and the area under the TU wave curve was calculated. The advantage of the area-based parameters is that they do not limit contribution of U wave (or second component of T wave) to the repolarization segment, and therefore allow quantification of changes in the entire TU complex. We applied the TU-area–derived parameters to quantify dispersion of repolarization in 34 affected LQTS patients and their 22 unaffected family members (Table 1).[36] The dispersion of time to accumulate first and median 50% of repolarization area was significantly higher in LQTS patients, indicating that the shape of repolarization (TU wave morphology and T loop morphology) is different in LQTS patients in comparison with healthy subjects, and possibly reflecting different pathway of repolarization in the myocardium. Interestingly, dispersion of the total (97%) repolarization duration was similar in LQTS patients and their unaffected family members. This observation suggests that evaluation of interlead dispersion of total repolarization duration might reflect inaccuracies in the measurement and projection phenomenon rather than representing magnitude of repolarization heterogeneity. The parameters describing dispersion of partial duration of repolarization may better reflect nonhomogeneity of repolarization than parameters quantifying QT dispersion or total-area–derived repolarization duration. However, the direct analysis of repolarization morphology (not only duration) seems

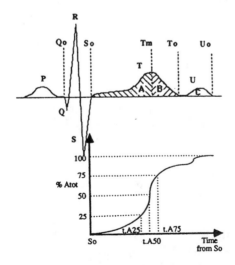

Figure 2. Schematic electrocardiographic complex (**top**) and normalized absolute integral of its repolarization segment. Reproduced from Reference 8, with permission.

Table 1
Dispersion of Repolarization Described
by Standard Deviation of Area-Derived Repolarization Parameters
in Affected LQTS Patients and Unaffected Family Members

Parameters	Unaffected Family Members (n=22)	Affected LQTS Patients (n=34)	P Value
T_{amp}(mV)	0.35±0.07	0.30±0.12	ns
A_{tot}-sd (mV*ms)	73.7±32.2	74.2±39.0	ns
t_{A97}-sd (ms)	53±19	44±20	ns
t_{A50}-sd (ms)	11±6	34±18	<0.001
t_{A25-75}-sd (ms)	24±15	44±19	<0.001
Pt_{A50}-sd (%)	6.5±2.3	8.0±2.9	0.055
Pt_{A25-75}-sd (%)	5.4±2.9	9.0±3.1	<0.001

T_{amp} = maximal amplitude of T wave (mV): A_{tot} = total absolute repolarization area (mV*ms); t_{A97} = time interval to accumulate 97% of area (ms); t_{A50} = time to accumulate 50% of area (ms); t_{A25-75} = time interval to accumulate the mid-50% of total area from 25% to 75% (ms); Pt_{A50} = percentage of repolarization time needed to accumulate first 50% of area, i.e., rate t_{A50}/t_{A97} (%); Pt_{A25-75} = percentage of repolarization time needed to accumulate middle 25-75% of area, i.e., rate t_{A25-75}/t_{A97} (%). Reproduced from Reference 36, with permission.

to be the most appropriate method for quantifying spatial heterogeneity of repolarization, and is in agreement with the vectorcardiographic principles of electrocardiography.

Principal Components Analysis

This technique, known before as principal factor analysis, was proposed to determine the redundancy of ECG information obtained in body surface mapping.[37,38] The principal component analysis (PCA) is a statistical method based on the calculation of eigenvectors from the correlation matrix describing correlation between leads. Eigen analysis, also known as single value decomposition, provides a summary of the data structure represented by a symmetrical matrix such as the correlation matrix of the lead system.

In 1991, De Ambroggi et al[29] used PCA to determine subtle changes in repolarization morphology in body surface mapping of LQTS patients. Priori and coworkers[16] applied the PCA concept to 12-lead ECGs and developed parameters describing relative contribution of single eigenvalues to the overall ECG signal. The ratio of the second to the first eigenvalue was found to reliably represent the complexity of the repolarization waveform. In this method the influence of T loop projection is partially avoided by using the eigenvalues that represent the mean square amplitude of the signal obtained from the two principal axes of the space of leads. This technique does not address the three-dimensional nature of repolarization, rather it provides information about repolarization morphology in two preferential planes.

In a study by Priori et al,[16] the PCA measured in a 24-hour 12-lead ECG recording identified LQTS patients with abnormal morphology of repolarization segment. Okin et al[39] analyzed the correlation of PCA and T wave area in 163 asymptomatic subjects with normal resting ECGs. They found independence between PCA and T wave area, suggesting that the ratio of eigenvalues may be a better measure of heterogeneity of repolarization than the time-domain parameters. PCA was also increased in patients with hypertrophic cardiomyopathy, in whom even higher values were found in symptomatic patients.[40] In our recent LQTS study comparing T wave complexity among carriers of mutated potassium (*KVLQT1*) and sodium (*SCN5A*) genes, we found that repolarization is more complex (heterogeneous) in the latter group.[41] Despite these encouraging observations, one must realize that the direct links between increased T wave complexity and repolarization heterogeneity, and between increased T wave complexity and ventricular arrhythmogenicity, have not been yet demonstrated. T wave complexity has been found to be independent of QT dispersion, suggesting that PCA measures provide different information about the repolarization process.

Reproducibility of PCA and the effect of various parameters such as heart rate, QT duration, T wave amplitude, and body position have not yet been studied extensively. Values of PCA ratio may vary substantially even in healthy subjects. Preliminary, as yet unpublished, work conducted in our laboratory indicates that low T wave amplitude could be a strong limitation of this method. Further studies are needed to identify technical limitations of the method and to determine clinical usefulness of PCA for diagnostic and prognostic purposes.

T Wave Loop Analysis

The analysis of T wave loop morphology seems to be the most direct approach in determining the complexity of repolarization pathway in the myocardium. Similar to PCA, there is no proof that the T wave loop reflects spatial heterogeneity of repolarization, but according to the vector-cardiographic concepts of electrocardiography, the shape of the T wave loop reflects the sequence and speed of the repolarization process in the myocardium. The main benefits of the vectorial approach are that it does not require identification of T wave endpoints and it avoids the distortion due to projection phenomena. However, accurate information about T wave loop morphology is not readily available from a standard ECG. Optimally, the orthogonal Frank lead system should be used to obtain vectorcardiographic loops. Since this lead configuration is rarely used in clinical practice, T wave loops must be derived from bipolar (Holter-recorded) X, Y, and Z leads or from standard 12-lead ECGs.[42,43]

The quantitative analysis of T wave loop morphology requires automation, and various parameters describing shape, position, and amplitude of the loop have been proposed. Badilini et al,[13] applying the CAVIAR program,[44] used roundness and planarity of T loop as two main parameters to differentiate LQTS patients and postinfarction patients from healthy subjects (Fig. 3). Increased roundness of T wave loop was associated with increased QT dispersion, although correlation between these parameters was relatively weak.

Recently Kors et al[15] explored the prognostic significance of the T axis for predicting cardiac death in an elderly community-based population. In the multivariate analysis, abnormal T axis was the most powerful predictor of follow-up cardiac events, and borderline T axis was the next significant parameter among many other clinical and ECG variables (Table 2).

New parameters describing details of T loop morphology are also being developed by our group.[44,45] Parameters based on the spherical

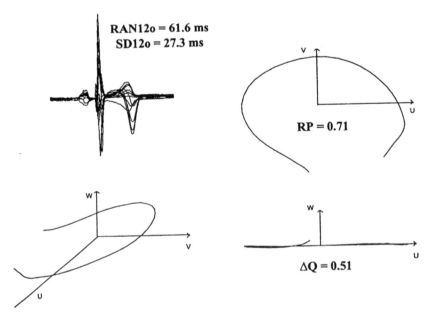

Figure 3. T wave loop morphology (the increased roundness of the loop) and superimposed 12-lead scalar electrocardiogram in a postinfarction patient. RAN12o = range of QT duration in 12 leads (maximal QT dispersion); SD12o = standard deviation of QT duration in 12 leads; RP = roundness parameter reflecting the shape of T wave loop; ΔQ = parameter reflecting the planarity of the loop. Reproduced from Reference 13, with permission.

Table 2
Hazard Ratios for Cardiac Death of Abnormal
and Borderline T Axis in Elderly People

Risk Factors		Hazard Ratio	96% Confidence Interval
Abnormal T axis		2.8	(1.8-4.5)
Borderline T axis		1.8	(1.1-2.4)
T wave inversion		1.4	(0.9-2.4)
QTc dispersion	>66 ms	1.9	(1.2-3.1)
	47-66 ms	1.8	(1.2-2.9)
MI by ECG		1.8	(1.3-2.6)
LVH by ECG		1.2	(0.7-1.9)
ST depression		0.8	(0.5-1.4)
QTc interval	>460 ms	1.5	(0.8-2.6)
	420-460 ms	1.2	(0.8-1.8)

MI = myocardial infarction; LVH = left ventricular hypertrophy.

coordinates of each point of the loop are computed: the difference between elevation and azimuth angles, and the ratio of magnitude of the maximum vector to the mean vector from the entire loop. These parameters aim to identify local singularities of the T wave and provide a semiautomatic quantification of T wave loop morphology for quantifying its degree of complexity. The field of T wave loop quantification for repolarization is in its infancy, and its usefulness in routine electrocardiology is yet to be determined.

Wavelet-Based Technique for Spatial Dispersion of Repolarization Morphology

Among other techniques currently being explored for the detection of morphological abnormalities of the repolarization segment, the wavelet-based technique provides insight into time-frequency components of the repolarization segment.[17,22,46] In the wavelet-based method, the distribution of the energy of repolarization in a dyadic time-frequency plane is computed in X, Y, and Z leads separately and compared among them. Changes in T wave morphology are emphasized by orthogonal decomposition, and the presence of notches, biphasic T wave, or U wave can be accurately detected and quantified. The wavelet-based methods can be applied to determine abnormalities of repolarization in a single beat in an individual lead,[46] in a single beat in multiple leads,[17] and in a series of consecutive beats.[22] This particular feature of wavelet-based analysis of repolarization signal makes this method particularly attractive for quantifying three-dimensional aspects of repolarization heterogeneity.

Table 3 summarizes main features of the above automatic methods used to quantify spatial heterogeneity of repolarization. In light of the vast clinical experience acquired with manual measurement of QT dispersion and preliminary experience with various automatic methods aiming to quantify spatial heterogeneity of repolarization, the following conclusions could be made: 1) automatic methods based on the comparison of QT interval duration (QT dispersion) are unlikely to succeed in every day clinical practice due to the limited reproducibility of T wave endpoint determination and the conceptual inconsistency of QT dispersion approach; 2) dispersion of TU-area–derived measures of partial repolarization duration reflecting shape of repolarization morphology may provide indirect information about abnormalities of repolarization morphology and are worth exploring; 3) the PCA of repolarization provides insight into the complexity of the repolarization process and should be considered as a promising approach, although it requires further testing; 4) T wave loop analysis, although in its infancy, seems to be the most appropriate approach for determining abnormalities in sequence of the repolarization process; and 5) wavelet analysis, revealing detailed abnormalities of repolarization, is promising particularly for analysis of three-dimensional features of heterogeneous repolarization, but this method also awaits validation and comparison with less complex approaches.

Automatic Methods Attempting to Determine Transmural Heterogeneity of Repolarization

In an experimental setting,[4] the T peak-T offset (TpTo, or T maximum-T offset; TmTo) duration was suggested to reflect the difference between

Table 3
Summary of Characteristics of Automatic Methods
Aiming to Detect Spatial Dispersion of Repolarization

	QT-Duration-Based Methods	Principal Component Analysis	T Loop Morphology Analysis	Wavelet-Based Method
Requires T wave end-points identification	Yes	No	No	No
Influenced by the lead projection effect	Yes	No	No	Yes
Reflects accurately repolarization morphology	No	No	Yes	Yes
Affected by low-amplitude T wave	Yes	Yes	No	Yes

action potential duration in epicardial and M cell zones. The automatic analysis of this ECG parameter was first performed by Merri et al[8] even before the concept linking T wave morphology with transmural heterogeneity of repolarization was proposed. Using the automatic detection of TmTo interval, Benhorin et al[10] found a significantly longer TmTo duration in LQTS patients than in healthy controls. However, the prognostic significance of TmTo duration and TmTo dispersion has not been confirmed in a large population of 252 LQTS probands.[19] Similarly, in an ischemic heart disease population, we were unable to find significant association between TmTo duration and dispersion and follow-up cardiac events.

Although analyzing just TmTo duration or dispersion in the standard ECG might not be the right approach for determining the magnitude of transmural heterogeneity of repolarization, it is accepted that the overall morphology of repolarization in the surface ECG reflects electrical contribution of a multitude of myocardial cells coming from various layers of myocardium. Computerized decomposition of T wave morphology could possibly describe differences in transmural spread of repolarization wave. Padrini et al[47] proposed a novel method which decomposes TU morphology into four major components that reflect the shape of the hypothetical action potential and contribution of T and U waves to the repolarization complex. The above mentioned techniques—principal component analysis and especially wavelet-based and T wave loop analyses of the repolarization segment—are also able to provide information about morphological abnormalities of repolarization, possibly reflecting transmural (combined with spatial) heterogeneity of repolarization. More studies are needed to determine the pathophysiological meaning and clinical usefulness of ECG parameters describing T wave morphology.

Automatic Detection of Temporal Heterogeneity of Repolarization: QT Variability, TWA, and T Wave Variability

Visible TWA, consisting of 2:1 beat-to-beat changes in repolarization duration and morphology, has been found to be associated with increased vulnerability to ventricular arrhythmias.[48-50] This association, further supported by the critical role of the QT–R-R relationship in action potential morphology,[5,6,34] created the conceptual background for computerized analysis of microvolt-level beat-to-beat changes in repolarization morphology. As shown recently by Shimizu and Antzelevitch[51] and Chinushi et al,[52] cycle length shortening precipitates an increased transmural heterogeneity of repolarization and contributes to a marked alternans of T wave morphology and polarity. Inappropriate adjustment of M cells to changing heart rate is responsible for the occurrence and polarity of TWA: a shorter action potential duration of M cells in comparison to epicardial and endocardial layers (opposite from normal conditions) contributes to alternans with changing T wave polarity. These observations, further supported by a study by Pastore et al,[27] confirmed that arrhythmogenicity attributed to TWA is due to increased spatial dispersion (heterogeneity) of repolarization. Therefore, beat-to-beat changes in repolarization can be recognized as a global reflection of static and dynamic characteristics of spatial heterogeneity of repolarization.

Computerized TWA Detection

In the 1980s, Adam et al[53] and Smith et al[24] developed a spectral method for computer detection of microvolt TWA and were the first to demonstrate that microvolt TWA is associated with propensity to ventricular fibrillation. Nearing et al[25] used a complex demodulation technique, which, similarly to the spectral method, detects the oscillatory nature of ECG signal during TWA. Recently, we developed a correlation method, the time-domain technique, which is particularly suitable for identifying transient (nonstationary) episodes of TWA.[26]

Spectral analysis identifies beat-to-beat ECG changes occurring at 0.5 cycle/beat frequency, distinguishing alternans-type ECG changes from other nonalternating ECG fluctuations. In spectral analysis, beat-to-beat changes in T wave amplitude are represented as power spectra by calculating the squared magnitude of the Fast-Fourier transformation of the beat-to-beat amplitude fluctuations of each sample points of 128 consecutive QRST complexes time-aligned by the R wave (Fig. 4).[24,54,55] Since TWA is more likely to occur at shorter cycle lengths (higher heart rates), cardiac pacing or exercise testing is used to induce TWA.[54] Preliminary clinical studies indicate that pacing- or exercise-induced TWA is predictive for arrhythmic events in various patient populations. Pastore et al[27] found that pacing-induced microvolt TWA detected in patients undergoing invasive electrophysiological testing was able to predict arrhythmic events with a prognostic accuracy similar to that of inducible ventricular tachycardia. A noninvasive exercise-induced TWA protocol implemented by Cambridge Heart, Inc. (Cambridge, MA) is currently being tested in several centers and preliminary data are very encouraging. In a study by Gold et al,[56] involving 201 patients undergoing invasive electrophysiology and exercise-induced TWA testing, TWA was positive in 19% of patients, negative in 55%, and indeterminate in 26%, whereas electrophysiology testing was positive in 23%, negative in 54%, and nonspecific or missing in 24%. During long-term follow-up, the presence of TWA was found to have superior prognostic value for predicting arrhythmic events compared with electrophysiological study. Recently, Hohnloser et al[55] evaluated the prognostic performance of exercise-induced TWA in 95 patients receiving

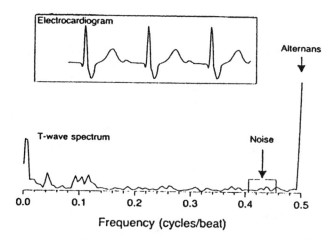

Figure 4. Spectral analysis method identifying T wave alternans, which is measured from the amplitude of spectral peak at 0.5 cycle/beat. Reproduced from Reference 54, with permission.

implantable cardioverter-defibrillators (ICDs). In the multivariate Cox model, TWA and ejection fraction were the only statistically significant predictors of defibrillator discharge during a mean 16-month follow-up. None of the other noninvasive tests (late potentials, QT dispersion, heart rate variability, and baroreflex sensitivity) were predictive for ICD discharge in this patient population.

In the complex demodulation method (proposed by Nearing et al[25]), beat-to-beat T wave amplitude fluctuations are modeled as a sinusoid with varying amplitude and phase, but with a constant frequency equal to the alternans frequency. In animal studies, Nearing et al[25] confirmed that both coronary artery occlusion and reperfusion increase TWA and that sympathetic nervous system exerts a prominent effect on TWA. They also reported that TWA levels increase significantly during Holter-recorded spontaneous ischemic episodes in patients with stable coronary disease.[57] A potential limitation of the widespread use of complex demodulation for TWA analysis is its intrinsic sophistication and complexity.

The correlation method is a time-domain technique that quantifies beat-to-beat changes in repolarization amplitude and morphology in resting or Holter-recorded ECGs.[26] After adjustment for R-R beat-to-beat variability, baseline wandering, and respiration modulation (signal processing needed to allow the detection of TWA from resting ECG recordings), an alternans correlation index is computed for each consecutive T wave. The alternans correlation index indicates morphological changes of each of the consecutive T waves in comparison with the median T wave (representative for a series of beats). This index is computed as the ratio of the maximum values of two correlation functions. The denominator is the maximum value of the autocorrelation function of the median beat, the numerator is the maximum value of the cross-correlation function between the median beat and the analyzed beat (Fig. 5). Since an alternans correlation index is computed for each individual T wave, this method is able to evaluate transient nonstationary TWA recorded in resting or ambulatory ECG recordings. Furthermore, this technique is able to quantify both amplitude and duration of TWA, whereas spectral and complex demodulation techniques do not provide insight into exact duration of TWA episodes. This new technique was used to determine the occurrence of microvolt TWA in resting Holter ECG recordings of 43 LQTS patients and 39 coronary artery disease patients.[26] Although TWA was detected in a similar proportion of LQTS and coronary patients (17 [44%] LQTS patients and 19 [44%] coronary artery disease patients), nonstationary TWA was more common in coronary than in LQTS patients (79% versus 47%, respectively; P=0.047). When the spectral method was applied to detect TWA in the above 17 LQTS patients with TWA detected by the correlation method, only three patients were identified as TWA-positive. This preliminary observation may suggest that the correlation method is more sensitive than the spectral method for detecting TWA.

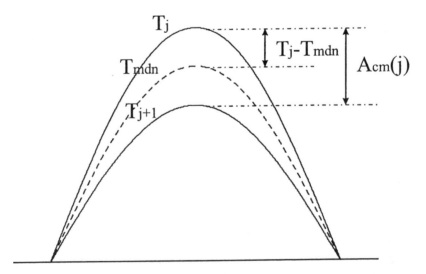

Figure 5. Alternans correlation index (ACI$_j$) for each of the consecutive T waves. Median T wave (Tmdn) is the reference for two consecutive T waves (T$_j$, T$_{j+1}$), and the value of Acm(j) represents the magnitude of alternans for these specific two beats.

Computer Detection of Beat-to-Beat QT Variability

Beat-to-beat non-2:1 changes in repolarization duration and morphology are also considered a marker of vulnerability to ventricular arrhythmias. Automatic beat-to-beat analysis of QT or QT-peak interval has been proposed as a measure of repolarization variability with full realization that this method is largely dependent on the accuracy of algorithms used to identify T wave endpoints.[31,58,59] T wave apex is usually identified by fitting a parabola, and the vertex of the parabola is used as the fiducial point for the apex of the T wave.[31] The end of the T wave is calculated by identifying the maximum slope of the latest descending part of the T wave, and the intersection between this slope and the baseline identifies the end of the T wave.[31,58,59] The limitation of QT-dependent algorithms quantifying beat-to-beat repolarization variability is that they are evaluating only duration of repolarization, whereas beat-to-beat variability of repolarization is primarily due to changes in morphology of ST-T wave complex. Recently Berger et al[21] described a novel computer algorithm that is based on QT interval duration analysis but also accounts for differences in T wave shape. After a visual identification of the QT interval template by the operator, the algorithm finds the QT interval of all other beats by determining how much each beat must be stretched or compressed in time to best match the template. The algorithm yields the measure of QT interval variability but does not provide direct measure of beat-to-beat changes in the amplitude of repolarization signal. In the preliminary study of 83 patients with dilated cardiomyopathy compared with 60 control subjects, Berger et al[21] found a significantly higher value of QT variability index (QTVI) in patients than in controls (-0.43 ± 0.71 versus -1.29 ± 0.51, respectively; $P<0.001$). The prognostic significance of QTVI for predicting arrhythmic events was recently investigated by Atiga et al[60] in 95 patients referred for electrophysiological study. During a mean 24 ± 14 months follow-up there were 14 arrhythmic events. The QTVI showed better predictive performance than heart rate variability, TWA, QT dispersion, and invasive electrophysiological study with induction of ventricular tachycardia (Fig. 6).

Computerized Methods to Quantify Beat-to-Beat Variability in Repolarization Morphology

Experimental and clinical observations indicate that repolarization variability is mainly due to beat-to-beat changes in the shape and amplitude (less in the duration) of action potential and repolarization segment.[5,6,61] The identification of T wave endpoints is a major limitation of current techniques. For these reasons there is a growing interest in new computerized methods that quantify beat-to-beat changes in repolariza-

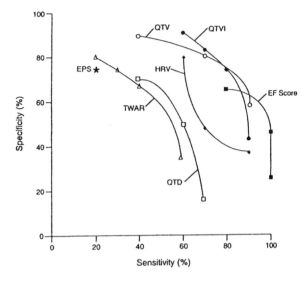

Figure 6. Receiver operating characteristic (ROC) plots for multiple cutoff values of studied variables. QTV = QT variability; QTVI = QT variability index; EF score = ejection fraction score; HRV = heart rate variability; QTD = QT dispersion; TWAR = T wave alternans ratio; EPS = inducibility of ventricular tachycardia during electrophysiological study. Reproduced from Reference 60, with permission.

tion morphology without a need to determine T wave endpoints. Two such algorithms were recently developed by our group: one method based on decomposition of repolarization segment using wavelet technique,[22,61,62] and the second method using the time-domain repolarization correlation index (RCI).[23]

The wavelet transformation method identifies amplitude changes between consecutive beats along the entire repolarization segment. A heart-rate–dependent interval from two consecutive beats (located between 100 ms after R peak and 220 ms prior to next R peak) are decomposed using wavelets. The estimation of beat-to-beat variability is obtained by comparing time-frequency components in the wavelet transformations of the two consecutive beats. Two parameters are computed: temporal variability in time (TVT) and temporal variability in amplitude (TVA). TVT describes a time shift between two consecutive beats by calculating the time needed to maximize the cross-correlation function between low-frequency wavelet components. The TVA value corresponds to the difference in amplitude distribution along the repolarization segment between a pair of beats. The overall magnitude of repolarization variability in duration (TVT) and amplitude (TVA) can be described on a beat-to-beat basis or as a median value from all pairs of beats in specific lead and, subsequently, as a median value for all leads analyzed.[22] This method can be used to evaluate beat-to-beat T wave variability in a standard 12-lead ECG, as well as in exercise testing and Holter ECGs.

The above wavelet-based method was used to evaluate the magnitude of beat-to-beat repolarization variability in LQTS patients with sodium channel gene mutation, who showed significantly higher values of TVT and TVA than their healthy relatives and unrelated control subjects.[62] The variability of T wave amplitude was found to be the dominating feature of repolarization variability in these patients. Our wavelet-based technique allows for quantitative comparison of repolarization morphology in each pair of beats (not comparison with a template or median beat). Ion channel kinetics of a given beat are dependent on ion channel kinetics and cycle length of the previous beat.[5,6,61] Therefore, tracking beat-to-beat changes in consecutive pairs of beats seems to provide better insight into the dynamic process of repolarization.

Our time-domain method for repolarization variability detection is based on the definition of a dimensionless RCI, which was described in our previous reports describing time-domain method for TWA detection.[23,26] The RCI compares each consecutive T wave with a template (median T wave) of the repolarization segment identified based on heart rate, regardless of T wave endpoint identification. The overall repolarization variability index globally quantifies repolarization variability in an ECG segment of chosen length (i.e., in 128 beats). Using this method, we analyzed repolarization variability in three-lead Holter recordings of 42 ischemic cardiomyopathy patients who showed significantly higher values of repolarization variability index than 36 healthy control subjects (0.045 ± 0.035 versus 0.024 ± 0.010, respectively; $P < 0.001$).[23]

Both techniques have two major advantages: first, they do not require identification of T wave endpoints (T wave end or apex); instead, they compute ECG changes inside a prespecified heart-rate–dependent window. Second, our methods allow for quantification of beat-to-beat changes throughout the entire repolarization segment, which allows for beat-to-beat analysis of both repolarization morphology and duration. The prognostic significance of repolarization variability quantified using our new methods is as yet unknown and further studies are required to determine whether the wavelet-based and correlation-based methods could be helpful in stratification of patients at risk for arrhythmic events.

Combined Three-Dimensional Approach to Determine Spatiotemporal Heterogeneity of Repolarization

Since spatial (regional and transmural) and temporal heterogeneity of repolarization are linked mechanistically, contributing to arrhythmogenic conditions in the myocardium, there is a need to determine automatically the magnitude of combined spatiotemporal heterogeneity of repolarization. Quantification of beat-to-beat changes in spatial dispersion of repolarization might provide insight into the three-dimensional nature of repolarization heterogeneity. Our preliminary experience with the wavelet-based method of quantifying beat-to-beat variability of spatial dispersion of repolarization shows that LQTS patients have higher spatiotemporal heterogeneity of repolarization than healthy subjects do. Figure 7 shows values of spatial dispersion of repolarization for each presented beat and variability

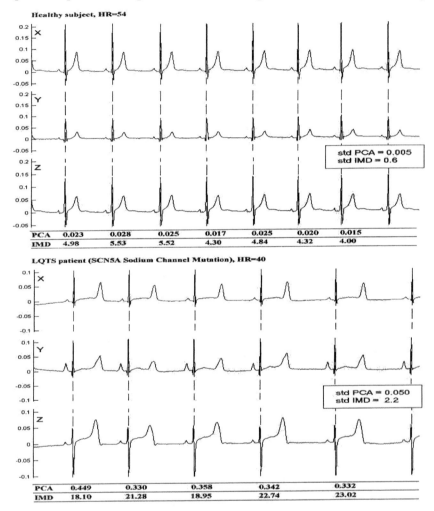

Figure 7. Beat-to-beat changes in spatial dispersion of repolarization morphology in a healthy subject **(top)** and a patient with the long QT syndrome (LQTS) **(bottom)**. Spatial dispersion for each consecutive beat is expressed as value of the principal component analysis (PCA) index and wavelet-based index of morphological difference (IMD). Beat-to-beat changes in spatial dispersion of repolarization morphology are expressed as standard deviation (std) of PCA and IMD parameters. Variability of spatial dispersion of repolarization (values of std PCA and std IMD) is substantially higher in an LQTS patient than in a control subject.

of spatial dispersion of repolarization in a series of beats (expressed using standard deviation) in an exemplary LQTS patient and a healthy subject. Standard deviation of PCA[16] and index of morphological difference (IMD)[17] values are increased in LQTS patients in comparison to healthy subjects. The clinical and prognostic significance of parameters describing spatio-temporal heterogeneity of repolarization requires further studies.

Summary

There is general agreement that the analysis of repolarization abnormalities in the ECG requires automation, since manual measurement of QT interval is not adequate due to its poor precision and insufficient yield of information about morphology of repolarization. Recently developed techniques for evaluating repolarization in a single lead or in multiple leads aim to obtain robust measurements of repolarization duration and morphology simultaneously. This approach is in agreement with current concepts of arrhythmogenesis, which emphasize the role of spatial and temporal heterogeneity of repolarization morphology in the mechanisms of ventricular arrhythmias. Spatial dispersion of repolarization is evaluated automatically using QT-based methods; however, the following techniques to identify interlead or spatial changes in repolarization morphology seem to be more appropriate: principal component analysis, T wave loop morphology analysis, and wavelet-based decomposition of repolarization segment. All of these techniques aim to determine repolarization abnormalities in a single beat; however, "static" spatial heterogeneity of repolarization is not sufficient to trigger arrhythmias. Spatial heterogeneity of repolarization must be disturbed by heart rate changes (due to sinus arrhythmia or premature beats) to generate arrhythmogenic response. For these electrophysiological reasons, the analysis of changes of repolarization in time (temporal heterogeneity of repolarization) is needed to provide full insight into both substrate of and vulnerability to arrhythmias. The computer detection of QT variability, TWA, and T wave variability addresses the dynamic behavior of repolarization, especially since these phenomena are mechanistically linked to spatial heterogeneity of repolarization. The three-dimensional (regional, transmural, and temporal) nature of repolarization heterogeneity calls for the computerized methods quantifying global spatiotemporal heterogeneity of repolarization. The beat-to-beat analysis of spatial dispersion of repolarization might be an option to determine contribution of spatial and temporal heterogeneity of repolarization to the mechanism of ventricular arrhythmias.

References

1. Kuo CS, Surawicz B. Ventricular monophasic action potential changes associated with neurogenic T wave abnormalities and isoproterenol administration in dogs. *Am J Cardiol* 1976;38:170-177.

2. Antzelevitch C, Shimizu W, Yan GX, Sicouri S. Cellular basis for QT dispersion. *J Electrocardiol* 1998;(30 suppl):168-175.
3. Lukas A, Antzelevitch C. Phase 2 reentry as a mechanism of initiation of circus movement reentry in canine epicardium exposed to simulated ischemia. *Cardiovasc Res* 1996;32:593-603.
4. Shimizu W, Antzelevitch C. Cellular basis for the ECG features of the LQT1 form of the long-QT syndrome: Effects of beta-adrenergic agonists and antagonists and sodium channel blockers on transmural dispersion of repolarization and torsade de pointes. *Circulation* 1998;98:2314-2322.
5. Marchlinski FE. Characterization of oscillations in ventricular refractoriness in man after an abrupt increment in heart rate. *Circulation* 1987;75:550-556.
6. Franz MR, Swerdlow CD, Liem LB, Schaefer J. Cycle length dependence of human action potential duration in vivo. Effects of single extrastimuli, sudden sustained rate acceleration and deceleration, and different steady-state frequencies. *J Clinic Invest* 1988;82:972-979.
7. Sylven JC, Horacek BM, Spencer CA, et al. QT interval variability on the body surface. *J Electrocardiol* 1984;17:179-188.
8. Merri M, Benhorin J, Alberti M, et al. Electrocardiographic quantitation of ventricular repolarization. *Circulation* 1989;80:1301-1308.
9. Day CP, McComb JM, Campbell RW. QT dispersion: An indication of arrhythmia risk in patients with long QT intervals. *Br Heart J* 1990;63:342-344.
10. Benhorin J, Merri M, Alberti M, et al. Long QT syndrome. New electrocardiographic characteristics. *Circulation* 1990;82:521-527.
11. Linker NJ, Colonna P, Kekwick CA, et al. Assessment of QT dispersion in symptomatic patients with congenital long QT syndromes. *Am J Cardiol* 1992;69:634-638.
12. Zareba W, Moss AJ, le Cessie S. Dispersion of ventricular repolarization and arrhythmic cardiac death in coronary artery disease. *Am J Cardiol* 1994;74:550-553.
13. Badilini F, Fayn J, Maison-Blanche P, et al. Quantitative aspects of ventricular repolarization: Relationship between three-dimensional T wave loop morphology and scalar QT dispersion. *Ann Noninvas Electrocardiol* 1997;2:146-157.
14. Zareba W. Ventricular repolarization measures: QT interval, RTm interval, or T wave loop morphology? *Ann Noninvas Electrocardiol* 1997;2:101-103.
15. Kors JA, de Bruyne MC, Hoes AW, et al. T axis as an indicator of risk of cardiac events in elderly people. *Lancet* 1998;352:601-605.
16. Priori SG, Mortara DW, Napolitano C, et al. Evaluation of the spatial aspects of T-wave complexity in the long-QT syndrome. *Circulation* 1997;96:3006-3012.
17. Couderc JP, Nomura A, Zareba W, Moss AJ. Heterogeneity of ventricular repolarization morphology measured using orthogonal wavelet time-scale decomposition of the surface ECG. *Computers in Cardiology* 1999;26:699-702.
18. Lubinski A, Lewicka-Nowak E, Kempa M, et al. New insight into repolarization abnormalities in patients with congenital long QT syndrome: The increased transmural dispersion of repolarization. *PACE* 1998;21:172-175.
19. Zareba W, Moss AJ, Locati E, et al. ECG predictors of follow-up cardiac events in long QT syndrome probands. *Circulation* 1997;96:I342. Abstract.
20. Merri M, Alberti M, Moss AJ. Dynamic analysis of ventricular repolarization duration from 24-hour Holter recordings. *IEEE Trans Biomed Eng* 1993;40:1219-1225.
21. Berger RD, Kasper EK, Baughman KL, et al. Beat-to-beat QT interval variability: Novel evidence for repolarization lability in ischemic and nonischemic dilated cardiomyopathy. *Circulation* 1997;96:1557-1565.

22. Couderc JP, Zareba W, Moss AJ. New-method for the quantification of beat-to-beat T wave temporal variability based on interscale changes in wavelet transform of the ECG: Application to simulated ECG signals. In Ruiz-Alzola J (ed): *Signal Processing and Communication.* 1999:213-216.

23. Burattini L, Zareba W. Time-domain analysis of beat-to-beat variability of repolarization morphology in patients with ischemic cardiomyopathy. *J Electrocardiol* 1999;32(suppl):166-172.

24. Smith JM, Clancy EA, Valeri CR, et al. Electrical alternans and cardiac electrical instability. *Circulation* 1988;77:110-121.

25. Nearing BD, Huang AH, Verrier RL. Dynamic tracking of cardiac vulnerability by complex demodulation of the T wave. *Science* 1991;252:437-440.

26. Burattini L, Zareba W, Rashban E, et al. ECG features of microvolt T-wave alternans in coronary artery disease and long QT syndrome patients. *J Electrocardiol* 1998;31(suppl):114-120.

27. Pastore JM, Girouard SD, Laurita KR, et al. Mechanism linking T-wave alternans to the genesis of cardiac fibrillation. *Circulation* 1999;99:1385-1394.

28. Mirvis DM. Spatial variation of QT intervals in normal persons and patients with acute myocardial infarction. *J Am Coll Cardiol* 1985;5:625-631.

29. De Ambroggi L, Negroni MS, Monza E, et al. Dispersion of ventricular repolarization in the long QT syndrome. *Am J Cardiol* 1991;68:614-620.

30. Kautzner J, Yi G, Camm AJ, Malik M. Short- and long-term reproducibility of QT, QTc, and QT dispersion measurement in healthy subjects. *PACE* 1994;17:928-937.

31. Merri M, Moss AJ, Benhorin J, et al. Relation between ventricular repolarization duration and cardiac cycle length during 24-hour Holter recordings. Findings in normal patients and patients with long QT syndrome. *Circulation* 1992;85:1816-1821.

32. Xue Q, Reddy S. new algorithm for QT dispersion analysis. *Comput Cardiol* 1996;23:293-296.

33. Alberti M, Merri M, Benhorin J, et al. electrocardiographic precordial interlead variability in normal individuals and patients with long QT syndrome. *Comput Cardiol* 1990;17:475-478.

34. Zareba W, Badilini F, Moss AJ. Automatic detection of spatial and dynamic heterogeneity of repolarization. *J Electrocardiol* 1994;27(suppl):66-72.

35. Caminal P, Blasi A, Vallverdu M, et al. New algorithm for QT dispersion analysis in YYZ-lead Holter ECG. Performance and applications. *Comput Cardiol* 1999;26:709-712.

36. Zareba W, Moss AJ, Konecki J. TU wave area-derived measures of repolarization dispersion in the long QT syndrome. *J Electrocardiol* 1998;30(suppl):191-195.

37. Haran LG, Flowers NC, Brody DA. Principal factors waveform of the thoracic QRS complex. *Circ Res* 1999;15:131-145.

38. Lux RL, Evans AK, Burgess MJ, et al. Redundancy reduction for improved display and analysis of body surface potential maps. I. Spatial compression. *Circ Res* 1981;49:186-196.

39. Okin P, Xue Q, Reddy S, et al. Electrocardiographic measures of heterogeneity of ventricular repolarization. *J Am Coll Cardiol* 1998;31:345A. Abstract.

40. Yi G, Prasad K, Elliott P, et al. T wave complexity in patients with hypertrophic cardiomyopathy. *PACE* 1998;21:2382-2386.

41. Zareba W, Konecki J, Timothy K, et al. Principal components analysis of spatial dispersion of repolarization in LQT1 and LQT3 gene carriers. *J Am Coll Cardiol* 1999;33:114A. Abstract.

42. Edenbrandt L, Pahlm O. Vectorcardiogram synthesized from a 12-lead ECG: Superiority of the inverse Dower matrix. *J Electrocardiol* 1988;21:361-367.
43. Kors JA, van Herpen G, Sittig AC, van Bemmel JH: Reconstruction of the Frank vectorcardiogram from standard electrocardiographic leads: Diagnostic comparison of different methods. *Eur Heart J* 1990;11:1083-1092.
44. Fayn J, Rubel P. CAVIAR: A serial ECG processing system for the comparative analysis of VCGs and their interpretation with auto-reference to the patient. *J Electrocardiol* 1988;21(suppl):S173-S176.
45. Kallert T, Couderc JP, Voss A, Zareba W. Semi-automatic method quantifying T wave loop morphology: Relevance for assessment of heterogeneous repolarization. *Comput Cardiol* 1999;26:153-156.
46. Couderc JP, Burattini L, Konecki JA, Moss AJ. Detection of abnormal time-frequency components of the QT interval using wavelet transformation technique. *Comput Cardiol* 1997;24;661-664.
47. Padrini R, Butrous G, Camm AJ, Malik M. Algebraic decomposition of the TU wave morphology patterns. *PACE* 1995;18:2209-2215.
48. Schwartz PJ, Malliani A. Electrical alternation of the T-wave: Clinical and experimental evidence of its relationship with the sympathetic nervous system and with the long Q-T syndrome. *Am Heart J* 1975;89:45-50.
49. Zareba W, Moss AJ, le Cessie S, Hall WJ. T wave alternans in idiopathic long QT syndrome. *J Am Coll Cardiol* 1994;23:1541-1546.
50. Navarro-Lopez F, Cinca J, Sanz G, et al. Isolated T wave alternans elicited by hypocalcemia in dogs. *J Electrocardiol* 1978;11:103-108.
51. Shimizu W, Antzelevitch C. Cellular and ionic basis for T-wave alternans under long-QT conditions. *Circulation* 1999;99:1499-1507.
52. Chinushi M, Restivo M, Caref EB, El-Sherif N. Electrophysiological basis of arrhythmogenicity of QT/T alternans in the long-QT syndrome: Tridimensional analysis of the kinetics of cardiac repolarization. *Circ Res* 1998;83:614-628.
53. Adam DR, Smith JM, Akselrod S, et al. Fluctuations in T-wave morphology and susceptibility to ventricular fibrillation. *J Electrocardiol* 1984;17:209-218.
54. Rosenbaum DS, Jackson LE, Smith JM, et al. Electrical alternans and vulnerability to ventricular arrhythmias. *N Engl J Med* 1994;330:235-241.
55. Hohnloser SH, Klingenheben T, Li YG, et al. T wave alternans as a predictor of recurrent ventricular tachyarrhythmias in ICD recipients: Prospective comparison with conventional risk markers. *J Cardiovasc Electrophysiol* 1998;9:1258-1268.
56. Gold MR, Bloomfield DM, Anderson KP, et al. A comparison of T-wave alternans, signal averaged electrocardiography and electrophysiology study to predict arrhythmia vulnerability. *J Am Coll Cardiol* 1999;33:145A. Abstract.
57. Nearing BD, Oesterle SN, Verrier RL. Quantification of ischaemia induced vulnerability by precordial T wave alternans analysis in dog and human. *Cardiovasc Res* 1994;28:1440-1449.
58. Pisani E, Pellegrini F, Ansuini G, et al. Performance evaluation of algorithms for QT interval measurements in ambulatory ECG recordings. *Comput Cardiol* 1999;11:459-462.
59. Laguna P, Thakor NV, Caminal P, et al. New algorithm for QT interval analysis in 24-hour Holter ECG: Performance and applications. *Med Biol Eng Comput* 1990;28:67-73.
60. Atiga WL, Calkins H, Lawrence JH, et al. Beat-to-beat repolarization lability identifies patients at risk for sudden cardiac death. *J Cardiovasc Electrophysiol* 1998;9:899-908.

61. Burgess MJ, Pollard AE, Spitzer KW, Yang L. Effects of premature beats on repolarization of postextrasystolic beats. *Circulation* 1995;92:1969-1980.
62. Couderc JP, Zareba W, Burattini L, Moss AJ. Beat-to-beat repolarization variability in LQTS patients with the SCN5A sodium channel gene mutation. *PACE* 1999;22:1581-1592.

Evaluation of Ventricular Activation-Recovery Coupling Using an Electroanatomical Mapping Technique

Lior Gepstein, Gal Hayam, and Shlomo A. Ben-Haim

Introduction

Functional heterogeneity in the electrophysiological substrate involving activation (slow conduction) or repolarization (increased dispersion) is a major prerequisite for the genesis and maintenance of various ventricular arrhythmias.[1-5] Ventricular tachycardia in patients with coronary artery disease and previous myocardial infarction is generally believed to be reentrant, and is accompanied by abnormal activation, namely the presence of a critical area of slow conduction within the scar.[3] Similarly, several clinical and experimental studies also support the role of augmented dispersion of repolarization in the generation of various types of cardiac arrhythmias.[4] Examples of experimental models in which increased dispersion of repolarization appears to play an important role include the circus movement tachycardia (leading circle reentry) induced by Allessie et al[5] in isolated segments of rabbit atrial muscle, and the ventricular arrhythmias elicited 3 to 5 days after coronary ligation in dogs.[2] It is generally believed, however, that in many cases both mechanisms are involved and that they often tend to be mutually interdependent.[2]

A major hurdle in the assessment of the spatial distribution of the activation and repolarization patterns in the clinical setting has been the inability to accurately associate endocardial spatial and electrophysiological information. Although endocardial activation patterns have been mea-

From Olsson SB, Amlie JP, Yuan S (eds): *Dispersion of Ventricular Repolarization: State of the Art.* ©Futura Publishing Company, Inc., Armonk, NY, 2000.

sured in numerous clinical studies, relatively little information exists regarding the spatial distribution of endocardial repolarization patterns and its role in arrhythmogenesis. Similarly, there is a paucity of data in the literature regarding the possible spatial interaction between these two processes in the global heart. Since both processes play an important role in generation of arrhythmias, such interactions may have crucial clinical implications.

The objectives of this chapter are twofold: 1) to describe a new electroanatomical mapping technique that enables to associate spatial and electrophysiological information, and may thus be used to assess the three-dimensional (3D) patterns of endocardial activation and repolarization, and 2) to provide recent results from our laboratory in mapping the endocardial activation, activation-recovery interval (ARI), and repolarization patterns of the healthy swine left ventricle (LV)[6] and to describe a unique mechanism by which tight spatial coupling of activation and repolarization may serve as a novel antiarrhythmic mechanism in normal tissue.

Nonfluoroscopic Electroanatomical Mapping Technique

To enable the regional and global spatial assessment of endocardial activation and repolarization patterns, we utilized a catheter-based, nonfluoroscopic, electroanatomical endocardial mapping technique.[6-8] This method (Carto, Biosense) uses ultralow magnetic fields to accurately determine the location and orientation of a miniature passive magnetic sensor incorporated just proximal to the tip of a 7F deflectable electrophysiological catheter. The mapping procedure is based on sampling the cardiac cycle-gated location of the tip of the roving mapping catheter simultaneous with the local electrogram recorded from its tip electrode, at a plurality of endocardial sites. This results in generation, in realtime, of a 3D electroanatomical map, with the electrophysiological information color-coded and superimposed on the chamber's geometry (Fig. 1).

Electroanatomical Mapping of LV Activation, ARI, and Repolarization Patterns

The 3D endocardial activation and repolarization patterns of the LV were assessed in 13 healthy male pigs during different activation patterns (sinus rhythm as well as atrial and ventricular pacing).

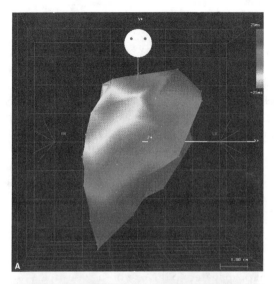

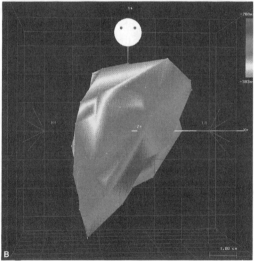

Figure 1. Right anterior oblique view of a three-dimensional electroanatomical map of the swine left ventricle during sinus rhythm. **A.** Activation map. The earliest activation site, represented by the red area, is located at the anterosuperior septum. The activation then spread to the rest of the endocardium, with the posterobasal area activated last (blue and purple areas). Yellow and green represent areas with intermediate local activation times. Total activation time of this ventricle was 47 ms. **B.** Activation-recovery interval (ARI) map of the same ventricle. Colors represent ARI values recorded at each site with red corresponding to sites with the longest ARIs, blue and purple indicating short ARIs, and yellow and green representing areas with intermediate values. Note the homogenous gradient of ARI resembling the activation sequence, with the longest ARIs (red) located along the septum (earliest activation). See color plate.

Activation Pattern

The local activation time (LAT) at each sampled site was determined from the intracardiac unipolar electrogram (filtered at 0.5 to 400 Hz). LAT was defined as the time interval between a fiducial point on the body surface electrocardiogram (peak of the R wave) and the steepest negative intrinsic deflection (dV/dt_{min}) in the local unipolar recording.

Panel A of Figure 1 and panel A of Figure 2 present right anterior oblique (RAO) views of typical activation patterns of the swine LV during sinus rhythm (or atrial pacing) and during right ventricular (RV) infero-septal pacing, respectively. Interestingly, the observed activation pattern during sinus rhythm agrees well with the endocardial activation pattern in humans previously described by Durrer et al.[9] The earliest activation site during sinus rhythm (represented in the map in Fig. 1, panel A as the red area) was noted at the anterosuperior septum, with a second endocardial breakthrough noted more posteriorly. The depolarization wavefront then propagated to the rest of the ventricle with the posteroba-sal and posterolateral areas activated last (colored blue and purple).

As anticipated, during RV septal pacing, the earliest LV activation site was noted at the inferior septum and then spread to the rest of the ventricle, with the basal and posterolateral areas activated last (Fig. 2, panel A). An interesting physiological phenomenon that can also be noted in this figure is the anisotropic properties of the myocardium, with faster conduction velocity along the longitudinal direction.

ARI Pattern

The local repolarization time (LRT) at each sampled site was deter-mined from the timing of the local T wave in the unipolar recording, using a method previously described by Wyatt et al[10] and later modified by Millar et al.[11] Using their methods, LRT was defined as the dV/dt_{max} in the local T wave for negative and biphasic T waves and as the dV/dt_{min} for positive T waves. The ARI at each site was then determined as the time difference between the corresponding LRT and LAT. Using this method, experimental studies in both humans and animals have shown high correlation between ARI and local action potential duration (APD) measured by transmembrane action potential, monophasic action poten-tial (MAP), and the effective refractory period determined by the extra-stimulus technique.[10-12]

Figure 1, panel B and Figure 2, panel B describe the typical ARI patterns of the LV during sinus rhythm and RV pacing, respectively. Colors represent the values of ARI measured at each site, with red repre-senting areas with long ARIs, blue and purple indicating areas with short ARIs, and green and yellow symbolizing sites with intermediate values.

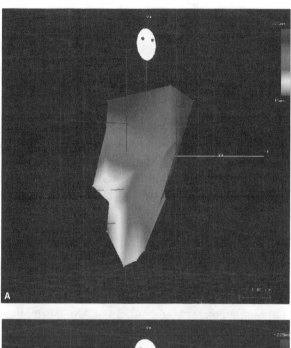

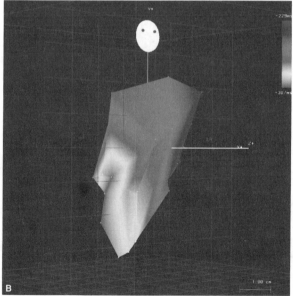

Figure 2. A. Activation map of the left ventricle during pacing from the right ventricular inferior septum (cycle length=350 ms). Total activation time was 61 ms. **B.** Activation-recovery interval (ARI) map of the same ventricle during pacing. Note again the inverse spatial correlation between ARI and activation time, with the longest ARIs (red) located at the sites of earliest activation and then shortening gradually as activation proceeds. See color plate.

Note that the ARI pattern closely resembles that of the activation (Fig. 1, panel A and Fig. 2, panel A). During sinus rhythm, a homogeneous gradient of ARIs was noted along the LV, with the longest ARIs observed at the septal area (corresponding to the site of earliest activation) and the shortest ARIs observed at the posterobasal region. The range of ARI distribution during sinus rhythm was 63 ± 7 ms (270 ± 16 ms [mean shortest ARI] to 331 ± 20 ms [mean longest ARI]).

Similarly, during RV septal pacing, the ARI maps resembled the corresponding activation maps, with the inferior septum having the longest ARIs, the posterolateral areas characterized by the shortest ARIs, and a gradual decrease in ARIs values between them. The range of LV ARI dispersion during ventricular pacing at a cycle length of 350 ms was 65 ± 5 ms (182 ± 8 to 247 ± 12 ms).

Relationship between the Spatial Distribution of LATs and ARIs

Independent of the specific depolarization pattern, sinus rhythm, or ventricular pacing, an inverse spatial correlation was noted such that sites activated earlier had longer ARIs than sites that were activated late. This resulted in a homogeneous spatial gradient of ARI shortening as activation proceeds.

The inverse correlation between the activation time and ARI was further evaluated when the pooled ARI values from all sampled sites were correlated with their respective LATs in each map. Figure 3 shows the typical relationship observed between the measured ARI and the corresponding LAT values in one animal. Note the inverse correlation between activation and ARI during both sinus rhythm and ARI, such that progressively later activation times are associated with shorter ARI values. Using linear regression analysis, a significant inverse correlation was noted between LAT and ARI for all rhythms in each of the maps ($r^2= 0.76\pm0.03$ and 0.77 ± 0.02 for sinus rhythm and ventricular pacing, respectively).

Repolarization Pattern

The LRT of a given endocardial site is a summation of the measured LAT and the ARI of the relevant site. The tight spatial coupling noted between the activation and ARI patterns, in which sites that are activated early are associated with longer ARIs and sites that are activated late are coupled with shorter ARIs, tends therefore to synchronize repolarization. Hence, total dispersion of repolarization in the LV was found to be relatively short, averaging less than 40 ms during the different depolarization patterns studied. Furthermore, the observed total dispersion of repolarization was significantly smaller than that of ARI and even than that of activation.

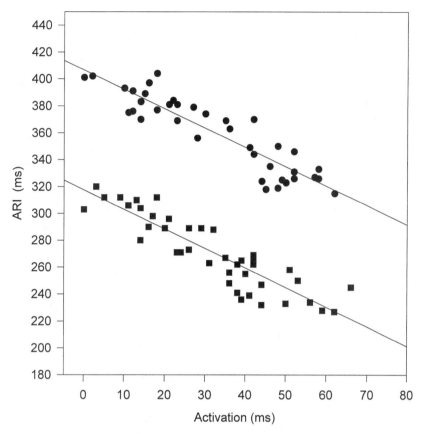

Figure 3. Linear regression analysis of the relationship between activation-recovery interval (ARI) and local activation time values pooled from all sampled sites in one animal during sinus rhythm and right ventricular pacing. A significant inverse correlation was noted in both rhythms, indicating that progressively later activation times are associated with progressively shorter ARIs.

Although in all the repolarization maps total dispersion was relatively narrow, three types of endocardial repolarization patterns were noted. In some maps the repolarization sequence resembled that of activation, in others it was reversed, whereas in some cases the earliest repolarization site was located between the earliest and latest activation sites.

Spatial Coupling between Activation and ARI: Significance and Possible Mechanisms

The results reported above present several intriguing findings. The first finding is the observed spatial coupling between the activation and ARI patterns. The inverse correlation found between activation and APD (estimated by the ARI) results in gradual shortening of the APD as the activation proceeds and consequentially in relatively narrow range of the termination of repolarization. The second interesting finding is that the inverse correlation between activation times and ARI was independent of the specific type of depolarization sequence. Hence, marked changes in the spatial distribution of ARI occurred when the activation pattern changed.

The inverse relationship between activation and APD was also noted previously in a number of in vitro and in vivo studies as well as in a number of computer simulations.[13-16] These studies, most of which were conducted in isolated tissue preparations or in a limited number of epicardial sites, also noted the shortening of APD as activation proceeds. Specifically, Zubair et al[13] noted marked effects of the activation sequence on the spatial dispersion of refractory periods at 36 sites within a 1-cm^2 region of the epicardial surface of the canine pulmonary conus. Similarly, Osaka et al[14] examined the influence of the activation sequence on action potential configuration in the epicardial surface of isolated pieces (2.5 cm^2) of canine ventricular myocardium. They found that APD shortened gradually as the recording site was moved further from the stimulation site. The spatial gradient of APD was found to be steeper, in their study, in the transverse than in the longitudinal direction.

One possible mechanism proposed to explain the effects of the activation sequence on repolarization is electrotonic interactions. Studies in isolated ventricular muscle and Purkinje fiber preparations have shown that repolarization (anodal) currents applied during repolarization shorten the action potential and that depolarization (cathodal) currents applied during repolarization prolong the action potential.[17-19] Thus, electrotonic currents flowing from sites that are activated late to neighboring sites activated earlier would tend to increase the APD in the latter sites and decrease the APD in the former sites.

The inverse correlation between activation and APD was also noted by Costard-Jäckle et al,[20] who studied the effect of ectopic pacing on the distribution of ventricular epicardial APDs (measured by MAP recordings) in the isolated Langendorff-perfused rabbit hearts. During both prolonged atrial and ventricular pacing they noted an inverse relationship between activation and APD (r=0.76, slope=−1.63 and r=0.68, slope=−0.68, during atrial and ventricular pacing, respectively). This resulted in a relatively synchronized epicardial repolarization time. Another important finding in their study was that abrupt changes in the activation sequence perturbed the inverse correlation between the activation and APD patterns. Thus, immediately after the activation sequence was changed from atrial to ventricular pacing, the inverse correlation disappeared. Nevertheless, continuation of the ventricular pacing produced slow changes that restored the inverse relationship. Similarly, immediately after switching back to atrial pacing the inverse relationship was lost again, but it reappeared slowly after 1 hour of pacing.

The latter results may suggest that additional factors other than electrotonic interactions alone may be responsible for the coupling between the sequence of activation and APD. The authors speculated that repeated current flow in the same direction through the intercellular gap junctions might have a modulating effect on the electrotonic interactions between the cells. This process might gradually decrease the gap junction resistance even further, thereby amplifying the electrotonic effects with time.

Clinical Implications

The results presented here may have a number of significant clinical implications. Augmented dispersion of repolarization has been shown in numerous studies to increase the propensity of ventricular arrhythmias both clinically and in experimental models. As discussed earlier, dispersion of repolarization is determined by the summation of regional differences in activation times and APD.

In humans, the mechanism of increased dispersion of repolarization may vary with the disease process. Vassalo et al[21] measured recovery of excitability at multiple LV endocardial sites in three groups of patients. In normal subjects the range of LV recovery times was 52 ms. In patients with previous myocardial infarction and ventricular tachycardia dispersion of recovery time was 90 ms, mainly due to prolonged activation times. In contrast, the increased dispersion of recovery times (114 ms) in patients with the long QT syndrome was primarily due to increased dispersion of refractory periods.

The tight spatial coupling between the activation and ARI patterns, resulting in an inverse correlation between the two processes, may serve as an important physiological mechanism in the prevention of ventricular arrhythmias. The shortening of APD as the activation proceeds tends to synchronize repolarization both globally and regionally, and may thus serve as an important antiarrhythmic mechanism. The tight dependency between the spatial distribution of activation and repolarization, as discussed earlier, may be caused by electrotonic interactions through intercellular gap junctions. One may therefore speculate that in the presence of a pathology that decreases cell-to-cell conductivity, this spatial coupling may be lost, resulting in an increased dispersion of repolarization and in an increased propensity to arrhythmogenesis. Further basic investigation as well as clinical studies would have to test this hypothesis.

The inverse relationship between APD and activation times may also provide insight into the paradox of T wave concordance in the normal electrogram, despite the fact that on the cellular level depolarization and repolarization produce deflections of opposite polarities. In a study published by Franz et al,[22] MAPs were recorded from 54 LV endocardial sites in seven patients and 23 epicardial sites in three patients. By plotting the APD measured at all sites as a function of the corresponding activation times, these authors also noted an inverse relationship. Interestingly, the average linear regression slope of this plot in the 10 patients was −1.32. The fact that the correlation between LAT and APD, found at both the endocardial and epicardial surfaces, had a negative slope that was greater than a unity may support the hypothesis that T wave concordance results from opposite directions of the repolarization and depolarization waves, at least in some parts of the myocardium. Their results may also support the concept of a transmural repolarization gradient in the human myocardium opposite to that of the depolarization.

Finally, the ability to accurately associate endocardial spatial and electrophysiological information may become a valuable clinical and research tool. The ability to study in vivo the 3D spatial interactions of different electrophysiological properties (e.g., the different properties of the action potential) in both healthy and variable disease states may improve our understanding of the mechanisms involved in arrhythmogenesis and may possibly identify patients at risk for ventricular arrhythmias.

References

1. Han J, Moe GH. Nonuniform recovery of excitability in ventricular muscle. *Circ Res* 1964;14:44-60.
2. Gough WB, Mehra R, Restivo M, et al. Reentrant ventricular arrhythmias in the late myocardial infarction period in the dog: Correlation of activation and refractory maps. *Circ Res* 1985;57:432-442.
3. Callans DJ, Josephson ME. Ventricular tachycardia in the setting of coronary artery disease. In Zipes DP, Jalife J (eds): *Cardiac Electrophysiology: From Cell to Bedside.* 2nd ed. Philadelphia: W.B. Saunders Co.; 1995:788-811.
4. Kuo CS, Munakata K, Reddy CP, Surawicz B. Characteristics and possible mechanism of ventricular arrhythmia dependent on the dispersion of action potential durations. *Circulation* 1983;67:1356-1367.
5. Allessie MA, Bonke FI, Schopman FJ. Circus movement in rabbit atrial muscle as a mechanism of tachycardia. II. The role of nonuniform recovery of excitability in the occurrence of unidirectional block, as studied with multiple microelectrodes. *Circ Res* 1976;39:168-177.
6. Gepstein L, Hayam G, Ben-Haim SA. Activation-repolarization coupling in the normal swine endocardium. *Circulation* 1997;96:4036-4043.
7. Ben-Haim SA, Osadchy D, Schuster I, et al. Novel, non-fluoroscopic, in vivo navigation and mapping technology. *Nat Med* 1996;2:1393-1395.
8. Gepstein L, Hayam G, Ben-Haim SA. A novel method for nonfluoroscopic, catheter-based, electroanatomical mapping of the heart: In vitro and in vivo accuracy results. *Circulation* 1997;95:1611-1622.
9. Durrer D, van Dam RT, Freud GE, et al. Total excitation of the isolated human heart. *Circulation* 1970;41:899-912.

10. Wyatt RF, Burgess MJ, Evans AK, et al. Estimation of ventricular transmembrane action potential duration and repolarization times from unipolar electrograms. *Am J Cardiol* 1981;47:488. Abstract.
11. Millar CK, Kralios FA, Lux RL. Correlation between refractory periods and activation-recovery intervals from electrograms: Effects of rate and adrenergic interventions. *Circulation* 1985;72:1372-1379.
12. Chen P-S, Moser KM, Dembitsky WP, et al. Epicardial activation and repolarization patterns in patients with right ventricular hypertrophy. *Circulation* 1991;83:104-118.
13. Zubair I, Pollard AE, Spitzer KW, Burgess MJ. Effects of activation sequence on the spatial distribution of repolarization properties. *J Electrocardiol* 1994;27:115-127.
14. Osaka T, Kodama I, Tsuboi N, et al. Effects of activation sequence and anisotropic cellular geometry on the repolarization phase of action potential of dog ventricular muscles. *Circulation* 1987;76:226-236.
15. Toyoshima H, Burgess MJ. Electrotonic interaction during canine ventricular repolarization. *Circ Res* 1978;43:348-356.
16. Lesh MD, Pring M, Spear JF. Cellular uncoupling can unmask dispersion of action potential duration in ventricular myocardium: A computer modeling study. *Circ Res* 1989;65:1426-1440.
17. Weidman S. Effect of current flow on the membrane potential of cardiac muscle. *J Physiol (Lond)* 1951;115:227-236.
18. Cranfield PF, Hoffman BF. Propagated repolarization in heart muscle. *J Gen Physiol* 1958;41:633-649.
19. Vassalle M. Analysis of cardiac pacemakers potentials using a "voltage clamp" technique. *Am J Physiol* 1966;210:1335-1341.
20. Costard-Jäckle A, Goetsch B, Antz M, Franz MR. Slow and long-lasting modulation of myocardial repolarization produced by ectopic activation in isolated rabbit hearts: Evidence for cardiac memory. *Circulation* 1989;80:1412-1420.
21. Vassallo JA, Cassidy DM, Kindwall KE, et al. Nonuniform recovery of excitability in the left ventricle. *Circulation* 1988;78:1365-1372.
22. Franz MR, Bargheer K, Rafflenbeul W, et al. Monophasic action potential mapping in human subjects with normal electrocardiograms: Direct evidence for the genesis of the T wave. *Circulation* 1987;75:379-386.

8

Global Dispersion of Ventricular Repolarization:
Findings from Monophasic Action Potential Mapping Using the CARTO System

*Shiwen Yuan, Ole Kongstad, Eva Hertervig,
Magnus Holm, and S. Bertil Olsson*

It has long been recognized that an increased dispersion of ventricular repolarization (DVR) may create an electrophysiological environment that favors reentry.[1-4] Accumulated evidence in recent years has highlighted the role of increased DVR in the genesis of tachyarrhythmias.[5-11]

To date, DVR has mainly been evaluated by measuring the QT intervals from the surface electrocardiogram (ECG) or the local refractoriness and/or repolarization time course from a limited number of intracardiac recordings.[1,5,8,9,12,13] The global DVR has, however, not been well evaluated.

In this chapter we present a novel method for exploring the global DVR, the monophasic action potential (MAP) mapping technique that combines the MAP recording and the electroanatomical mapping techniques, with our preliminary findings in healthy pigs and in patients with cardiac arrhythmias.

Previously Used Methods for Evaluation of DVR

The most frequently used method for DVR evaluation is the measurement of QT dispersion on the surface ECG. This method has important

This study is supported in part by funds from the Swedish Heart-Lung Foundation and Biosense Webster Europe.

121

limitations associated with low-amplitude and/or distorted T waves. More importantly, the correlation between QT dispersion and global DVR has not yet been verified. Zabel et al[14] recorded MAPs from seven epicardial sites in isolated rabbit hearts and reported close correlations of the QT dispersion with the dispersions of the MAP duration and the recovery time. However, MAP recordings from seven sites over both ventricles, three on the right and four on the left ventricle, were not sufficient to reflect the global status of the DVR.

Sequential measurement of the myocardial effective refractory period from multiple myocardial sites is another way of evaluating the DVR that has been widely used. Vassallo et al[4] measured the effective refractory period from 10 ± 2 endocardial sites of the left ventricle and found that the dispersion of the effective refractory period was significantly different in patients with different kinds of ventricular arrhythmias. However, the method is very time consuming and therefore the global data from sufficient number of sites were difficult to obtain. Besides, the refractoriness is not always parallel to the repolarization.[15]

The activation-recovery intervals, or "QT" intervals, on the intracardiac unipolar electrogram have also been used to evaluate the DVR.[16-18] Gepstein et al[18] recorded unipolar electrograms from 50 to 70 left ventricular endocardial sites in pigs using an electroanatomical mapping system, the CARTO system (Biosense Webster), and evaluated the dispersion of the activation-recovery intervals. Similar to the measurement of QT dispersion, the accuracy of this unipolar electrogram technique was limited by the low-amplitude, multiphasic, and/or distorted pattern of the local "T" waves.[18-20]

A high-resolution optical mapping technique with voltage-sensitive dyes could accurately determine the local repolarization times and evaluate the DVR among hundreds of simultaneously recorded action potentials in the same cardiac cycle.[10,11,21] This technique has limitations associated with noises and motion artifacts, and, more importantly, it is only applicable to visible areas and thereby unable to acquire global information of DVR.[10,11,21]

The MAP recording technique can accurately reproduce the time course of the local repolarization and is therefore generally accepted as the method of choice in the evaluation of myocardial repolarization in vivo.[22-25] In the early 1980s, Kuo et al[1] studied DVR using MAPs simultaneously recorded from six left ventricular sites in canine models. In the clinical setting, however, simultaneous MAP recordings were limited to two to three sites due to ethical and/or technical limitations.[5,8,9,26] In practice, MAPs can also be sequentially recorded from multiple sites and synchronized according to a fixed time reference. In this way, the global DVR can be explored in patients without the need to introduce multiple catheters. However, the most detailed information on the DVR evaluated using this method was based on sequential MAP recordings from eight to 10 epicardial sites[12,13] and five to 11 endocardial sites in the left ventricle[12] and from 11 to 14 endocardial sites in the right ventricle.[5] Due to the limited number of recording sites, the global DVR was not clearly delineated.

Methodological Aspect of the MAP Mapping Technique

To evaluate the global DVR, recording from a sufficient number of sites is crucial. Moreover, an accurate correlation of the acquired signal to its original recording site is important for the evaluation of the spatial distribution of the MAP duration and the regional differences in the DVR, etc.

The introduction of the CARTO system, a computerized, electroanatomical mapping system, has provided the possibility of rapid endocardial activation assessment with high spatial accuracy.[27-29] It is not necessary to follow any anatomical scheme since the system accurately memorizes the recording sites and the acquired signals. If the MAP, instead of the intracardiac electrograms, could be recorded using the CARTO system, not only the activation map but also a repolarization map and the spatial distribution of the MAP duration could be obtained. This idea motivated our effort in the development of the MAP mapping technique using the CARTO system.

A prerequisite for use of the CARTO system to evaluate repolarization is that the MAP recording catheter must be locatable by the system. We first validated the possibility of recording MAPs using a conventional platinum electrode ablation catheter (Yuan S et al, unpublished data) and then verified the feasibility of recording MAP using a CARTO sensor-equipped catheter (Navi-Star, Biosense Webster).[30] To improve the quality of the MAP recordings and to facilitate the mapping procedure, a special Navi-Star catheter with a modified tip was developed for MAP mapping using the CARTO system.[31] Based on these developments, we have successfully integrated the MAP recording technique with the CARTO system's electroanatomical mapping capability.

The CARTO System

The system was previously described in detail.[28,29] In brief, a location pad consisting of three magnetic coils is placed under the torso of the patient. Each of the coils generates a magnetic field (10^{-6} to10^{-5} T) with specific frequency. The torso of the patient is thus covered by three magnetic fields of different frequencies. A location reference device (Ref-Star, Biosense-Webster) is fixed on the back of the patient, while a mapping catheter (Navi-Star) is navigating within the heart chamber. Both are equipped with a magnetic sensor embedded into the tip. The magnetic sensor continuously compares the intensities of the three magnetic fields, implying that the location of the mapping catheter can be accurately determined. The location and orientation of the mapping catheter tip is displayed in three dimensions and in real time on a screen, together with the local electrograms. Three-dimensional maps of endocardial activation can be constructed from the accurately localized electrograms. The location reference device compensates for the movements of the patient, and a cardiac cycle-gated technique allows for the sampling at a specific time during the cardiac cycle and thus compensates for the cyclic movement of the heart. The localization accuracy of the CARTO system has been verified to be 0.7 mm in vivo.[28,29]

MAP Recording

In the pigs, ventricular MAP mapping was performed using the modified tip Navi-Star catheter. In patients, the MAP mapping was performed using the ordinary Navi-Star catheter prior to a clinical electrophysiological study and/or catheter ablation. In brief, a 7F quadripolar Navi-Star catheter with a tip electrode of 4 mm, three ring electrodes of 2 mm, and the interpolar distances of 1, 7, and 4 mm, respectively, was percutaneously introduced into the right and/or the left ventricles. A MAP signal was recorded between the tip (exploring electrode) and the ring electrode proximal to the tip (indifferent electrode) at a filter bandwidth of 0.01 to 400 Hz. To indirectly monitor the contact pressure,[24] a unipolar electrogram was also recorded from the indifferent electrode, at a filter bandwidth of 0.1 to 120 Hz.

In the real time monitor window of the CARTO system, one lead ECG, the MAP, and the unipolar electrogram were displayed. When the amplitude and morphology of the MAP appeared satisfactory,[24,25] the signals were captured into a 3-second sampling window for further inspection. Accepted MAP signals, together with 12-lead ECG, were stored using a sampling frequency of 1 kHz. Caution was taken to put the mapping catheter perpendicularly against the endocardium and to avoid "ST segment" elevation, i.e., greater than 20% amplitude of the ventricular deflection on the unipolar electrogram from the indifferent electrode.[24]

In order to obtain a complete mapping of the ventricles, the right ventricular mapping was performed via both the femoral and jugular veins while the left ventricular mapping was mainly performed via the jugular artery in the pigs. In three patients the right ventricular mapping was performed via the right femoral vein, and in two patients via both the femoral and the jugular veins, while the left ventricular mapping was performed via the right femoral artery in all of the three patients for five maps.

The endpoint of the MAP mapping was that all of the areas in which MAP recording was possible were mapped, the activation maps were complete using a triangle filling threshold of 45 mm, or termination of the mapping was requested by the clinical situation of the patient.

MAP Analysis

The MAP analysis was performed off-line using the feature of double annotations of the CARTO system. The first annotation was set at the onset of the MAP upstroke, representing the local activation, while the second was set at the intersection between the baseline and the tangent to the steepest slope on phase 3 of the MAP,[32-34] representing the local end of repolarization (EOR). The two annotation lines were both manually set and carefully checked under a time scale of 200 mm/s and 100 mm/s, respectively. When there was a baseline disturbance and/or MAP distortion, the MAP of the previous beat was also measured for necessary corrections.

The activation time (AT) was defined as the time interval from the recorded earliest ventricular activation to the local activation, the MAP duration as from the local activation to the local EOR, and the EOR time as from the earliest ventricular activation to the local EOR. The EOR time is equal to the sum of the AT and the MAP duration at that recording site. Taking the peak of the QRS complex as a time reference, the relative values of AT and the EOR time were obtained (Fig. 1). Based on these relative values, three-dimensional maps of the right or left ventricular activation sequence, EOR sequence, and the spatial distribution of MAP durations were constructed. The relative measurement values were also converted into the actual measurement values of AT, EOR time, and MAP duration, according to the above definitions, as presented in the Tables 1 and 2.

The maximal differences in the AT, EOR time, and MAP duration, i.e., the total ranges of the scales of these maps, represent the total magnitude of the disparity between the measurement values, and are called the maximal dispersion of these parameters. The variances in these parameters were also obtained to represent the disparity among all the sampling sites in each map.

In order to evaluate the difference between the global and the local dispersions of repolarization, the dispersion parameters were also measured from all the areas that were ≤ 1 cm^2 and had at least three MAPs recorded.

Linear correlation and regression analyses were also used to study the relation between the MAP duration and AT as well as between the EOR time and AT. Thus, all the MAP durations and EOR times in a map were plotted against the ATs, regardless of the original recording sites.

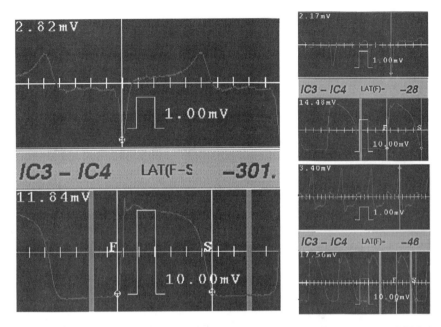

Figure 1. Representative recordings of the monophasic action potentials (MAPs) and the reference electrocardiogram (ECG) from the sampling window of the CARTO system. **Left:** Signals from the left ventricle during sinus rhythm in a healthy pig. Time scale 100 mm/s. **Right top:** Signals from the right ventricle during sinus rhythm in a patient with ventricular tachycardia (50 mm/s). **Right bottom:** Signals from the left ventricle during a monomorphic ventricular tachycardia in another patient with ventricular tachycardia (50 mm/s). On the MAP recordings, the first annotation line (F, first thin vertical line) was set on the onset of the MAP upstroke, representing the local activation and the second annotation line (S, second thin vertical line) on the intersection between the baseline and the tangent to the steepest slope on phase 3 of the MAP, representing the local end of repolarization. The MAP duration was measured as the interval between the two annotation lines. On the ECG traces, the time reference line was set on the peak of the QRS complex.

Preliminary Findings of Our MAP Mapping Study

Data Obtained from Healthy Pigs

Ten healthy pigs of 50 to 55 kg were studied under anesthesia of pentobarbital and catamine. In three of the 10 pigs, both the right and the left ventricular mapping were performed, with the MAPs recorded from 132±33 endocardial sites. In the other seven pigs, only the left ventricle was mapped, from 57±11 sites (Table 1). In total, 10 sets of left ventricular maps and three sets of right ventricular maps were constructed. In the three pigs with mapping performed in both ventricles,

Table 1
Analysis of Dispersion of Ventricular Repolarization on the 13 Maps from 10 Pigs

Groups	n	Sites	Activation Time		End of Repolarization		MAP Duration	
			Max. Disp.	Variance	Max. Disp.	Variance	Max. Disp.	Variance
In pigs with biventricular maps								
RV+LV maps	3	132±33	58±16	137±62	68±11*	197±75	52±3	130±60
RV maps	3	83±24	34±15	57±39	44±9	106±45	37±15	73±50
LV maps	3	49±11	46±10	138±28	47±7	135±38	40±10	108±48
In the whole group								
LV maps in the other 7 pigs	7	57±11	48±6	124±29	43±11	107±44	45±12	124±54
All LV maps	10	55±11	47±7§	128±28||	44±10‡	115±42†	44±11	119±50
All maps	13	61±18	44±11	112±42	44±9	113±41	42±12	108±52

M±1SD in ms. Max. Disp. = maximal dispersion, i.e., the maximal difference in these parameters over the endocardium in the mapped chamber; RV and LV = the right and left ventricles; MAP = monophasic action potential. *P<0.05, versus RV maps and LV maps in the same 3 pigs; †P<0.05, ‡P<0.005 versus RV+LV maps; §P<0.05; || = P<0.005 versus RV maps.

Table 2

Analyses on Dispersion of Repolarization on the 10 Maps from 8 Patients

Groups	n	Chamber	Sites	Activation Time		End of Repolarization		MAP Duration	
				Max. Disp.	Variance	Max. Disp.	Variance	Max. Disp.	Variance
All maps	10	5 RV, 5 LV	44±16	71±29	388±369	66±30	317±286	65±27	261±200
All maps in SR	8	5 RV, 3 LV	42±14	60±15	249±130	57±23	237±184	65±30	265±227
RV maps	5	RV	49±11	62±17	250±135	63±28	283±222	64±33	241±240
LV maps	5	LV	38±19	80±38	526±490	68±35	351±362	66±23	280±178
Concordant T	4	2 RV, 2 LV	38±16	53±9	191±39	45±10	145±70	59±30	217±248
ST-T changes	6	3 RV, 3 LV	48±15	84±32	520±438	80±31	432±323	70±26	290±181
VF (SR)	1	RV	62	61	213	106	636	120	634
VT, VPB	2	LV	52±24	116±35	947±572	99±38	638±491	67±4	245±21
VF/VT/VPB	3	1 RV, 2 LV	55±20	97±40	702±586	101±27	637±348	85±31	374±225
VT/SVT(SR)	7	4 RV, 3 LV	39±13	60±17	254±140	51±12*	180±96*	57±22	212±184

M+1SD in ms. SR = sinus rhythm; RV and LV = right and left ventricles; VF = ventricular fibrillation; VT = ventricular tachycardia; SVT = supraventricular tachycardia; VPB = ventricular premature beats; MAP = monophasic action potential; Max. Disp. = maximal dispersion; Concordant T = the polarity of T waves is concordant with that of the QRS in I, II, a VR, V_3 through V_6. ST-T changes = ST depression, low-amplitude and/or inverted T waves secondary to bundle branch block, VPBs, VT, or preexcitation. VF/VT/VPB = the map during SR from the VF patient and the map during VT and that during VPBs. VT/SVT (SR) = the 7 maps during SR from VT or SVT patients. *P<0.01 as compared with that in the VF/VT/VPB group.

the overall transventricular dispersion of activation, repolarization, and spatial distribution of the MAP duration were available for analysis (Table 1, Fig. 2).

Data Obtained from Patients with Cardiac Arrhythmias

Eight patients with ventricular (n=5) or supraventricular (n=3) tachyarrhythmias referred for an electrophysiological study/catheter ablation were recruited. In these patients, MAPs were recorded from 44±16 sites in the right or the left ventricle for 10 sets of maps (Table 2). Five left ventricular maps were obtained in three patients. In a patient with Wolff-Parkinson-White syndrome, the maps were obtained both before and after the ablation of the accessory pathway, and in a patient with monomorphic ventricular tachycardia the MAPs were obtained during the ventricular tachycardia and during sinus rhythm. Right ventricular maps were obtained in five patients.

DVR in Healthy Pigs

The maximal dispersions and variances of the AT, EOR time, and MAP duration among the 13 maps from the 10 pigs are presented in Table 1. The maximal dispersion and variance of the AT were significantly greater in the 10 left ventricular maps than in the three right ventricular maps. The dispersion parameters and their variances appeared greater in the biventricular maps in the three pigs than in the 10 left ventricular maps and than in the three right ventricular maps. However, the differences were statistically significant only in the dispersion and variance of the EOR between the three biventricular maps and the left ventricular maps (Table 1). In the three pigs with both ventricles mapped, the maximal and the minimal values of the EOR and the MAP duration were located within the left ventricle in one pig and in different sides of the two ventricles in two pigs.

DVR in the Eight Patients

The maximal dispersions and variances of the AT, EOR time, and MAP duration among the 10 maps from the eight patients are presented in Table 2. There was no significant difference in the dispersion parameters between the five right ventricular maps and the five left ventricular maps. The dispersions and variances in the six maps associated with secondary ST-T changes appeared relatively larger than in those four with concordant T waves. However, the differences were not statistically significant in this small group of patients (Table 2).

The maximal dispersion and variance of the EOR time were significantly larger in the map during sinus rhythm from a patient with ventricu-

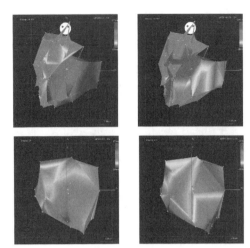

Figure 2. Maps during sinus rhythm from a healthy pig. **Top:** Biventricular maps, posterior-anterior views. **Bottom:** Left ventricular maps, right-lateral views. **Left:** End-of-repolarization (EOR) maps showing the earliest EOR at the upper septum of the left ventricle (red) and a few isolated long EOR areas over the posterior septum and along the right ventricular anteroparaseptal areas. The full range of the EOR times, i.e., the maximal dispersion, was 74 ms. **Right:** Monophasic action potential (MAP) duration map, showing that MAPs with the longest durations (red) were recorded at the left ventricular anteroparaseptal area with isolated long MAP areas on the upper septum of the left ventricle and the short MAP areas (dark blue) at the right anteroparaseptal and the left ventricular apex. The full range of the MAP durations, i.e., the maximal dispersion, was 55 ms. Note that the MAP map was plotted using negative values of the MAP durations. See color plate.

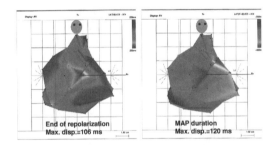

Figure 3. Right ventricular maps during sinus rhythm from the patient with ventricular fibrillation, 20° right anterior oblique views. **Left:** End-of-repolarization (EOR) map. The pattern of the EOR sequence started from the anterior free wall and ended along the paraseptal and apical areas, while the lateral basal region, the outflow tract and the septum showed isolated late and intermediate EOR areas. The maximal dispersion of the EOR was 106 ms. **Right:** Monophasic action potential (MAP) duration map. The longest MAPs were recorded at two anteroparaseptal sites, while the posterobasal region recorded the shortest MAPs. The maximal dispersion of the MAP duration was 120 ms. See color plate.

lar fibrillation (Fig. 3) and in the two maps during ventricular tachycardia and ventricular premature beats, respectively, from patients with ventricular tachycardia as compared with those in the other seven maps during sinus rhythm (Table 2). The increased dispersion of EOR time was mainly due to the increase in the dispersion of the AT in the ventricular tachycardia and the ventricular premature beat maps, but mainly due to the increase in the dispersion of the MAP duration in the map from the patient with ventricular fibrillation (Table 2). The dispersion of repolarization during sinus rhythm was not significantly different in the maps from patients with monomorphic ventricular tachycardia than in the maps from patients with supraventricular tachycardias (Table 2).

Besides the quantitative analyses, the color-coded, three-dimensional maps outlined accurately the magnitudes, spatial distributions, and other characteristics of the dispersions such as isolated short or long duration islands (Figs. 2 and 3).

Local Dispersion of Repolarization in Small Areas

The local dispersion parameters were measured among three to seven MAPs in small areas of less than 1 cm^2 in all of the 13 maps from the healthy pigs. A total of 72 areas were selected, mean 5.8 ± 1.2 (range 4 to 8) areas from each maps. The dispersion of repolarization among three to seven MAPs in these small areas was calculated and taken as the dispersion of local repolarization to compare with those of the global repolarization. In these healthy pigs, the mean dispersion of the EOR and that of the MAP duration were 13 ± 3 ms and 12 ± 3 ms, respectively, as compared with the global dispersions of these two parameters, 44 ± 9 ms and 42 ± 12 ms, respectively (P<0.0001 for both comparisons) in the 13 maps. An example of condensed MAP recordings from an area of approximately 0.7 cm^2 in size at the left lateral ventricle is shown in Figure 4. The dispersion of the EOR time and that of the MAP duration were 9 ms and 6 ms, respectively, which is much smaller than the global dispersion of these two parameters, 34 ms and 41 ms, respectively, in the same case.

The AT-Dependent Shortening of the MAP Duration

Our correlation and regression analysis between the AT and the MAP duration revealed a significant negative correlation between the AT and MAP duration in the healthy pigs and in our patients with arrhythmias. The slope of the linear regression between the MAP duration and the AT was negative in all the 13 maps from the pigs and in nine of the 10 maps from our patients. Two typical examples are shown in Figure 5, and the sum-up findings of the correlation analysis are presented in Table 3. Thus, progressively later activation was associated with progressively shorter MAP duration in all the maps.

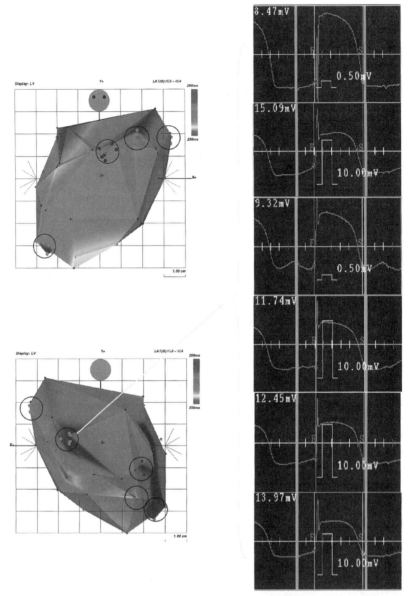

Figure 4. Left: End of repolarization (EOR) map from the left ventricle in a healthy pig, anterior-posterior (top) and posterior-anterior (bottom) views, showing seven selected areas of ≤1 cm² within which three to seven monophasic action potentials (MAPs) were recorded. The dispersion of repolarization was measured in each of the seven areas. **Right:** In one of the areas, the dispersion of EOR was 9 ms and that of the MAP duration 6 ms among the six MAPs in this area, which were markedly smaller than the global dispersion in the whole ventricle, 34 ms and 41 ms respectively, in this case. See color plate.

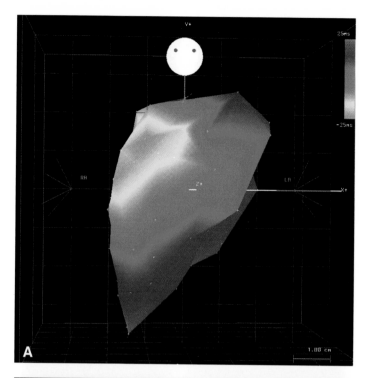

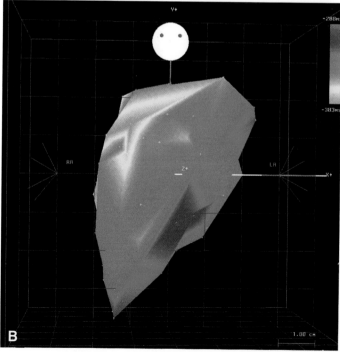

Figure 7-1. See page 111 for legend.

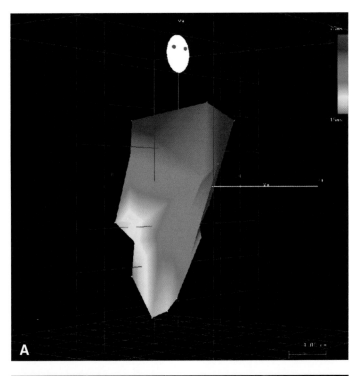

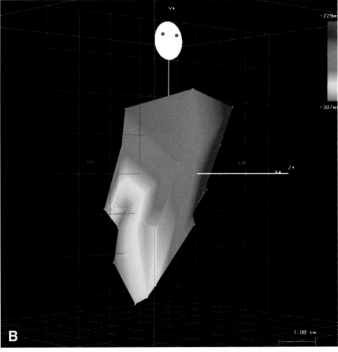

Figure 7-2. See page 113 for legend.

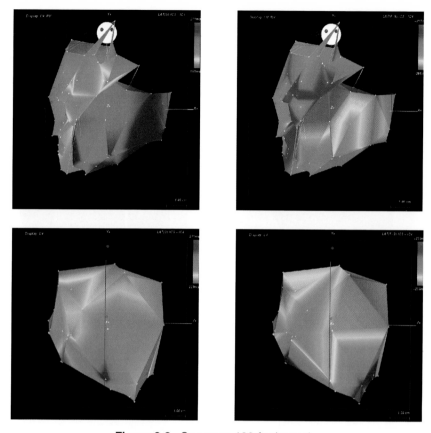

Figure 8-2. See page 130 for legend.

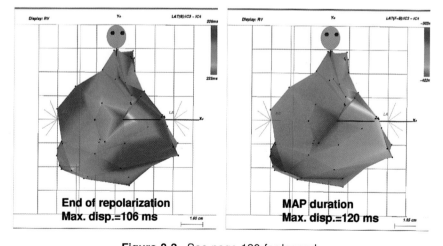

Figure 8-3. See page 130 for legend.

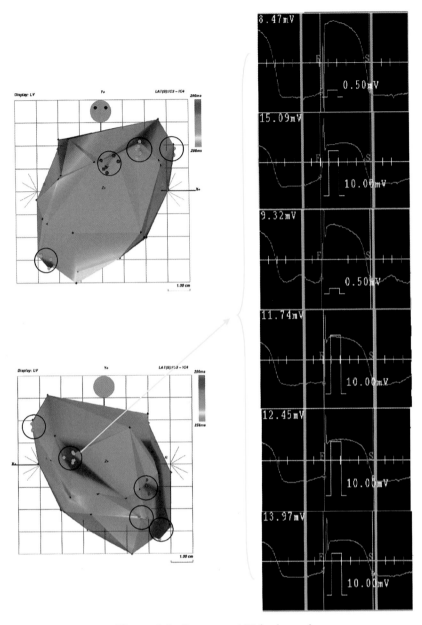

Figure 8-4. See page 132 for legend.

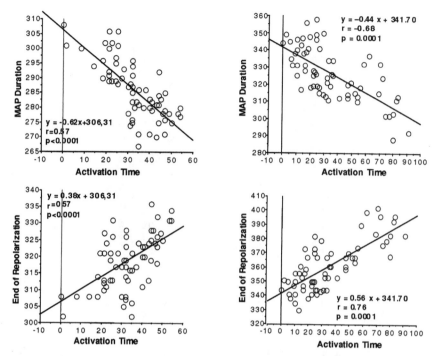

Figure 5. Linear regression analysis of two typical maps: the left plots are from a left ventricular map during sinus rhythm in a pig and the right from a right ventricular map during sinus rhythm in a patient. Both showing a negative correlation between the monophasic action potential duration and the activation time (**top**) and a positive correlation between the end-of-repolarization time and the activation time (**bottom**). Note the correlations were statistically significant and the slopes of the linear regression were less negative than −1, the negative unity, for the upper and less than +1, the positive unity, for the lower plots.

Implications of the Global Dispersion of Ventricular Repolarization

In the current study, the dispersion of repolarization was mapped using MAP recordings in both the left and right ventricles from a markedly higher number of sites than that in previous studies. These data, though from a limited number of animals and patients, represent the first attempts of detailed mapping of dispersion of repolarization using the MAP recording technique and the CARTO system.

We found that in healthy pigs the dispersion of AT was significantly greater in the left than in the right ventricular maps, while the dispersion of the EOR and that of the MAP duration were not different between the two ventricles. This may reflect that longer AT is needed for the relatively larger mass of the left ventricle than that of the right. The dispersion of

Table 3

Linear Regression Analysis between the MAP Duration and Activation Time and between the End-of-Repolarization Time and Activation Time in Healthy Pigs and in Patients

Groups	Chamber	Sites	MAPd/AT		EOR/AT	
			Slope	r	Slope	r
In pigs						
All LV maps	10 LV	55±11	−0.29±0.17	−0.54±0.13	0.48±0.18	0.51±0.18
All RV maps	3 RV	83±24	−0.52±0.18	−0.22±0.04	0.71±0.17	0.53±0.32
All LV + RV maps	3 LV + RV	132±33	−0.31±0.21	−0.29±0.19	0.69±0.21	0.58±0.21
Sum 16 maps		75±35	−0.44±0.20	−0.43±0.19	0.56±0.20	0.53±0.20
In patients						
All RV maps	5 RV	48±11	−0.53±0.21	−0.53±0.21	0.47±0.21	0.51±0.30
All LV maps	5 LV	38±19	−0.57±0.60	−0.45±0.25	0.69±0.17*	0.65±0.21*
All maps	5 RV, 5 LV	44±16	−0.58±0.40	−0.63±0.18	0.53±0.19*	0.66±0.28*

MAPd = monophasic action potential duration; AT = activation time; EOR = end of repolarization time; RV or LV maps = right or left ventricular maps; LV+RV maps = biventricular maps. The correlation coefficient r is statistically significant in all individual maps. *The correlation is negative in one map, which is not included in these calculations.

the EOR and that of the MAP duration were markedly larger in the biventricular maps than in single-sided ventricular maps, 68 ± 11 and 52 ± 3 ms as compared with 44 ± 10 ms and 44 ± 11 ms in the left ventricle, respectively. More interestingly, the magnitudes of the dispersion parameters were markedly greater in a global extent than in local areas. Condensed mapping within 1-cm^2 areas revealed that the dispersion parameters were only about 13 ± 3 ms and 12 ± 3 ms in the same group of animals. These findings suggest that in normal hearts the magnitude of the dispersion of repolarization is related to the size of the involved area, i.e., a relatively greater dispersion of repolarization is expected in relatively larger areas. This is not consistent with the previously reported observations in cardiac arrhythmia patients that the MAP duration varied as much over small areas as over the entire right ventricular endocardial surface.[5] Our measurements of the dispersion of EOR are, however, consistent with the maximal dispersion of the left ventricular activation-recovery intervals, 40 to 50 ms during sinus rhythm in healthy pigs measured by Gepstein et al,[18] and with the dispersion of the total recovery time approximately 50 ms in the normal left ventricle in patients measured by Vassallo et al.[4]

We also found that progressively later activation was associated with progressively shorter MAP duration and this AT-dependent shortening of the MAP duration reduces the magnitude of the maximal dispersion of EOR, a mechanism that protects the normal myocardium from the genesis of reentrant arrhythmias.

In our patients, the magnitude of the dispersion of EOR time and that of MAP duration were markedly greater than those reported in the previous clinical studies.[12,13] In our four maps during sinus rhythm with concordant T waves, the maximal dispersions of EOR time and MAP duration were 46 ± 10 and 55 ± 34 ms, as compared with 26 ± 14 and 41 ± 16 ms in the study by Franz and colleagues,[12] and 24 ± 6 and 34 ± 10 ms in the study by Cowan and colleagues,[13] respectively. In our six maps during sinus rhythm with ST-T changes, these two parameters were 80 ± 31 and 70 ± 26 ms, while they were 24 ± 6 and 34 ± 10 ms in Cowan and colleagues' four patients with inverted T waves.[13] Even though the electrophysiological status of our patients may differ from that of the patients in the above mentioned studies, the obvious difference in number of sampling sites may possibly be a cause of the difference in parameters of dispersion of repolarization. In this respect, the global dispersion of repolarization is more accurately and reliable evaluated using the current method than the previously reported methods with limited number of recording sites.[1,5,8,9,12,13,26]

Previous studies have shown that different magnitudes of the dispersion of repolarization are associated with different types of tachyarrhythmias.[4,5,26] Our earlier studies suggested that the increase in dispersion of repolarization was more pronounced in patients with polymorphic ventricular tachycardia/fibrillation than in those with monomorphic ventricular tachycardia, and that the increased dispersion of repolarization was mainly caused by an increased dispersion of MAP duration in the former, but mainly by that of the AT in the latter patients.[8,9] In this study, we found that the maximal dispersions of EOR time and MAP duration were both significantly increased in the patient with ventricular fibrillation. In the two patients who had the mapping performed during either monomorphic ventricular tachycardia or ventricular premature beats, the maximal dispersion of repolarization was also markedly increased. However, the latter associated only with an increased dispersion of AT, but not that of MAP duration. Thus, data obtained from detailed MAP mapping in this study support our earlier findings. However, it is clear that the observation in this study is far from sufficient to delineate the differences in global dispersion of repolarization underlying different types of tachyarrhythmias.

Limitations of this Mapping Technique

The time-dependent changes of the MAP configuration were observed in epicardial MAP recordings in patients undergoing routine cardiac surgery.[35] Beat-to-beat T wave alternans was also found in some patients with long QT syndrome, which may account for a dynamic, or time-dependent, heterogeneity of repolarization.[7] The present study was based on sequentially recorded MAPs that might have been influenced by the potential dynamic changes of repolarization. However, the above mentioned beat-to-beat changes were found only in approximately one third of the patients under pacing and different surgical interventions,[35] while our recordings were taken mainly during sinus rhythm without any intervention. Besides, our observations during the on-line monitoring of the MAP pattern and the off-line measurement of the recorded MAPs and the 12-lead ECG did not reveal any alternans. The constant time intervals between our reference signal and the two annotation points suggest that the time-dependent changes had no crucial influence on our findings.

It is also worth mentioning that myocardial repolarization is a complicated electrophysiological process and, besides, the transventricular repolarization gradients, the epicardial gradients, and especially the transmural gradients are very important factors influencing the global sequence and dispersion of repolarization.[36,37] The electrotonic interaction among cells, which tends to synchronize the repolarization of the neighboring cells, could also influence the repolarization sequence.[38] Our data, however, do not permit evaluation of these factors, especially the interaction between the transmural and the endocardial gradients.

Summary

The dispersion of repolarization was mapped on a global basis in healthy pigs and, for the first time, in humans, thus verifying the feasibility of this MAP mapping technique using the CARTO system for experimental and clinical applications. This novel technique may have potential usefulness in the areas of T wave genesis and its abnormalities, the interaction between activation and repolarization, and the dispersion of repolarization, as well as the underlying mechanism of arrhythmias.

In healthy pigs, the maximal dispersion of AT was 47 ± 7 ms, that of MAP duration 44 ± 11 ms, and that of EOR 44 ± 10 ms over the left ventricular endocardium in this study. The AT-dependent shortening of the MAP duration, i.e., progressively later activation associated with progressively shorter MAP duration, reduces the magnitude of the maximal dispersion of EOR.

The dispersion and variance of the EOR were slightly smaller in the right than in the left ventricular maps, but were markedly greater in the biventricular maps, while the dispersion parameters within small areas were significantly smaller than the global dispersion parameters.

In our patients with cardiac arrhythmias, the magnitude of the dispersion of EOR time and that of MAP duration were markedly greater than those in healthy pigs and in patients from the previous studies. These dispersion parameters were further augmented in maps associated with ST-T changes or during ventricular tachycardia or premature beats. In a patient with ventricular fibrillation, the dispersion of repolarization was obviously increased even during sinus rhythm.

The color-coded, three-dimensional maps outlined the magnitudes, area differences, and other characteristics of dispersion of repolarization.

References

1. Kuo CS, Atarashi H, Reddy CP, Surawicz B. Dispersion of ventricular repolarization and arrhythmia: Study of two consecutive ventricular premature complexes. *Circulation* 1985;72(2):370-376.
2. Mitchell L, Wyse D, Duff H. Programmed electrical stimulation for ventricular tachycardia induction in humans. I. The role of ventricular functional refractoriness in tachycardia induction. *J Am Coll Cardiol* 1986;8:567-575.
3. Downar E, Harris L, Mickelborough L, et al. Endocardial mapping of ventricular tachycardia in the intact human ventricle: Evidence for reentrant mechanisms. *J Am Coll Cardiol* 1988;11:783-791.
4. Vassallo JA, Cassidy DM, Kindwall KE, et al. Nonuniform recovery of excitability in the left ventricle. *Circulation* 1988;78:1365-1372.
5. Morgan JM, Cunningham D, Rowland E. Dispersion of monophasic action potential duration: Demonstrable in humans after premature ventricular extrastimulation but not in steady state. *J Am Coll Cardiol* 1992;19(6):1244-1253.

6. Kurz RW, Xiao LR, Franz MR. Increased dispersion of ventricular repolarization and ventricular tachyarrhythmias in the globally ischaemic rabbit heart. *Eur Heart J* 1993;14(11):1561-1571.

7. Zareba W, Badilini F, Moss AJ. Automatic detection of spatial and dynamic heterogeneity of repolarization. *J Electrocardiol* 1994;27(suppl):66-72.

8. Yuan S, Wohlfart B, Olsson SB, Blomström-Lundqvist C. The dispersion of repolarization in patients with ventricular tachycardia. A study using simultaneous monophasic action potential recordings from two sites in the right ventricle. *Eur Heart J* 1995;16(1):68-76.

9. Yuan S, Blomström-Lundqvist C, Pehrson S, et al. Dispersion of repolarization following double and triple programmed stimulation—A clinical study using the monophasic action potential recording technique. *Eur Heart J* 1996;17:1080-1091.

10. Laurita KR, Girouard SD, Rosenbaum DS. Modulation of ventricular repolarization by a premature stimulus. Role of epicardial dispersion of repolarization kinetics demonstrated by optical mapping of the intact guinea pig heart. *Circ Res* 1996;79(3):493-503.

11. Laurita KR, Rosenbaum DS. Implications of ion channel diversity to ventricular repolarization and arrhythmogenesis: Insights from high resolution optical mapping. *Can J Cardiol* 1997;13(11):1069-1076.

12. Franz MR, Bargheer K, Rafflenbeul W, et al. Monophasic action potential mapping in human subjects with normal electrocardiograms: Direct evidence for the genesis of the T wave. *Circulation* 1987;75(2):379-386.

13. Cowan JC, Hilton CJ, Griffiths CJ, et al. Sequence of epicardial repolarisation and configuration of the T wave. *Br Heart J* 1988;60(5):424-433.

14. Zabel M, Portnoy S, Franz MR. Electrocardiographic indexes of dispersion of ventricular repolarization: An isolated heart validation study. *J Am Coll Cardiol* 1995;25(3):746-752.

15. Lee RJ, Liem LB, Cohen TJ, Franz MR. Relation between repolarization and refractoriness in the human ventricle: Cycle length dependence and effect of procainamide. *J Am Coll Cardiol* 1992;19:614-618.

16. Chen PS, Moser KM, Dembitsky WP, et al. Epicardial activation and repolarization patterns in patients with right ventricular hypertrophy. *Circulation* 1991;83(1):104-118.

17. Lux RL, Ershler PR, Taccardi B. Measuring spatial waves of repolarization in canine ventricles using high-resolution epicardial mapping. *J Electrocardiol* 1996;29(suppl):130-134.

18. Gepstein L, Hayam G, Ben-Haim S. Activation-repolarization coupling in the normal swine endocardium. *Circulation* 1997;96(11):4036-4043.

19. Witkowski FX, Penkoske PA. A completely automated activation-repolarization interval algorithm for directly coupled unipolar electrograms and its three-dimensional correlation with refractory periods. *J Electrocardiol* 1988;21(3):273-282.

20. Steinhaus BM. Estimating cardiac transmembrane activation and recovery times from unipolar and bipolar extracellular electrograms: A simulation study. *Circ Res* 1989;64(3):449-462.

21. Efimov IR, Ermentrout B, Huang DT, Salama G. Activation and repolarization patterns are governed by different structural characteristics of ventricular myocardium: Experimental study with voltage-sensitive dyes and numerical simulations. *J Cardiovasc Electrophysiol* 1996;7(6):512-530.

22. Olsson SB. Estimation of ventricular repolarization in man by monophasic action potential recording technique. *Eur Heart J* 1985;6(suppl D):71-79.
23. Franz MR. Method and theory of monophasic action potential recording. *Prog Cardiovasc Dis* 1991;33(6):347-368.
24. Olsson SB, Yuan S. Technique and use of monophasic action potential recordings. In Mandel WJ (ed): *Cardiac Arrhythmias. Their Mechanisms, Diagnosis, and Management.* 3rd ed. Philadelphia: J. B. Lippincott Company; 1995:785-810.
25. Franz MR. Monophasic action potential recordings: What are they, how can they be recorded, what is their use? In Franz MR, Schmitt C, Zrenner B (eds): *Monophasic Action Potentials.* Berlin: Springer; 1997:22-39.
26. Shimizu W, Ohe T, Kurita T, et al. Early afterdepolarizations induced by isoproterenol in patients with congenital long QT syndrome. *Circulation* 1991;84(5):1915-1923.
27. Ben-Haim S, Osadchy D, Schuster I, et al. Nonfluoroscopic, in vivo navigation and mapping technology. *Nat Med* 1996;2(12):1393-1395.
28. Shpun S, Gepstein L, Hayam G, Ben-Haim S. Guidance of radiofrequency endocardial ablation with real-time three-dimensional magnetic navigation system. *Circulation* 1997;96(6):2016-2021.
29. Gepstein L, Hayam G, Ben-Haim S. A novel method for nonfluoroscopic catheter-based electroanatomical mapping of the heart. In vitro and in vivo accuracy results. *Circulation* 1997;95(6):1611-1622.
30. Yuan S, Kongstad O, Hedin E, et al. Global repolarization sequence and its dispersion: Preliminary findings of monophasic action potential mapping using the CARTO system. *Circulation* 1998;98(suppl-I):I842. Abstract.
31. Yuan S, Kongstad O, Hertervig E, et al. Global and local dispersion of ventricular repolarization: A study using the MAP mapping technique and the CARTO system. *Europace* 2000;1(suppl B):B33. Abstract.
32. Shabetai R, Surawicz B, Hammill W. Monophasic action potentials in man. *Circulation* 1968;38:341-352.
33. Autenrieth G, Surawicz B, Kuo CS. Sequence of repolarization on the ventricular surface in the dog. *Am Heart J* 1975;89(4):463-469.
34. Yuan S, Wohlfart B, Olsson SB, Blomström-Lundqvist C. Clinical application of a microcomputer system for recording and measuring monophasic action potentials. *PACE* 1996;19:297-308.
35. Sutton PM, Taggart P, Lab M, et al. Alternans of epicardial repolarization as a localized phenomenon in man. *Eur Heart J* 1991;12(1):70-78.
36. Yan G-X, Antzelevitch C. Cellular basis for the normal T wave and the electrocardiographic manifestations of the long-QT syndrome. *Circulation* 1998;98:1928-1936.
37. Yan G-X, Shimizu W, Antzelevitch C. Characteristics and distribution of M cells in arterially perfused canine left ventricular wedge preparations. *Circulation* 1998;98:1921-1927.
38. Antzelevitch C, Sun ZQ, Zhang ZQ, Yan G-X. Cellular and ionic mechanisms underlying erythromycin-induced long QT and torsade de pointes. *J Am Coll Cardiol* 1996;28:1836-1848.

Dispersion of Ventricular Repolarization and Ventricular Arrhythmias

9

Increased Dispersion of Repolarization:

A Major Mechanism Behind the Genesis of Malignant Ventricular Arrhythmias in Cardiac Diseases

Jan P. Amlie

Introduction

For many years, textbooks have claimed that the classic mechanisms behind ventricular arrhythmias are reentry, increased automaticity, influence of autonomic transmitters, and diseased cardiac substrate. These pathophysiological factors have been demonstrated and characterized at a cellular level in isolated heart strips or in intact animals.

In clinical practice reentry is well established in many types of clinical arrhythmias; a classic example is Wolff-Parkinson-White syndrome. Increased automaticity is observed as extrasystoles. Triggered activity has been more difficult to demonstrate but is obviously present after treatment with Class III antiarrhythmic drugs. Disturbances in the autonomic system are well known as pathogenic factors for ventricular arrhythmias together with the state of the myocardium.

Ventricular fibrillation and ventricular tachycardias in humans are electrical events and it is therefore of considerable interest to find out how action potentials and conduction in different parts of the beating human heart are affected by different stimuli and heart diseases.

Until now, the knowledge in this field has been scarce and many theories have been postulated on the basis of data from basic electrophysiological studies in normal myocardium taken from animals. This gap

From Olsson SB, Amlie JP, Yuan S (eds): *Dispersion of Ventricular Repolarization: State of the Art.* ©Futura Publishing Company, Inc., Armonk, NY, 2000.

between basic electrophysiology and clinical electrophysiology observed over the last 15 years now seems to have been filled by studies of excised heart tissue studied by multiple electrodes[1] or by sophisticated noninvasive and invasive methods.

Many of our pharmacological treatments for arrhythmias have been based on thinking from simple basic electrophysiological experiments over the last 20 years. These data have not been as helpful as earlier believed for decision making in clinical medicine and have even led clinicians to do harmful studies.[2,3] Now in the beginning of the 21st century, treatment of clinical arrhythmias has a better rationale due to many nonpharmacological treatment modalities and the introduction of other drugs not originally made for arrhythmias, such as β-blockers.[4]

In clinical arrhythmology much focus has been on conduction velocity in different parts of the heart, because it could be measured simply in the beating human heart. The repolarization phase of the impulse was characterized by measurements of refractoriness. The dispersion of refractoriness, however, could not be measured and was forgotten or not understood by many leading clinical electrophysiologists.

Disturbances in the repolarization phase of the action potentials as an arrhythmogenic mechanism have received increased attention over the last few years, mainly because of the proposition that QT dispersion may give a picture of global dispersion of refractoriness of the heart.[5]

Dispersion of Repolarization

Human ventricular cardiac cells have long action potentials and thus long refractory periods that can be considered a safety mechanism protecting the heart against excessively high heart rates. The principle of prolongation of the action potentials slightly and uniformly has been accepted as an antiarrhythmic effect rather than an arrhythmogenic effect. The refractory periods in the ventricles are not constant but are dependent on the heart rate and adapt gradually to an increase in heart rate.[6]

Increased dispersion of refractoriness and, thus, electrical heterogeneity, are closely linked to malignant ventricular arrhythmias in different kinds of heart diseases.[7] This is evident from many experimental and clinical studies. The dispersion of refractoriness and disturbed conduction of extrasystoles in the setting of increased dispersion of refractoriness seem to be the main electrophysiological mechanisms behind the two most important clinical arrhythmias, ventricular tachycardia and ventricular fibrillation.

Spatial inhomogeneity of the repolarization phase of action potentials (dispersion of repolarization) can be caused by different durations of action potentials and also by some action potentials appearing late due to slow conduction. Therefore, dispersion of refractoriness can be due to the presence of nonhomogenous refractoriness, nonhomogenous conduction, or both.

The normal beating heart has a certain dispersion of repolarization. Action potentials in the endocardium last longer than do those in the epicardium. They are even different in appearance due to different ionic movements. The sum of the action potentials can be observed in the normal electrocardiogram (ECG) as concordant QRS and T deflections (similar QRS and T axis). Gradients of long to short repolarization durations from the apex to the base have also been demonstrated in humans by us and others. In experimental animals a large transmural heterogeneity has been found, and the change in repolarization times can be rather abrupt due to high adjacent dispersion.[8] To my knowledge, this has not been measured in the beating human heart.

The duration of an action potential of an extrasystole is dependent on the proximity to the preceding action potential—the so-called proximity effect.[6] This effect has been characterized in humans (Fig. 1). A very short action potential can be observed very close to refractoriness (Fig. 2) (see page 150). A premature impulse shows subnormal conduction when the extrasystole occurs close to the refractory period (Fig. 3). If the repolariza-

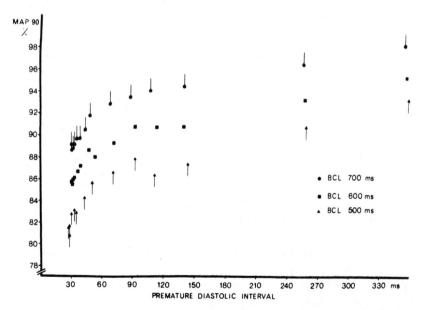

Figure 1. Electrical restitution curves showing monophasic action potential at 90% repolarization (MAP$_{90}$) durations of premature betas at basic cycle lengths (BCL) 700, 600, and 500 ms. All values are normalized to the individual steady state MAP$_{90}$ durations at CL of 700 ms, and related to premature diastolic intervals to the preceding beat. A hump of the restitution is observed at CL of 500 ms. Mean values (SE) are shown.

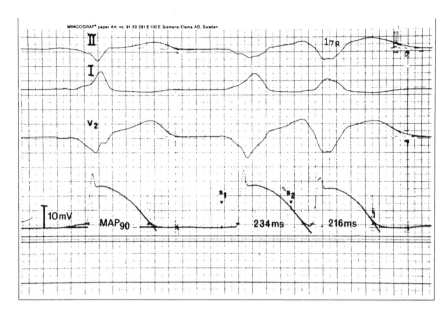

Figure 2. Monophasic action potential (MAP) and electrocardiogram (leads I and V₂) at a paper speed of 200 ms⁻¹, where MAP at 90% repolarization is measured. Two regular beats and one premature beat are shown.

tion phase is unsynchronized, the impulses may disorganize and a ventricular fibrillation can occur. Such experiments have not been performed in humans, but from our open chest dog experiments we could observe that ventricular fibrillation can be initiated locally and thereafter spread to the whole heart (Fig. 4).[9-11] In our experiments six monophasic action potential recordings were performed on the epicardium of the heart.

While disturbances of the conduction play an important, if not the dominant, role in the ventricular arrhythmias of patients with structural heart disease, e.g., due to myocardial ischemia or cardiomyopathy, asynchronous repolarization appears to be the underlying cause of serious arrhythmias in patients without obvious morphological derangement of the heart. The latter include patients with the long QT time syndrome.

ECGs recorded at the characteristic polymorphous ventricular tachycardia or ventricular fibrillation show that these arrhythmias are precipitated by a ventricular premature complex (VPC) sometimes interrupting the T wave.[9] If we assume that the onset of premature ventricular depolarization corresponds to the repolarization phase in some portions of the ventricle, while the end of the T wave corresponds to late action potentials,[10] we may consider the interval between the onset of VPC and the end of QT as the minimum duration of the dispersion of repolarization. It has, until recently, been impossible to study in detail dispersion of

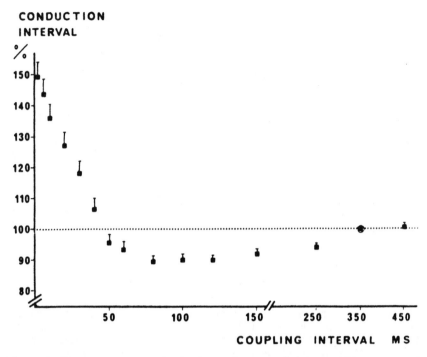

Figure 3. The premature conduction intervals at a cycle length of 600 ms normalized as percentages of the values of individual steady state conduction intervals. Mean values (SE) are shown as a function of coupling intervals from refractoriness.

repolarization of the beating human heart. Therefore, our knowledge must be based on animal experiments and on some data from the human heart.

In our studies, an animal model was created in which dispersion of repolarization was mainly due to differences in the ventricular action potential durations, without any appreciable conduction disturbances or structural lesions in the myocardium. Kuo and colleagues[10-12] produced a dog heart model with general hypothermia (29°C to 30°C) due to a decrease in temperature in the left atrium. We were therefore able to study the effect of general hypothermia and general action potential prolongation on dispersion of repolarization at regular sinus rhythm, during ventricular pacing, and after premature stimuli in different parts of the heart (Fig. 5).[11] With perfusion with warm blood in the left anterior descending coronary artery, we could create a large dispersion of repolarization and easily create ventricular fibrillation by an extrastimuli with a fixed localization (Fig. 4).[9,10]

General hypothermia did not increase dispersion of repolarization significantly during sinus rhythm.[11] Action potential duration and refractoriness were independent of the stimulation site. However, we could

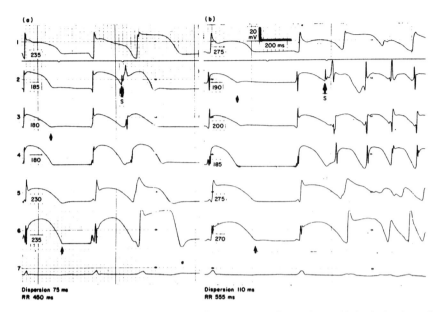

Figure 4. Effect of atrial pacing rate on maximum dispersion and the induction of ventricular fibrillation. In **a**, the cycle length during atrial pacing is 450 ms and in **b** 555 ms. Note that ventricular fibrillation was induced only at a slower atrial pacing rate when the maximum dispersion was greater. The stimulus in **a** represents the most premature stimulus that elicited a ventricular premature complex. In each panel, short vertical arrows show the ends of the monophasic action potential (MAP). The maximum dispersion, as defined by the maximal differences between the ends of any of six MAPs, is shown at the bottom of each panel. Numbers within each MAP represent their durations in milliseconds. In each panel, the first two complexes are the basic complexes during atrial pacing, and the third complex is the premature complex in response to ventricular premature stimulus. Reproduced from Reference 12, with permission.

observe that during ventricular pacing conduction velocity in the specialized conducting system was impaired during hypothermia.

When a large dispersion was created with perfusion of the left anterior descending coronary artery with warm blood, it was apparent that a premature extrasystole in the area with short action potentials created ventricular fibrillation (Fig. 4) while an extrasystole in the area with long action potentials did not. The critical maximal dispersion ranged from 95 to 145 ms between six monophasic action potentials obtained on the epicardial surface when ventricular fibrillation could occur.[10]

We could therefore demonstrate that increased dispersion of repolarization was a substrate for ventricular fibrillation, and an extrasystole in the area with short action potentials was the triggering factor.

Juxtapositions of two such action potentials might be expected to create a potential difference during repolarization and generate an excit-

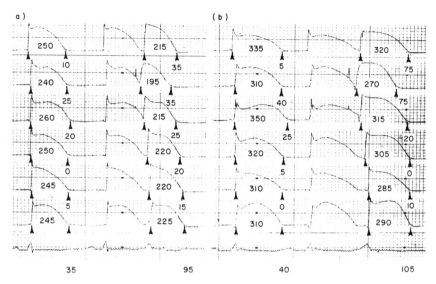

Figure 5. Effect of hypothermia on basic and premature dispersion. Six monophasic action potentials (MAPs) and Y lead of the electrocardiogram during atrial and premature ventricular stimulation in **(a)** control, and **(b)** during hypothermia. The arrows point to the onset and the end of each MAP. The numbers within the MAPs designate their duration in ms. The numbers to the right of the MAP designate the interval between the ends of two MAPs at adjacent sites in ms. The numbers at the bottom of the figure show the maximum dispersion between any of two of the six sites. Note, that hypothermia prolongs each nonpremature MAP by 65 to 90 ms but increases the maximum basic dispersion by only 5 ms and the premature dispersion by only 10 ms. However, at the adjacent sites, the difference between basic and premature dispersion ranges from –20ms (between sites 4 and 5) to 40 ms (between sites 2 and 3). Reproduced from Reference 11, with permission.

atory current of sufficient grade to reexcite the fiber with the shorter action potential duration. No such activity was detected in our experiments. In the presence of critical dispersion, the conduction of premature impulses in the area with short action potentials was inhibited while more rapid impulse conduction was observed from the area with long action potentials.

Thus, it was reasonably clear from our experiment and from other experiments that dispersion of repolarization of action potentials is a substrate for ventricular fibrillation in the dog heart in situ when a certain value is reached and that a type of microreentry is created leading to ventricular fibrillation. ECG recordings from patients with long QT time support that the same mechanism is present in humans.[9] A large difference in action potential duration has been found in those patients.[13]

Dispersion of repolarization can be classified as maximal, which is the difference between the earliest and the latest repolarization measured, or as adjacent from two action potentials obtained from two close sites.[10,11]

When maximal dispersion of repolarization is increased, adjacent dispersion must of course be increased in some areas.

In a study by Yuan et al,[14] monophasic action potentials were obtained from the right ventricle in patients with a history of monomorphic ventricular tachycardia, polymorphic ventricular tachycardia, and ventricular fibrillation. In these patients, where structural heart disease was common the local dispersion in the right ventricle was increased mainly due to activation time differences. This was evident both during pacing and when premature extrastimuli were given. In patients with induced ventricular tachycardia, differences in action potential duration did not contribute to the local dispersion of repolarization. This is in agreement with the common theories that nonhomogenous conduction is the most important factor for induction of ventricular tachycardia. In patients with polymorphic ventricular tachycardia or ventricular fibrillation induced during the electrophysiological study, differences in the action potential durations probably contribute to the increase in dispersion of refractoriness.

Extrasystoles and Dispersion of Refractoriness

Premature impulses play probably a crucial role in the pathogenesis of ventricular fibrillation. The conduction of the premature impulses is dependent on the proximity to the steady state action potential. Closer than 40 ms to the refractory period, the conduction velocity of premature impulses is markedly depressed, while from 40 to 150 ms, a more rapid conduction, named supernormal conduction, is observed (Fig. 3).

Thus, changes in conduction velocity affect dispersion of repolarization of premature impulses. Increased excitability of Purkinje fibers might be a cause of the supernormal conduction. These effects on the conduction velocity of extrasystoles have secondary effects on dispersion of repolarization of premature beats. Lidocaine inhibits mainly supernormal conduction[15] in addition to its effects in ischemic tissue.

Premature action potentials are shortened markedly close to the preceding beat, described as the proximity effect. This effect has been described at different heart rates in humans.[6] Shorter action potentials decrease less than longer action potentials at close proximity; this is in agreement with studies in animals (Fig. 6).[16] A homogenization of premature action potentials is therefore expected at higher heart rates. In agreement with that, a decrease in dispersion of repolarization has been observed in humans at higher heart rates, even in patients suffering from coronary artery disease,[17] but at levels without clinical signs of ischemia (see below).

In experimental models the electrical restitution is of importance for the dispersion of excitability[11] and, thus, for the possibility of inducing malignant arrhythmias by premature beats.[6] An increased dispersion due

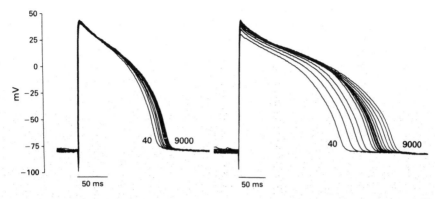

Figure 6. Superimposed action potentials from guinea pig right ventricular papillary muscle recorded when the diastolic interval prior to the extra stimulus increased from 40 to 9000 ms. **Left** at 37°C; **right** at 27°C. Note the increased range of premature action potential durations at wider action potentials. Reproduced from Reference 16, with permission.

to a small difference in coupling intervals has been shown at sites and times where the restitution curves were steep. It increased to critical values when the effects of great differences in action potential duration were added to conduction differences of premature impulses.[12]

QT dispersion has, in past years, been adopted by many as a noninvasive measure of the "maximal" dispersion of ventricular repolarization[18,19] and thus as an index of arrhythmia susceptibility.[19] Available experimental data support this concept with many reservations.[5]

Physiological Stimuli Affecting Dispersion of Repolarization

Heart Rate

Action potential duration is gradually decreased at increasing heart rates. A certain action potential duration is gradually reached when the heart rate is increased to a certain higher level.[6] It takes approximately 2 minutes before steady state is reached in humans. Some difference in cycle length dependence of repolarization between right and left muscle cells is possible. During the initial beats of a new faster heart rate, before a steady state is reached, there are marked alterations in the duration of the refractory periods, especially in the bundle branches. This has also been observed in patients in our electrophysiology laboratory. Thus, in the steady state of the slower heart rate, refractory periods of the specific conduction system are longer than those of the myocardium. After the first beat of the fast rate, this situation is reversed, and recovery of excitability occurs faster in the bundle branches than in the papillary muscles.[21]

The normal dispersion of repolarization in the human heart decreases at increasing paced steady state heart rates.[17] This can be due to a homogenization of action potentials and also some slight enhancing effect on the conduction velocity. The slight increase in conduction velocity during ventricular pacing at high heart rates observed in our experience in patients with coronary artery disease, contrary to what was expected from single cell studies (Fig. 7),[17] may be due to some release of catecholamines before ischemia occurs.

It must be mentioned that during severe ischemia in patients, a decrease in heart rate often inhibits malignant ventricular arrhythmias. This effect is probably due to lesser inhomogeneity of depolarization and repolarization due to better conduction in ischemic areas.

When ischemia is not present, it has been observed repeatedly in clinical situations that increase in heart rate can inhibit incessant ventricular arrhythmias, including ventricular fibrillation and torsade de pointes arrhythmias.

However, during ischemia a decrease in heart rate may inhibit malignant ventricular arrhythmias due to lesser inhomogeneity, which is probably due to lesser ischemia.[21]

Autonomic Activity

Neural mechanisms are importantly involved in the regulation of ventricular repolarization, and that process itself is a significant factor in both normal cardiac physiology and a variety of disease states. Although

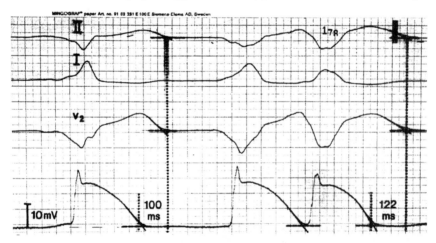

Figure 7. Monophasic action potential (MAP) and surface electrocardiogram leads I, II, and V₂. The terminations of the MAPs at 90% repolarization and T waves are shown by the vertical dotted lines. The duration of basic and premature dispersion are measured as the distance between these lines, in the present examples 100 and 122 ms, respectively.

neural influences on ventricular repolarization are both definite and significant, their detailed definition has been limited by the methods available for study of that process. Sympathetic innervation has been shown to be localized but overlapping, and provides an anatomical basis for sympathetic effects on repolarization in disease states. As shown by Kralios and others,[22] dispersion of refractoriness may increase 25 ms after sympathetic stimulation. An uneven distribution of sympathetic nerve endings has also been shown in humans.[23] β-Blockade increases ventricular refractoriness with approximately the same values in dogs with high sympathetic activity due to barbiturate anesthesia.[24] Stimulation of the vagus has the same prolonging effect on ventricular repolarization during high sympathetic tone,[25] and even digitoxin has this effect,[26] counteracting the direct shortening effect of digitoxin.

It is therefore reasonable to believe that β-blockade and vagus stimulation may decrease dispersion of repolarization at high sympathetic tone and therefore decrease the vulnerability to ventricular fibrillation. This is well in agreement with the Norwegian timolol study and other β-blocker studies dealing with sudden cardiac death in different types of patients.[4,27]

Sympathetic stimulation induces T wave changes in the ECG, which may reflect increased dispersion of repolarization. The malignant ventricular arrhythmias and the ECG changes observed during cerebral strokes may be due to increased dispersion of refractoriness induced by autonomic imbalance.

Chronic β-blockade may have additional effects on myocardial electrophysiology. Necrosis and degeneration of myocardial cells have been observed after prolonged sympathetic stimulation. This process has recently been characterized in more detail in experimental animals[28] and can probably be inhibited by β-blockade.

Prolonged β-blockade seems to give rise to prolonged action potential duration in the ventricles in humans,[29] in agreement with acute effects in animals with high sympathetic activity.[24]

Available evidence indicates therefore that β-blockade inhibits malignant ventricular arrhythmias in different kinds of heart diseases by several electrophysiological mechanisms.

Pathophysiological Stimuli

Ventricular Pacing

Ventricular pacing increases dispersion of repolarization compared with sinus rhythm. This was well documented in our dog experiments (Fig. 5).[11] From a theoretical point of view, atrial pacing should be used in patients with sinus node disease when possible to avoid malignant ventricular arrhythmias in patients after myocardial infarction. Clinical data support this concept.[30]

Smoking

From a study in our electrophysiological laboratory we found that smoking a cigarette decreased action potential duration in the right ventricle in patients with coronary artery disease with an average of 30 ms at the level of 90% repolarization (Fig. 8).[31] If this shortening appears unevenly in the ventricles, an increase in dispersion of refractoriness may occur. This has not until now been studied. The supernormal conduction velocity increased also after smoking.[31] Smoking may therefore have a direct arrhythmogenic effect.

Left Ventricular Hypertrophy

Left ventricular hypertrophy is observed in many different heart diseases, among them aortic valvular stenosis, hypertrophic obstructive cardiomyopathy, and essential systemic hypertension. Left ventricular hypertrophy attenuates the damaging effect on the ventricular wall and augments pump function, yet its presence is associated with a substantial increase in cardiovascular risk. This cardiac hypertrophy is associated

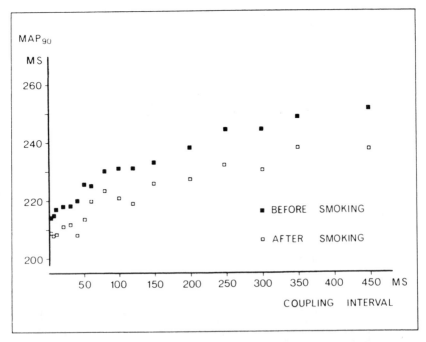

Figure 8. The median monophasic action potential at 90% repolarization duration of the premature beats from 10 patients studied before and after smoking, plotted as coupling interval from ventricular effective refractory period. Reprinted from Reference 29, with permission.

with alterations in ventricular action potentials, which are not homogenous throughout the left ventricle.[32] The difference in action potential duration between subendocardial and subepicardial myocytes seen in normal hearts seems to be lost in hypertrophy. This should lead to ST-T changes in ECG in humans, which are probably an indicator of increased dispersion of refractoriness.[29,33] A calcium-insensitive transient outward current may be involved in this process.[34]

The fact that left ventricular hypertrophy is detectable on electrocardiography confers a risk that is several times greater than that attributed to the associated blood pressure level.[35,36] The risk is similar to that associated with a history of myocardial infarction. All of the clinical sequelae of coronary artery disease are worsened in patients with evidence of left ventricular hypertrophy on ECG, and there is a sixfold increase in the risk of sudden cardiac death from cardiac causes.[37] Electrophysiological testing has not revealed sustained ventricular tachycardia in these patients. It is therefore reasonable to suspect that increased dispersion of repolarization is present and that the changes in ST and T waves on the ECG are a sign of this.[33]

Increased QT dispersion has been found in patients with mild hypertension.[38] QT dispersion has also been shown to increase during follow-up in patients with borderline hypertension, and to decrease after treatment with drugs.[36,39] When QT dispersion increased to more than 80 ms in patients with hypertension, sudden cardiac death was more common.[40] Ischemia[41] and/or sympathetic stimulation[23] may be the provoking factor for ventricular fibrillation.

Echocardiography is considered a more accurate and sensitive means of detecting left ventricular hypertrophy than electrocardiography is. However, ECGs provide additional prognostic information, probably because they reflect more closely the electrical activity of the heart; ECG should probably not be replaced by echocardiography but should be used additionally.[42]

Antihypertensive therapy improves the cardiovascular autonomic regulation in systemic therapy, and even enalapril and hydrochlorothiazid can reduce sympathetic activity.[43] This can partially explain the reduced cardiac mortality seen in patients with intensified antihypertensive therapy after different antihypertensive drugs.[44]

Left Ventricular Pressure Load

It is well known that many patients with aortic stenosis die suddenly due to malignant ventricular arrhythmias. In 1% to 3% of these patients, it may be the first and only symptom of aortic stenosis.[45]

The relationship between hypertrophy of the heart and QT dispersion is discussed above. An increase in QT dispersion has been found with a linear relationship to the pressure gradients.[46] Implantation of an artificial valve should therefore reduce the risk of ventricular fibrillation; this is well in agreement with clinical observations.

Myocardial Ischemia

Experimental studies show that profound changes in activation times and action potential duration occur during ischemia, leading to increased dispersion of refractoriness and to malignant ventricular arrhythmias.[21]

In patients with coronary artery disease QT dispersion is increased by atrial pacing.[47] The increased QT dispersion observed during exercise in patients with coronary artery disease can be inhibited by a successful angioplasty[48] and β-blockade.[49] In a coronary risk population increased QT dispersion was a risk factor for sudden cardiac death and myocardial infarction.[50] In women with possible coronary artery disease exercise QT dispersion is an easily measurable ECG variable that significantly increases the accuracy of exercise testing.[51] In vasospastic angina induction of a coronary spasm increases QT dispersion and may be a marker for prognosis.[52]

The logical treatment for patients with significant stenosis of the coronary arteries and ventricular tachycardia and ventricular fibrillation should therefore probably be to revascularize them before treating them with antiarrhythmic drugs or antiarrhythmic devices. Clinical data from our hospital and from other hospitals indicate that this is the best policy. A combination of a defibrillator and revascularization seems to be optimal; however this has not been confirmed in adequately large series.

Myocardial Infarction

After the acute phase the conduction velocity is decreased in some parts of the heart due to scars and disorganization of the myocardial fibers. In healed myocardial infarction normal action potential is often found in the border zone while changed fiber orientation and connective tissue impair conduction. Impaired depolarization of the myocardium can be reflected by an increased QRS time with possible secondary increase in dispersion of repolarization if action potential duration is not changed. In a large patient group that underwent coronary bypass surgery the QRS time was an independent marker of sudden cardiac death.[53] The extent of the viable myocardium seems to determine the magnitude of QT dispersion.[54] In addition to that, the extent of the reperfusion status seems to play a role.[55]

In patients with ventricular tachycardia or ventricular fibrillation after myocardial infarction an increase in QT dispersion is often found.[56,57] However, in a study of 280 consecutive infarct survivors, a multivariate analysis showed that QT dispersion was not an independent marker of sudden cardiac death.[58] This chapter may however be subject to a subtle statistical failure. An earlier myocardial infarction is a well-known independent marker for sudden cardiac death.

Myocardial Failure

The two main causes of death in patients with cardiac insufficiency have been recognized as malignant ventricular arrhythmias or pump failure. In New York Heart Association functional Class II, the proportion of patients who die of ventricular fibrillation is high. In Class IV many die simply of pump failure.[59] It was recently shown that patients with cardiac insufficiency suffering an arrhythmic death present initially with a ventricular tachycardia that may be monomorphic or polymorphic. Thereafter, the arrhythmia disintegrates into ventricular fibrillation. The transition from ventricular tachycardia to ventricular fibrillation is probably dependent on dispersion of refractoriness similar to ventricular fibrillation.[60]

In patients with chronic heart failure, changes in action potentials and local conduction may occur. Action potentials have been shown to be shortened if they are subject to stretch.[61] It is well known from animal studies that stretch and hypertrophy increase dispersion of refractoriness and thus create a substrate for ventricular fibrillation. In patients with cardiac insufficiency stretch can be observed as an increase in left ventricular end-diastolic dimension by echocardiography or simply as an increase in cardiac size on an x-ray. Both variables have been shown to be independent predictors of sudden cardiac death in patients with cardiac insufficiency.[62]

It has been known for a long time that changes in potassium levels have a profound effect on cardiac electrophysiology and also on the risk of sudden cardiac death. Hypopotassemia is an independent predictor for sudden cardiac death in these patients.[62] Hypopotassemia prolongs rate-corrected QT and changes the T waves, and polymorphic ventricular tachycardias are easily initiated. Hypopotassemia causes an uneven prolongation of action potential duration by influencing different potassium channels in addition to its effect on the membrane potentials.

In patients with cardiac insufficiency increased QT dispersion correlates with decreased magnesium and may therefore represent a significant risk factor.[63]

Increased QT dispersion has been found in many patients waiting for a cardiac transplantation. A very high mortality was found in patients with QT dispersion above 140 ms.[64] All of these data indicate that therapy in patients with cardiac insufficiency should be aimed at reduction of left ventricular stretch and correction of electrolytes, preferably by spirono-lactone.[65]

Right Ventricular Overload

Dispersion of repolarization is probably increased in tetralogy of Fallot and may be due to disturbances in conduction locally and also due to changes in action potentials in the right ventricle subject to stretch. In tetralogy of Fallot both increased QRS time and increased dispersion of QT intervals have predictive value for occurrence of ventricular tachycardia.[66]

Right Ventricular Degeneration, Necrosis, and Apoptosis

Right ventricular arrhythmogenic dysplasia is of considerable interest because in this setting a general apoptosis is probably taking place in the right ventricle. Many signs of increased dispersion of refractoriness have been found in these patients.[67] The patients have positive late potentials and increased QRS time, indicating disturbed conduction of electrical impulses giving rise to unsynchronized depolarization with secondary increased dispersion of refractoriness. However, the action potentials may be affected by the conduction in such a way that a synchronizing of the repolarization may occur. While this occurs in the normal heart,[68] it is uncertain if it occurs in diseased hearts. The increased duration of QRS time has been shown to be correlated to increased fibrosis.[69] The negative T waves in the precordial leads also indicate increased dispersion of refractoriness, as described earlier. In patients with right ventricular hy-perplasia and malignant ventricular arrhythmias a significantly higher QT dispersion has been found in comparison with controls.[70]

Congenital Defects of Ionic Channels

Recent research has shown many genotypes in the long QT syndrome that have different effects on ionic channels.[71] This is described in another chapter of this book. These channels are also affected by many different drugs such as some antiarrhythmic drugs, antibiotics, psykopharmaca, and an antiemetic drug. All of these drugs may provoke ventricular fibrillation under certain circumstances. In patients with a genetically uniform type of LQT1, QT dispersion was significantly higher in symp-tomatic patients compared with unaffected relatives, but not in asymp-tomatic patients.[72] Epinephrine but not norepinephrine increases QT dis-persion in these patients, suggesting that β-adrenergic stimulation may increase dispersion of refractoriness in patients with the long QT syn-drome, while α-adrenergic stimulation is less important for arrhythmic vulnerability.[13,73] The Brugada syndrome also belongs to this category and is now under intense investigation.

Acknowledgment After some years with basic electrophysiological studies in Oslo I met Borys Surawicz, who led me into this important part of electrophysiology more than 20 years ago. I want to express my thanks to him and also to CS Kuo who, together with us, performed the technically almost impossible dog experiments during the early 1980s in Lexington, Kentucky. Furthermore, I will thank Knut Endresen who, together with me, did the basic electrophysiological studies in patients with coronary artery disease in Oslo, confirming that the same electrophysiological mechanisms are probably present in patients with coronary artery disease.

References

1. Hwang C, Hrayr S, Karagueuzian S, et al. Re-entrant wavefronts in human ventricular tissue. *J Cardiovasc Electrophysiol* 1999;10:419.
2. Bigger JT Jr, Rolnitzky LM, Steinman RC, Fleiss JL. Predicting mortality after myocardial infarction from the response of RR variability to antiarrhythmic drug therapy. *J Am Coll Cardiol* 1994;23:733-740.
3. Pratt CM, Camm AJ, Cooper W, et al. Mortality in the Survival With Oral D-sotalol (SWORD) trial: Why did patients die? *Am J Cardiol* 1998;81:869-876.
4. The Norwegian Multicenter Study Group. Timolol induced reduction in mortality and reinfarction in patients surviving myocardial infarction. *N Engl J Med* 1981;304:801-809.
5. Amlie JP. QT dispersion and sudden cardiac death. *Eur Heart J* 1996;18:189-190.
6. Endresen K, Amlie JP. Electrical restitution and conduction intervals of ventricular premature beats in man: Influence of heart rate. *PACE* 1989;12:1347-1354.
7. Han J, Moe GK. Non-uniform recovery of excitability in ventricular muscle. *Circ Res* 1964;14:44-60.
8. Antzelevitch C, Shimuzu W, Yan GX, Sicouri S. Cellular basis for QT dispersion. *Electrocardiography* 1998;30(suppl):168-175.
9. Jervell A. The surdo-cardiac syndrome. *Eur Heart J* 1985;6(suppl D):97-102.
10. Kuo CS, Amlie JP, Munakata K, et al. Basic and premature dispersion of repolarization on ventricular surface in dog heart. *Cardiovasc Res* 1983;17:152-161.
11. Amlie JP, Kuo CS, Munakata K, et al. Effect of uniformly prolonged, and increased basic dispersion of repolarization on premature dispersion on ventricular surface in dogs: Role of action potential duration and activation time differences. *Eur Heart J* 1985;6(suppl D):15-30.
12. Kuo CS, Munakata K, Reddy PS, Surawicz B. Characteristics and possible mechanisms of ventricular arrhythmias dependent on dispersion of action potential durations. *Circulation* 1983;67:1356-1367.
13. Priori SG, Napolitano C, Diehl L, Schwartz PJ. Dispersion of the QT interval: A marker of therapeutic efficacy in the idiopathic long QT syndrome. *Circulation* 1994;89:1681-1689.
14. Yuan S, Blomstrøm-Lundqvist C, Pripp CM, et al. Signed value of monophasic action potential duration difference. A useful measure in evaluation of repolarization in patients with ventricular arrhythmias. *Eur Heart J* 1997;18:1329-1338.
15. Endresen K, Amlie JP. Acute effects of lidocaine on repolarization and conduction in patients with coronary artery disease. *Clin Pharmacol Ther* 1989;45:387-395.
16. Bjørnstad H, Tande PM, Lathrop DA, Refsum H. Effects of temperature on cycle length dependent changes and restitution of action potential duration in guinea pig ventricular muscle. *Cardiovasc Res* 1993;27: 946-950.

17. Endresen K. Rate dependent change in dispersion of repolarisation during ventricular pacing in man. *Int J Cardiol* 1989;23:199-206.
18. Day CP, McComb JM, Campbell RWF. QT dispersion: An indication of arrhythmia risk in patients with long QT intervals. *Br Heart J* 1990;63:342-344.
19. Hii JTY, Wyse GD, Gillis AM, et al. Precordial QT interval dispersion as a marker of torsade de pointes. *Circulation* 1992;86:1376-1382.
20. Zabel M, Lichtlen PR, Haverich A, Franz MR. Comparison of ECG variables of dispersion of ventricular repolarisation with direct myocardial repolarization measurements in the human heart. *J Cardiovasc Electrophysiol* 1998;9:1279-1284.
21. Janse MJ, Capucci A, Coronel R, Fabius MAW. Variability of recovery of excitability in the normal and ischaemic porcine heart. *Eur Heart J* 1985;6(suppl D):41-52.
22. Kralios FA, Martun L, Burgess MJ, Miller K. Local ventricular repolarization changes due to sympathetic nerve branch stimulation. *Am J Physiol* 1975;228:1621-1626.
23. Calkins H, Allman K, Bolling S, et al. Correlation between scintigraphic evidence of regional dysfunction and ventricular refractoriness in the human heart. *Circulation* 1993;88:172-179.
24. Amlie JP, Refsum H, Landmark K. Prolonged ventricular refractoriness and action potential duration after beta-adrenergic blockade in the dog heart in situ. *J Cardiovasc Pharmacol* 1982;4:157-162.
25. Amlie JP, Refsum H. Vagus-induced changes in ventricular electrophysiology of the dog heart with and without β-blockade. *J Cardiovasc Pharmacol* 1981;3:1203-1210.
26. Amlie JP. The modifying effect of autonomic blockade on digitoxin-induced changes in monophasic action potential and refractoriness of the right ventricle of the dog heart. *Acta Pharmacol Toxicol* 1980;47:112-118.
27. MERIT-HF Study Group. Effect of metoprolol CR/XL in chronic heart failure. Metoprolol CR/XL Randomised Intervention Trial in Heart Failure(MERIT-HF). *Lancet* 1999;353:2001-2007.
28. Iaccarino G, Tomhave ED, Lefkowitz RJ, Koch WJ. Reciprocal in vivo regulation of myocardial G protein-coupled expression by beta-adrenergic receptor stimulation and blockade. *Circulation* 1998;98:1783-1789.
29. Edvardsson N, Olsson SB. Effects of acute and chronic beta-receptor blockade on ventricular repolarisation in man. *Br Heart J* 1981;45:628-636.
30. Andersen HR, Nielsen JC, Thomsen PE, et al. Long term follow-up of patients from a randomised trial of atrial versus ventricular pacing for sick sinus syndrome. *Lancet* 1997;350:1210-1216.
31. Endresen K, Forfang K. Acute effects of smoking one cigarette on monophasic action potentials and intraventricular conduction in coronary artery disease. *Am J Cardiol* 1989;63:1522-1526.
32. Bryant SM, Shipsey SJ, Hart G. Regional differences in electrical and mechanical properties of myocytes from guinea pig hearts with mild hypertrophy. *Cardiovasc Res* 1997;35:315-323.
33. Shipsey SJ, Bryant SM, Hart G. Effect of hypertrophy on regional action potential characteristics in the rat left ventricle: A cellular basis for T-wave inversion. *Circulation* 1997;96:2061-2068.
34. Bailly P, Benitah JP, Mouchoniere M, et al. Regional alteration of the transient outward current in human left ventricular septum during compensated hypertrophy. *Circulation* 1997;96:1266-1274.

35. Kannel WB, Gordon T, Offutt D. Left ventricular hypertrophy by electrogram: Prevalence, incidence and mortality in the Framingham Study. *Ann Intern Med* 1969;71:89-105.
36. Solokow M, Perloff D. The prognosis of essential hypertension treated conservatively. *Circulation* 1961;23:697-713.
37. Kreger BE, Cupples LA, Kannel WB. The electrocardiogram in prediction of sudden death. Framingham Study experience. *Am Heart J* 1987;113:377-382.
38. Perkiömäki JS, Ikaheimo MJ, Pikkujamsa SM, et al. Dispersion of the QT interval and autonomic modulation of heart rate in hypertensive men with and without left ventricular hypertrophy. *Hypertension* 1996;28:16-21.
39. Tomiyama H, Doba N, Fu Y, et al. Left ventricular geometric patterns and QT dispersion in borderline and mild hypertension: Their evolution and regression. *Am J Hypertens* 1998;11:286-292.
40. Galinier M, Bakanescu S, Fourcade J, et al. Prognostic value of ventricular arrhythmias in systemic hypertension. *J Hypertens* 1997;15:1779-1783.
41. Prible SD, Dunn FG, Tweddel AC. Symptomatic and silent myocardial ischaemia in hypertensive patients with left ventricular hypertrophy. *Br Heart J* 1992;67:377-382.
42. Dunn FG, McKenachan J, Isles CG, et al. Left ventricular hypertrophy and mortality in hypertension: An analysis from data from the Glasgow Blood Pressure Clinic. *J Hypertens* 1990;8:775-782.
43. Ylitalo A, Airaksinen KE, Selin L, Huikuri HV. Effects of combination antihypertensive therapy on baroreflex sensitivity and heart rate variability in systemic hypertension. *Am J Cardiol* 1999;83:885-889.
44. Hansson L, Lindholm LH, Ekbom T, et al, for the STOP-Hypertension 2-Study Group. Randomised trial of old and new antihypertensive drugs in elderly patients: Cardiovascular mortality and morbidity the Swedish Trial in Old Patients with Hypertension-2 Study. *Lancet* 1999;354:1751-1756.
45. Wagner HR, Ellison RC, Keane JF, et al. Clinical course in aortic stenosis. *Circulation* 1997;56(2 suppl I):147-156.
46. Ducceschi V, Sarubbi B, D{{quotesingle}}Andrea A, et al. Increased QT dispersion and other repolarization abnormalities as a possible cause of electrical instability in isolated aortic stenosis. *Int J Cardiol* 1998;64:57-62.
47. Sporton SC, Taggart P, Sutton PM, et al. Acute ischaemia: A dynamic influence on QT dispersion. *Lancet* 1997;349:306-309.
48. Naka M, Shiotani I, Koretsune Y, et al. Occurrence of sustained increase in QT dispersion following exercise in patients with residual myocardial ischemia after healing of anterior myocardial infarction. *Am J Cardiol* 1997;80:1528-1531.
49. Roukema G, Singh JP, Meijs M, et al. Effect of exercise-induced ischemia on QT dispersion. *Am Heart J* 1998;135:88-92.
50. Mantari M, Oikarinen L, Manninen V, Viitasalo M. QT dispersion as a risk factor for sudden cardiac death and fatal myocardial infarction in a coronary risk population. *Heart* 1997;78:268-272.
51. Stoletniy LN, Pai RG. Value of QT dispersion in the interpretation of exercise stress test in women. *Circulation* 1997;96:904-910.
52. Suzuki M, Nishizaki M, Arita M, et al. Increased QT dispersion in patients with vasospastic angina. *Circulation* 1998;98:435-440.
53. Abdelnoor M, Nitter-Hauge S, Risum Ø, et al. Duration of preoperative electrocardiographic QRS complex and the incidence of heart arrest after aorto coronary by-pass surgery. *Scand Cardiovasc J* 2000;34:186-191.

54. Schneider CA, Voth E, Baer FM, et al. QT dispersion is determined by the extent of viable myocardium in patients with chronic Q-wave myocardial infarction. *Circulation* 1997;96:3913-3920.
55. Karagounis LA, Abderson JL, Moreno FL, Sorensen SG. Multivariate associates of QT dispersion in patients with acute myocardial infarction: Primary of patency status of the infarct-related artery. TEAM-3 Investigators. Third trial of thrombolysis with eminase in acute myocardial infarction. *Am Heart J* 1998;135:1027-1035.
56. Perkiömäki JS, Huikuri HV, Koistinen JM, et al. Heart rate variability and dispersion of QT interval in patients with vulnerability to ventricular tachycardia and ventricular fibrillation after previous myocardial infarction. *J Am Coll Cardiol* 1997;30:1331-1338.
57. Oikarinen L, Viitasalo M, Toivonen L. Dispersion of the QT interval in post-myocardial infarction patients presenting with ventricular tachycardia or ventricular fibrillation. *Am J Cardiol* 1998;81:694-697.
58. Zabel M, Klingenheben T, Franz MR, Hohnloser S. Assessment of QT dispersion for prediction of mortality or arrhythmic events after myocardial infarction: Results of a prospective, long-term follow-up study. *Circulation* 1998;97:2543-2550.
59. Uretsky BF, Sheahan RG. Primary prevention of sudden cardiac death in heart failure: Will the solution be shocking? *J Am Coll Cardiol* 1997;30:1589-1597.
60. Misier AR, Opthof T, Van Hemel NM, et al. Dispersion of "refractoriness" in noninfarcted myocardium of patients with ventricular tachycardia or ventricular fibrillation after myocardial infarction. *Circulation* 1995;91:2566-2572.
61. Riemer TL, Sobie EA, Tung L. Stretch induced changes in arrhythmogenesis and excitability in experimental based heart models. *Am J Physiol* 1998;275(2 Pt. 2):H431-H442.
62. Brooksby P, Batin PD, Nolan J, et al. The relation between QT intervals and mortality in ambulant patients with chronic heart failure: The United Kingdom failure evaluation and assessment of risk trial (UK-Heart). *Eur Heart J* 1999;20:1335-1341.
63. Haigney MC, Berger R, Schulman S, et al. Tissue magnesium and the arrhythmic substrate in humans. *J Cardiovasc Electrophysiol* 1997;8:980-986.
64. Pinsky DJ, Sciacca RR, Steinberg JS. QT dispersion as a marker of risk in patients awaiting heart transplantation. *J Am Coll Cardiol* 1997;29:1576-1584.
65. Pitt B, Zannad F, Remme WJ, et al. The effect of spironolactone on morbidity and mortality in patients with severe heart failure. *N Engl J Med* 1999;341:709-717.
66. Gatzoulis MA, Till JA, Redington AN. Depolarization-repolarization inhomogeneity after repair of tetralogy of Fallot. The substrate for malignant ventricular tachycardia. *Circulation* 1997;95:401-406.
67. Amlie JP. Increased dispersion of repolarization in patients with arrhythmogenic right ventricular hyperplasia—a major electrophysiological factor responsible for malignant ventricular arrhythmias. *Eur Heart J* 1999;20:703-705.
68. Gepstein L, Hayam G, Ben-Haim SA. A novel method for nonfluoroscopic, catheter, electromechanical mapping of the heart: In vitro and in vivo accuracy results. *Circulation* 1997;95:1611-1622.
69. Kazmierczak J, De Sutter J, Tavernier R, et al. Electrocardiographic and monomorphic features in patients with ventricular tachycardia of right ventricular origin. *Heart* 1998;79:388-393.

70. Benn M, Steen Hansen P, Pedersen AK. QT dispersion in patients with ARVD. *Eur Heart J* 1999;20:764-770.
71. Lubinski A, Lewicka-Nowak E, Kempa M, et al. New insights into repolarization abnormalities in long QT syndrome: The increased transmural dispersion of repolarization. *PACE* 1998;21:172-175.
72. Swan H, Saarinen K, Kontula K, et al. Evaluation of QT interval duration and dispersion and proposed clinical criteria in diagnosis of long QT syndrome in patients with a genetically uniform type of LQT1. *J Am Coll Cardiol* 1998;32:486-491.
73. Sun ZH, Swan H, Viitasalo M, Toivonen L. Effects of epinephrine on QT interval dispersion in congenital long QT syndrome. *J Am Coll Cardiol* 1998;31:1400-1405.

10

Dispersion of "Refractoriness" and Ventricular Tachycardia or Fibrillation After Myocardial Infarction

Michiel J. Janse

Introduction: How to Measure Dispersion of Refractoriness

It has long been recognized that differences in refractory periods in adjacent areas in the ventricles could be responsible for the occurrence of reentrant arrhythmias, especially fibrillation.[1-3] The study by Han and Moe[3] was the first in which refractory periods were measured at multiple sites, and these authors expressed the notion that a series of premature beats could be arrhythmogenic because it would increase the temporal dispersion in refractoriness: "It is likely that the degree of non-uniformity of recovery of excitability should become greater and greater after each successive train of repetitive premature beats. Because of the danger of ventricular fibrillation, direct demonstration of this was not attempted."[3] At the time of this study, it was thought that the refractory period was determined only by the length of the immediately preceding cycle.[4] Later it became clear that the heart has a long "memory" and that changes in refractory period brought about by transient changes in rate or rhythm persist for many beats.[5-7] For this reason the determination of refractory periods at multiple sites is a lengthy procedure. In our experiments,[5,6] premature test pulses were applied during a regularly paced rhythm only after every eighth beat, so that the effect of a premature impulse elicited

From Olsson SB, Amlie JP, Yuan S (eds): *Dispersion of Ventricular Repolarization: State of the Art.* ©Futura Publishing Company, Inc., Armonk, NY, 2000.

by a test pulse would have disappeared when the next test pulse was applied.

In our experiments, the determination of refractory periods at 12 sites lasted between 30 and 40 minutes (to ensure that the heart was in a stable condition, refractory periods at the same site were often determined twice at varying times). In the experiments of Han and Moe,[3] approximately 5 minutes were needed to determine refractory periods at 12 sites, and the possibility exists that test pulses were given too quickly in succession.

I emphasize this point because it may explain the differences in results between their study and ours, in which no differences in dispersion were found after one or more premature beats. Figure 1 shows the results of an experiment in an open chest dog, in which refractory periods were determined at 12 intramural sites in the left ventricle during a regularly paced rhythm with a basic cycle length of 600 ms, and after one, two, three, and four consecutive premature beats, each preceded by the shortest possible interval. No significant differences in the standard deviations of the refractory periods were found between the refractory periods of a

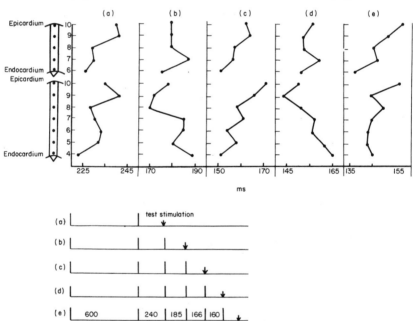

Figure 1. Refractory periods at 12 different intramural sites of the normal canine left ventricle during steady state conditions (regular driving at a cycle length of 600 ms: **(a)**, and after one **(b)**, two **(c)**, three **(d)**, and four **(e)** premature beats. Note alternation in the pattern of distribution of refractory periods throughout the ventricular wall in the subsequent premature beats. Diagram shows the stimulation pattern (numbers are in milliseconds). Reproduced from Reference 6, with permission.

regular rhythm and those following one or multiple premature beats. However, since the refractory period is shortened considerably by the induced premature beats, the range of variation in refractory period is relatively larger after a series of premature impulses.

Figure 2 shows refractory periods at 12 intramural sites during a regular rhythm and after a long pause, following a series of premature impulses. This experiment was performed to mimic the short-long-short interval that so often precedes torsade de pointes, and which is thought to be arrhythmogenic because of an increase in dispersion of refractoriness. Again, no differences in the range of variation in refractory period could be detected. The dispersion in refractoriness is relatively smaller after the long pause because the average refractory period has lengthened. Apparently, in the normal dog heart changes in rhythm do not result in an increased dispersion of ventricular refractoriness.

Another feature worth mentioning is that there is no indication that the refractory period in midmural layers is longer than in subendocardial

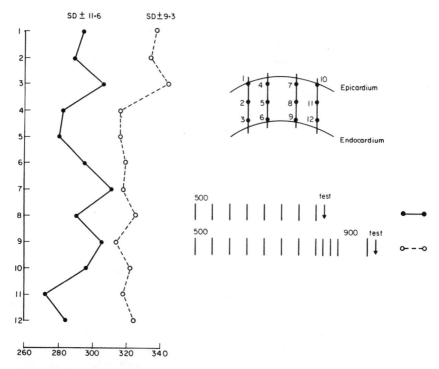

Figure 2. Refractory periods at 12 intramural sites during a regularly driven rhythm (basic cycle length 500 ms, solid dots, solid lines) and after a long pause following a series of three premature beats (open circles, dotted lines). Standard deviations indicate dispersion in refractoriness. Diagrams show the intramural electrode terminals and the stimulation pattern. Reproduced from Reference 19, with permission.

or subepicardial layers. This is in contrast to the findings of Sicouri and Antzelevitch,[8] who found a subpopulation of midmural cells, the so-called M cells, in which action potential duration was much longer than that of subendocardial or subepicardial cells, especially at very long cycle lengths. A possible explanation for this discrepancy could be that in the intact ventricular wall, where the cells are very well coupled to each other via low-resistance gap junctions, intrinsic differences in action potential duration are attenuated because of electrotonic current flow. This would shorten the action potentials of M cells and prolong those of subendocardial and subepicardial cells.

From the above it is clear that an accurate determination of dispersion in refractoriness is a time consuming procedure and requires that the heart remains in a perfectly stable condition during this procedure. To determine dispersion in refractoriness in situations where conditions change over brief periods of time (e.g., during acute ischemia or during brief periods of sympathetic nervous stimulation) or when time for measurements is limited (e.g., open heart surgery in patients), alternative methods must be used. One such method is the determination of the so-called fibrillation interval. The averaged interval between local activations during fibrillation correlates well with local refractoriness in atrium and ventricle[9-12] and may therefore be used as an index of local refractoriness. For that reason, we sought to determine dispersion in "refractoriness" in patients with a myocardial infarction and ventricular tachycardia or fibrillation who underwent antiarrhythmia surgery.[13]

Intraoperative Determination of Fibrillation Intervals in Patients with Ventricular Tachycardia or Fibrillation

A small subset of patients who survive the acute phase of myocardial infarction develop in subsequent months or years sustained monomorphic ventricular tachycardias which sometimes degenerate into ventricular fibrillation. The anatomical substrate for the reentrant tachycardias is formed by the network of surviving myocardial fibers within the infarct. These small bundles are separated from each other by septae of fibrous tissue, and the impulse often follows a tortuous route via "zig-zag" conduction.[14-16] The arrhythmia is in essence caused by anatomical reentry. It is likely that the electrophysiological properties of the noninfarcted part of the left ventricle determine whether or not the tachycardia will degenerate into fibrillation. We hypothesized that dispersion in refractoriness might be greater in patients in whom fibrillation occurred compared with patients with stable tachycardia. We therefore determined the ventricular fibrillation interval in a group of patients who underwent antiarrhythmia surgery for symptomatic, drug-refractory, postinfarction ventricular tachycardia. Group 1 consisted of seven patients with hemodynamically tolerable sustained monomorphic tachycardia, group 2 of seven patients with cardiac arrest and documented ventricular fibrillation. A multiterminal grid electrode, with an interelectrode distance of 7 mm, was used to simultaneously record unipolar epicardial electrograms from up to 64 sites from the noninfarcted left ventricle. During cardiopulmonary bypass at normothermia, ventricular fibrillation was induced by multiple premature stimulation of the ventricles, and recordings were made during 4 seconds and stored on disk. An interactive computer program allowed determination of local activation times, defined as a negative deflection with a steepness of at least 0.5 V/s over an 8-ms period. Subsequently, histograms of the intervals between local activation were made. The ventricular fibrillation interval was defined as the mean of the first (or only) peak in the histogram (see Fig. 3).

Table 1 summarizes the results. In the ventricular tachycardia group, reliable recordings were made from 195 sites, in the ventricular fibrillation group from 207 sites. The average ventricular fibrillation intervals were not significantly different between the two groups, but various indices for spatial dispersion in "refractoriness" were. The coefficient of variation (standard deviation times 100, divided by the mean) was 1.55±0.40 in the ventricular tachycardia group, and was approximately two and a half times greater, at 3.63±0.56, in the ventricular fibrillation group. The same was true for the mean difference between the longest and shortest interval and for the largest difference between adjacent recording sites (statistical significance was determined by applying the Wilcoxon test).

Figure 4 shows the spatial distribution of ventricular fibrillation intervals in one patient from the ventricular tachycardia group and one from the fibrillation group. Although these data indicate that dispersion in "refractoriness" is significantly larger in patients who develop ventricular fibrillation than in patients in whom the tachycardia remains stable, the question arises whether the observed dispersion is large enough to explain the transition of anatomical reentry (tachycardia) into functional multiple wavelet reentry (fibrillation). Previous studies[10] in which a correlation was made between the ventricular fibrillation interval and the refractory period determined by the extrastimulus technique during a regularly paced rhythm with a cycle length of 300 ms showed that one must multiply the dispersion in fibrillation intervals by a factor three to arrive at the corresponding dispersion in refractoriness during a regular rhythm. When we apply this to the present data, the mean difference between longest and shortest refractory period would be approximately 50 ms in the fibrillation group, and the largest difference between adjacent electrodes about 30 ms.

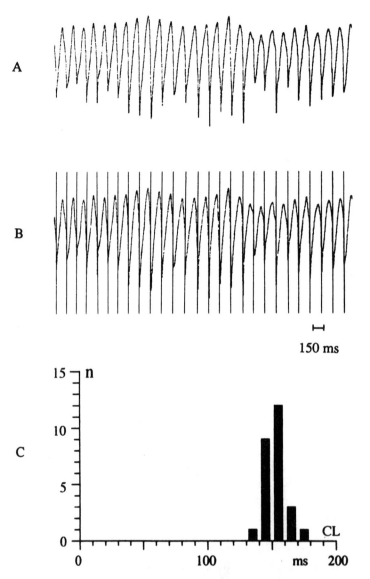

Figure 3. A. Local electrogram during a 4-s period of ventricular fibrillation in one patient from the ventricular tachycardia group. **B.** Same signal as in **A** with the activation moments superimposed. These were determined by an interactive computer program. **C.** Histogram of the intervals indicated in **B**. The mean of the peak of the histogram was 151.7±1.63 (SEM) ms and it was considered as the ventricular fibrillation interval of this particular site. This procedure was followed at all 32 or 64 sites in each heart. Only ventricular fibrillation intervals with SEM values less than 2.5 ms were accepted. Reproduced from Reference 13, with permission.

Table 1
Recording Sites and VF Intervals in Patients from VT and VF Groups

	VT	VF	P Value
Patients (n)	7	7	—
Recording sites (n)	195	207	—
VF interval (ms)	136±5.50	129±3.40	ns
Coefficient of variation	1.55±0.40	3.63±0.56	<0.01
Mean difference longest and shortest interval (ms)	8.9±2.27	17.4±2.66	<0.02
Largest difference between adjacent electrodes (ms)	5.9±1.74	10.3±2.20	<0.05

Values are means ±1 SEM. VF = ventricular fibrillation; VT = ventricular tachycardia.

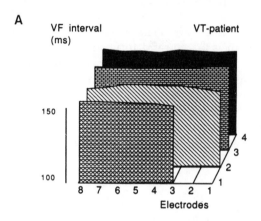

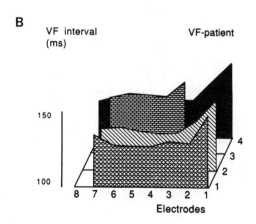

Figure 4. A. Ventricular fibrillation (VF) intervals at 30 sites in one patient from the ventricular tachycardia group (VT-patient). Interelectrode distance was 7 mm. Measurements were restricted to the noninfarcted myocardium. The mean ventricular fibrillation interval at all sites was 155.3 ms. The standard deviation was 1.37 ms and the coefficient of variation amounted to 0.88. **B.** Ventricular fibrillation intervals at 27 sites in one patient from the ventricular fibrillation group (VF-patient). The mean ventricular fibrillation interval at all sites was 131.9 ms. The standard deviation was 8.34 ms and the coefficient of variation amounted to 6.33. Reproduced from Reference 13, with permission.

Usually a reentrant arrhythmia is initiated by a premature impulse that causes unidirectional block. Unidirectional block is a prerequisite for reentry, leaving a return pathway through which the impulse conducts to reexcite previously excited areas. In rabbit atrial tissue, Allessie et al[17] found that the minimal difference in refractory period needed to cause unidirectional block of an appropriately timed stimulated premature impulse was between 11 and 16 ms, well within the physiological range of variation of refractory period durations. The regions of long and short refractory periods must be close to one another for block to occur. In addition, the area with long refractory periods must be large so that the impulse traveling around the area of unidirectional block will be sufficiently delayed to reexcite the previously activated areas.

In the normal canine ventricle, the dispersion in refractory periods is in the order of 20 ms, and this is not sufficient to cause unidirectional block and reentry.[6] When dispersion of refractoriness is increased by local cooling of the ventricles, and a critical difference between shortest and longest refractory period ranging from 95 to 145 ms is reached, premature stimuli delivered at the site with the shortest refractory period can induce repetitive activity in the canine left ventricle, presumably because of unidirectional block and reentry.[18] This critical dispersion was found at regular pacing cycle lengths varying from 450 to 580 ms.

It is possible, but as yet unproven, that at more rapid rates, such as during monomorphic ventricular tachycardia, the critical dispersion in refractory periods needed to cause multiple wavelet reentry and fibrillation might be less.

References

1. Mines GR. On dynamic equilibrium in the heart. *J Physiol* 1913;46:349-383.
2. Mines GR. On circulation excitations in heart muscles and their possible relation to tachycardia and fibrillation. *Trans R Soc Can* 1914;section IV:43-53.
3. Han J, Moe GK. Nonuniform recovery of excitability of ventricular muscle. *Circ Res* 1964;14:44-60.
4. Mendez C, Gruhzit CC, Moe GK. Influence of cycle length upon refractory period of auricles, ventricles and A-V node in the dog. *Am J Physiol* 1956;184:287-295.
5. Janse MJ, Van der Steen ABM, Van Dam RTH, Durrer D. Refractory period of the dog's ventricular myocardium following sudden changes in frequency. *Circ Res* 1969;24:251-261.
6. Janse MJ. *The Effect of Changes in Heart Rate on the Refractory Period of the Heart.* PhD thesis; University of Amsterdam. Amsterdam, Mondeel Offset Drukkerij; 1971.
7. Han J, Moe GK. Cumulative effects of cycle length on refractory period of cardiac tissues. *Am J Physiol* 1969;217:106-112.
8. Sicouri S, Antzelevitch C. Subpopulation of cells with unique electrophysiological properties in the deep subepicardium of the canine ventricle. The M cell. *Circ Res* 1991;68:1729-1741.

9. Lammers WJEP, Allessie MA, Rensma PL, et al. The use of fibrillation cycle length to determine spatial dispersion in electrophysiological properties used to characterize the underlying mechanism of fibrillation. *New Trends Arrhyth* 1986;2:109-112.

10. Opthof T, Ramdat Misier AR, Coronel R, et al. Dispersion of refractoriness in canine ventricular myocardium. Effects of sympathetic stimulation. *Circ Res* 1991;68:1204-1215.

11. Opthof T, Coronel R, Vermeulen JT, et al. Dispersion in refractoriness in normal and ischaemic canine ventricle: Effects of sympathetic stimulation. *Cardiovasc Res* 1993;27:1954-1960.

12. Ramdat Misier AR, Opthof T, Van Hemel NM, et al. Increased dispersion of "refractoriness" in patients with idiopathic paroxysmal atrial fibrillation. *J Am Coll Cardiol* 1992;19:1531-1535.

13. Ramdat Misier AR, Opthof T, Van Hemel NM, et al. Dispersion of 'refractoriness' in noninfarcted myocardium of patients with ventricular tachycardia or ventricular fibrillation after myocardial infarction. *Circulation* 1995;91:2566-2572.

14. De Bakker JMT, Van Capelle FJL, Janse MJ, et al. Reentry as a cause of ventricular tachycardia in patients with chronic ischemic heart disease: Electrophysiologic and anatomic correlation. *Circulation* 1988;77:598-606.

15. De Bakker JMT, Coronel R, Tasseron S, et al. Ventricular tachycardia in the infarcted, Langendorff-perfused human heart: Role of the arrangement of surviving cardiac fibers. *J Am Coll Cardiol* 1990;15:1594-1607.

16. De Bakker JMT, Van Capelle FJL, Janse MJ, et al. Slow conduction in the infarcted human heart. "Zigzag" course of activation. *Circulation* 1993; 88:915-926.

17. Allessie MA, Bonke FIM, Schopman FJG. Circus movement in rabbit atrial muscle as a mechanism of tachycardia. II. The role of nonuniform recovery of excitability in the occurrence of unidirectional block, as studied with multiple microelectrodes. *Circ Res* 1976;39:168-177.

18. Kuo C-S, Munakato K, Reddy CP, Surawicz B. Characteristics and possible mechanism of ventricular arrhythmia dependent on the dispersion of action potential duration. *Circulation* 1983;67:1356-1367.

19. Janse MJ, Capucci A, Coronel R, et al. Variability of recovery of excitability in the normal canine and the ischaemic porcine heart. *Eur Heart J* 1985;6(suppl D):41-52.

11

The Electrophysiological Mechanism of Torsade de Pointes in the Long QT Syndrome

Nabil El-Sherif, Gioia Turitto,
Dmitry O. Kozhevnikov, and Mark Restivo

Introduction

Both the congenital and acquired long QT syndromes (LQTS) are due to abnormalities (intrinsic, acquired, or both) of the ionic currents underlying repolarization. Prolongation of the repolarization phase acts as a primary step for the generation of early afterdepolarizations (EADs).[1] EAD-induced triggered beats arise predominantly from the Purkinje network.[1] In the LQTS, prolonged repolarization is associated with increased spatial dispersion of repolarization.[2,3] The focal EAD-induced triggered beat(s) can infringe on the underlying substrate of inhomogeneous repolarization to initiate polymorphic reentrant ventricular tachycardia (VT).[3] Torsade de pointes (TdP) is an ear-pleasing term that describes an eye-catching form of polymorphic VT. The term was first coined by Dessertenne,[4] who described its electrocardiographic (ECG) pattern of continuously changing morphology of the QRS complexes that seem to twist around an imaginary baseline. The quasi-musical term and the intriguing ECG pattern have caught the attention of electrophysiologists for years and have been, to some extent, a driving force behind the recent focused interest in the role of genetics and cardiac ion channel pathophysiology in cardiac arrhythmias in general.[5] More importantly, it is helping to

Supported in part by Veterans Administration Medical Research Funds.
From Olsson SB, Amlie JP, Yuan S (eds): *Dispersion of Ventricular Repolarization: State of the Art.* ©Futura Publishing Company, Inc., Armonk, NY, 2000.

refocus attention on the role of dispersion of ventricular repolarization in the genesis of malignant ventricular tachyarrhythmias.

There is more than one electrophysiological mechanism for polymorphic VT, and an understanding of these mechanisms can be of valuable help in the proper treatment of individual patients. The most appropriate way to classify polymorphic VT is based on whether it is associated with normal or prolonged QT (or QTU) segment. The electrophysiological mechanisms of these two types of polymorphic VT may be different. The term TdP should be reserved for use with LQTS. However, not all patients with LQTS have polymorphic VT with a characteristic TdP configuration,[6] and this classic configuration can be seen in some cases without a prolonged QT interval.[7]

Ionic Basis of LQTS

Multiple ion currents contribute to the repolarization phase of the action potential (AP).[8] Under normal physiological conditions, inward currents during phase 2 could be carried by Na through a Na "window" current or a slowly inactivating Na current, by Ca through the Ca channel and a Ca "window" current, and by the electrogenic Na/Ca exchange. Outward currents include a number of K currents, of which the two delayed rectifiers I_{kr} and I_{ks} are the two most commonly involved (i.e., depressed) when Class III pharmacological agents result in a prolonged repolarization. Other outward currents are generated by the inward rectifier (I_{k1}), the transient outward current (I_{to}), and by the Na-K pump (I_p). The importance of the I_{to} varies with cardiac tissue and species. The role of nonspecific cation channels that may appear in response to increased intracellular Ca is not clear.

The congenital LQTS is caused by mutations of at least six genes (Table 1).[9] Four disease genes have been identified and a number of mutations have been described for each gene. KVLQT1,[10] MinK,[11,12] and HERG[13] encode for K channels. SCN5A[14] encodes for the cardiac Na chan-

Table 1
Currently Recognized LQTS Disease Genes

Disease	Gene	Chromosome	Ion channel
LQT1	KVLQT1*	11p15.5	I_{KS}subunit
LQT2	HERG	7q35–36	I_{Kr}
LQT3	SCN5A	3p21–24	Na
LQT4	Unknown	4q25–27	Unknown
LQT5	MinK	21	I_{KS}subunit

*Homozygous carriers of novel mutations of KVLQT1 have Jervell and Lange-Nielsen syndrome. KVLQT1 and MinK coassemble to form the I_{KS} channel. LQT = long QT; LQTS = long QT syndrome.

nel. *KVLQT1* and *MinK* coassemble to form the I_{ks} (the slowly activating delayed rectifier K channel).[11,12] *HERG* forms the I_{kr} (the rapidly activating delayed rectifier K channel).[15] A fifth gene locus at chromosome 4q 25-27 has been found in one family,[16] but the gene itself has not yet been reported. In addition, there are other families with the long QT phenotype that do not link to any of these gene loci. They must have mutations of one or more other genes, so at least six genes can cause LQTS, and there may be many more. For example, there are yet no described abnormalities in the Ca channel, the I_{to}, or I_p in patients with the LQTS.

The most recent discovery involves the Jervell and Lange-Nielsen form of the syndrome. It was thought for many years to be an autosomal recessive disorder. Recently it was shown to be due to novel mutations in the *KVLQT1* gene.[17] The cardiac ion channel dysfunction and QT prolongation are inherited as an autosomal dominant disease, like the Romano-Ward variant. The hearing deficit is inherited as an autosomal recessive trait. The Jervell and Lange-Nielsen phenotype occurs when both parents have the mutant *KVLQT1* gene and an offspring inherits the abnormal gene from both parents. The child is therefore homozygous for the mutant gene and manifests severe LQTS. The *KVLQT1* gene also encodes for elements of the hearing mechanism, and deafness occurs when the patient is homozygous but not heterozygous (i.e., the parents are not deaf) for the mutant *KVLQT1* gene. The concept that the more severe phenotype in the Jervell and Lange-Nielsen syndrome reflects a "double dose" of a mutant gene is further confirmed by a report of a Lebanese family in whom the syndrome was due to compound heterozygous mutation in *KCNE1* inherited from both the father and mother of affected children.[18] The *KCNE1* enclosed the cardiac K⁺ channel protein *minK*. As mentioned above, coexpression of *KCNE1* and *KVLQT1* induces the I_{ks} current. Therefore, the combination of the *KVLQT1* proteins with mutant *minK* subunit could form abnormal I_{ks} channels. It is interesting to note that *KCNE1* is also expressed in vestibular cells. The "double dose" mutation of the Jervell and Lange-Nielsen syndrome requires unusual circumstances; therefore, it is rare.

The majority of pharmacological agents that can produce prolonged repolarization and acquired LQTS could be grouped as acting predominantly through one of four different mechanisms[8]: 1) a delay of one or both K currents, I_{ks} and I_{kr}, as in the case of quinidine, N-acetylprocainamide, cesium, sotalol, bretylium, clofilium, and other new Class III antiarrhythmic agents (this action could possibly be specifically antagonized by drugs that activate the K channel such as pinacidil and cromakalin); 2) suppression of I_{to}, as in the case of 4-aminopyridine, which was shown to prolong repolarization and induce EADs preferentially in canine subepicardial M cells, which are reported to have prominent I_{to}; 3) an increase of I_{Ca}, as in case of Bay K 8644 (this action could be reversed by Ca channel blockers; 4) a delay of I_{Na} inactivation, as in the case of aconitine, veratridine, batrachotoxin, DPI, and the sea anemone toxins anthopleurin-A (AP-A) and ATX-II (this action could be antagonized by drugs that block I_{Na}, and/or the slowly inactivating Na current such as lidocaine and mexiletine). Since these drugs can shorten prolonged repolarization, they can also suppress EADs induced by the first two mechanisms.

The ionic mechanisms of pharmacologically induced prolonged repolarization and EAD formation can be complex. Several pharmacological agents act by affecting more than one ionic current either in synergistic or opposing directions. More importantly, the synergistic effects of other interventions are frequently required for critical lengthening of repolarization and the generation of EADs. A slow driving rate as well as a low extracellular K usually have a significant synergistic effect. The slow driving rate probably acts by reducing the I_p. Low extracellular K will decrease K conductance, which in turn will affect a number of currents, including I_k, I_{k1}, and I_f.

The list of drugs that causes LQTS and TdP is continually increasing (Table 2). Literally any pharmacological agent that can result in prolonged QT can induce LQTS. The incidence of TdP has not been correlated with the plasma concentrations of drugs known to precipitate this arrhythmia. However, high plasma concentrations, resulting from excessive dose or reduced metabolism of some of these drugs, may increase the risk of precipitating TdP. Such reduced metabolism may result from the concomitant use of other drugs that interfere with cytochrome P_{450} enzymes. Medications reported to interfere with the metabolism of some drugs associated with TdP include systemic ketoconazole and structurally similar drugs

Table 2
Abbreviated List of Drugs Reported to Cause
Prolongation of the QT Interval or Tosade de Pointes

Category of Drug	Drugs
Antiarrhythmic	
Class Ia	Disopyramide, procainamide, quinidine
Class III	Amiodarone, bretylium, sotalol
Antimicrobial	Erythromycin, trimethoprim-sulfamethoxazole
Antifungal	Fluconazole, ketoconazole, itraconazole
Antimalarial or antiprotozoal	Chloroquine, halofantrine, mefloquine, pentamidine, quinine
Antihistamine	Astemizole, terfenadine, diphenhydramine
Gastrointestinal prokinetic	Cisapride
Psychoactive	Chloral hydrate, haloperidol, lithium, phenothiazines, pimozide, tricyclic antidepressants
Miscellaneous	Amantadine, indapamide, probucol, tacrolimus, vasopressin

(fluconazole, itraconazole, metronidazole); serotonin reuptake inhibitors (fluoxetine, fluvoxamine, sertraline) and other antidepressants (nefazodone); HIV protease inhibitors (indinavir, ritonavir, saquinavir); dihydropyridine calcium-channel blockers (felodipine, nicardipine, nifedipine); and erythromycin and other macrolide antibiotics.[19] Grapefruit and grapefruit juice may also interact with some drugs by interfering with cytochrome P_{450} enzymes. Some of the drugs listed in Table 2 have been associated with TdP not so much because they prolong the QT interval but because they are inhibitors primarily of P4503A4, and thereby increase plasma concentration of other QT prolonging agents. The best example is ketoconazole and itraconazole, which are potent inhibitors of the enzyme and thereby account for TdP during terfenadine, astemizole, or cisapride therapy. On the other hand, the incidence of drug-associated TdP has been very low with some of the drugs listed in Table 2: diphenhydramine, fluconazole, quinine, lithium, indapamide, and vasopressin. It should also be noted that TdP may result from the use of drugs that cause QT prolongation in patients with medical conditions such as hepatic dysfunction or congenital LQTS or in those with electrolyte disturbances (particularly hypokalemia and hypomagnesemia). Electrolyte disturbances may be induced by corticosteroids, diuretic therapy, liquid protein diet, severe diarrhea, or vomiting. Although it is difficult to predict which patients are at risk for TdP, careful assessment of the risk-benefit ratio is important before prescribing drugs known to be able to cause QT prolongation.

A Paradigm of TdP from Ion Channels to ECG

An in vivo canine model of LQTS and TdP was developed using the neurotoxins AP-A[20] or ATX-II.[21] These agents act by slowing Na channel inactivation resulting in a sustained inward current during the plateau and prolongation of the AP duration (APD).[22,23] The model anticipated the more recent discovery of a genetic mutation of the Na channel subunit (SCN5A) in patients with LQT3.[14] The mutant channels were shown to generate a sustained inward current during depolarization quite similar to the Na channel exposed to AP-A or ATX-II.[24] Although the model is a surrogate of LQT3, which is a relatively uncommon form of congenital LQTS, the basic electrophysiological mechanism of TdP in this model seems to apply, with some necessary modifications, to all forms of congenital and acquired LQTS. In a series of reports, a paradigm of the mechanisms of TdP that extends from an ion channel abnormality to an arrhythmia with a characteristic ECG morphology was elucidated.[3,20-23,25]

Figures 1 to 3 illustrate this paradigm in a logical, uninterrupted sequence. Figure 1, panel A illustrates the behavior of single Na channels exposed to AP-A. Figure 1, panel B demonstrates the effects of AP-A on

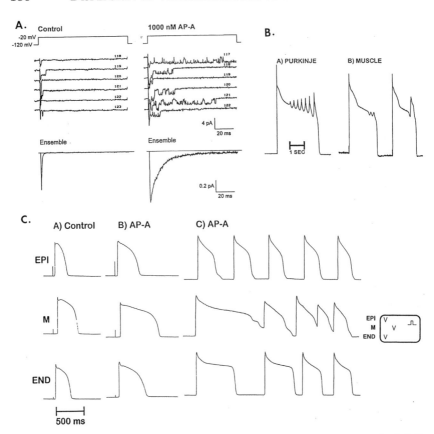

Figure 1. A. The behavior of single Na channels exposed to anthopleurin-A (AP-A). Sequential recordings of single Na channel current responses during depolarizing steps from −120 to −20 mV from two rabbit cardiac myocytes. **Left:** Recordings under control conditions; **right:** recordings from a patch exposed to 1000 nM of AP-A. At −20 mV, control Na channels opened briefly, on average only once, very soon after the potential step. In contrast, Na channels exposed to AP-A showed long-lasting bursts consisting of repetitive long openings interrupted by brief closures. Some of the bursts lasted for the entire duration of the potential step. The ensemble currents from both patches are shown on the bottom. The control ensemble current shows fast relaxation. Conversely, the ensemble current of the Na channel exposed to AP-A shows markedly slowed relaxation, with the current failing to relax completely by the end of the 95-ms step. Kinetic analysis suggested that AP-A results in modal gating behavior of the Na channel. **B.** Action potential recordings from a Purkinje fiber in an endocardial preparation and from a midmyocardial M cell, from a transmural strip; both isolated from the left ventricle of a 10-week-old puppy and placed in the same chamber and perfused with 50 mg/L AP-A. The two preparations were stimulated at a cycle length (CL) of 3000 ms. The Purkinje fiber shows a series of early afterdepolarizations (EADs) that increased gradually in amplitude before final repolarization. On the other hand, the first action potential of the midmyocardial M cell showed marked prolongation of action potential duration (APD) and low-amplitude EADs at the end of phase 2. The

the AP of a canine Purkinje fiber (PF) from an endocardial preparation and a midmyocardial (M) cell from a transmural strip that were placed in the same chamber and superfused with the same concentration of AP-A. Administration of the drug resulted in prolongation of the APD of the PF and the development of a series of EADs. On the other hand, the drug resulted in marked prolongation of APD of the M cell and low-amplitude EADs at the end of phase 2. The subsequent AP showed the occurrence of a potential at the end of phase 2 that is more representative of an electrotonic interaction than an EAD. This observation is emphasized in Figure 1, panel C, which shows simultaneous recordings from a subepicardial (Epi) cell, an M cell, and a subendocardial (End) cell from a transmural strip isolated from the left ventricular free wall of a 12-week-old puppy and transfused with AP-A. The recording illustrates the differential marked lengthening of the AP of the M cell compared with both Epi and End cells—the development of conduction block between the Epi and M cells and the occurrence of asynchronous activation in the slice suggestive of reentrant excitation.

Figure 2 further investigates the effects of AP-A in the in vivo canine heart using high-resolution tridimensional isochronal mapping of both activation and repolarization. To map tridimensional repolarization in vivo, activation-recovery intervals (ARIs)[26] were measured from unipolar extracellular electrograms recorded by multielectrode plunge needles. The ARI was shown to correspond to local repolarization.[3,26] Microelectrode studies in transmural preparations have shown that Epi, M, and End cell respond differently to changes in cycle length (CL): the M cells had the steepest APD-CL relationship, followed by End cells. The least relation-

---

Figure 1 *(continued)*. subsequent action potential showed the occurrence of a potential at the end of phase 2 that is more representative of an electrotonic interaction rather than an EAD. This observation is emphasized in **C**, which shows simultaneous recordings from a subepicardial (EPI) cell, midmyocardial (M) cell, and a subendocardial (END) cell from a transmural strip isolated from the left ventricle of a 12-week-old puppy and transfused with 50 μg/L AP-A. The preparation was stimulated at a CL of 4000 ms. Control recordings show the characteristic prolongation of APD of the M cell compared to EPI and END cells. AP-A resulted in prolongation of all three cell types, but the effect was more marked in the M cell. In **C**, spontaneous regular activity arose in the preparation at a CL of 1200 ms. There was a 1:1 response in the EPI cell but irregular responses in the M and END cells. In particular, the M cell which had a markedly prolonged APD, showed an inflection on phase 3, suggestive of electrotonic interaction. There was also evidence of asynchronous activation in the preparation (possible substrate for reentrant excitation). In four other transmural preparations, midmyocardial M cells showed a steep relation between APD and CL. However, it was uncommon to see oscillatory responses characteristic of EAD in these cells compared to PF at similar CL and concentration of AP-A.

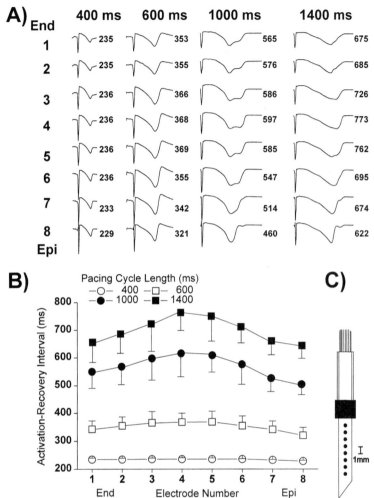

Figure 2. A. Recordings of eight transmural unipolar electrograms, 1 mm apart, across the basolateral wall of the left ventricle at cycle lengths (CLs) of 400, 600, 1000, and 1400 ms, from a canine heart following anthopleurin-A (AP-A) infusion. The calculated activation-recovery interval (ARI) is shown next to each electrogram (in ms). The figure illustrates the steep ARI-CL relation of midmyocardial sites compared with subepicardial (Epi) and subendocardial (Endo) sites, resulting in steep gradients of ARI at the transition zones at the longer CL. **B.** Composite data of ARI distribution collected from 12 unipolar plunge needle recordings in the basolateral wall of the left ventricle in a 4×10-mm section from the same experiment. After AP-A, ARIs increased two to three times compared with control at similar CLs. The steepest increase occurred at midmyocardial zones. At 600 ms, ARIs were slightly longer in midmyocardial zones, but the differences were not statistically significant. At 1000 and 1400 ms, a significant increase in ARIs was apparent in midmyocardial electrodes 3 to 6 compared with both subendocardial electrodes

ship was observed in Epi cells.[27,28] Figure 2, panel A illustrates eight transmural unipolar electrograms recorded across the basolateral wall of a canine left ventricle during AP-A infusion at four different CLs. The figure shows that as the CL increased, the calculated ARI at M sites (#3 to #6) increased significantly more, compared with End sites (#1 and #2) and Epi sites (#7 and #8). This resulted in a steep gradient of ARI, especially between Epi and M sites. This behavior is illustrated graphically in Figure 2, panel B, which shows composite data of ARI distribution collected from 12 unipolar plunge needle recordings from the same heart.

Figure 3 illustrates the final step in the synthesis of the in vivo electrophysiological mechanism of TdP. The figure shows the tridimensional activation pattern of a 12-beat run of nonsustained TdP. Panel A shows that the initiating beat of TdP arose from a focal subendocardial activity. The activation wavefront encountered multiple zones of functional conduction block that developed at contiguous sites with disparate refractoriness as shown in Figure 2. The wavefront proceeded in a very slow counter-clockwise circular pathway around the left ventricular cavity before reactivating sites in sections 3 and 4 at isochrone #20 to initiate the first reentrant cycle. Figure 3, panels B through E show that all subsequent beats of TdP were due to reentrant excitation with varying tridimensional activation pattern. The TdP VT terminated when the reentrant wavefront blocked, thus ending the reentrant activity. The twisting of the QRS axis during this run of TdP was more evident in the inferior lead, aVF. The initial transition in QRS axis (between V7 and V10) correlated with the bifurcation of a predominantly single rotating wavefront (scroll) with two separate simultaneous wavefronts rotating around the left ventricular and right ventricular cavities. The final transition in QRS axis (between V10 and V11) correlated with the termination of the right ventricular circuit and the reestablishment of a single left ventricular circulating wavefront. In this and other examples of TdP, the initiating mechanism for the bifurcation of the single wavefront frequently was the development of functional conduction block between the anterior or posterior right ventricular free wall and the interventricular septum. The termination of the right ventricular wavefront was also frequently associated with the development of functional conduction block ahead of the circulating wavefront between the right ventricular free wall and the anterior or

---

Figure 2 *(continued)*. 1 and 2 and subepicardial electrodes 7 and 8. There was, however, marked variation in ARI dispersion at the two transitional zones between midmyocardial sites and both Epi and Endo sites. Differences in ARIs of up to 80 ms (at a CL of 1400 to 1500 ms) between contiguous sites, 1 mm apart, at the transition zones were not uncommon. **C.** Diagrammatic illustration of the plunge needle electrode used to collect ARI data. Modified from Reference 3, with permission.

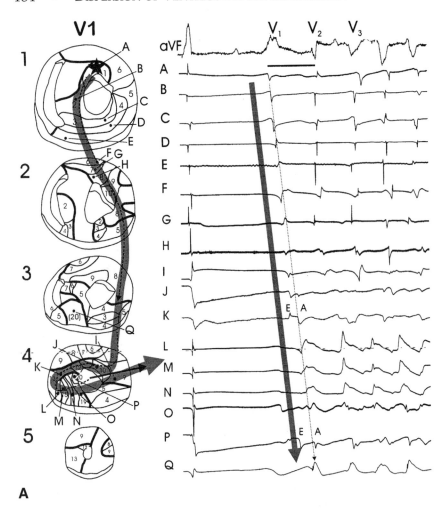

Figure 3. Tridimensional ventricular activation patterns of a 12-beat nonsustained torsade de pointes (TdP) ventricular tachycardia (VT). The maps are presented as if the heart was cut transversely into five sections, oriented with the basal section on top and the apical section on bottom and labeled 1 to 5. In **B** to **E**, section 1 was deleted. The activation isochrones were drawn as closed contour at 20-ms intervals and labeled as 1, 2, 3, and so on to make it easier to follow the activation patterns of successive beats of the VT. Functional conduction block is represented in the maps by heavy solid lines. The thick bars under the surface electrocardiogram lead mark the time intervals covered by each of the tridimensional maps. The V1 beat arose as a focal subendocardial activity (marked by a star in section 1). **A.** Selected local electrograms recorded along the reentrant pathway during the V1, which illustrates complete diastolic bridging during the first reentrant cycle of 400-ms duration. Bipolar electrograms recorded from the very slow conducting component of the circuit in section 4 had a wide multicomponent configuration. Electrograms recorded in close proximity to arcs of functional

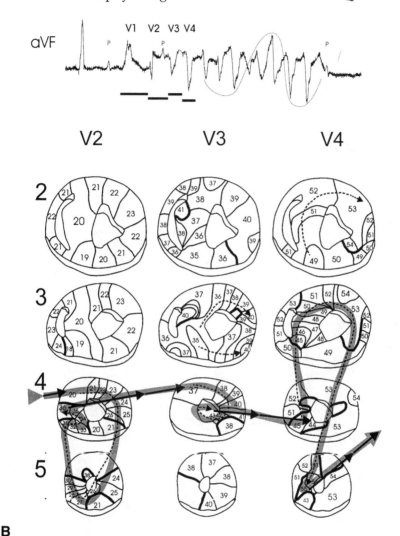

Figure 3 *(continued).* conduction block had double potentials representing an electrotonic potential (**E**) and an activation potential (**A**), respectively. Note that the electrotonic potentials were synchronous with activation at the opposite side of arcs of functional block (electrograms J, K, and Q). All subsequent beats of TdP were due to reentrant excitation with varying configuration of the reentrant circuit (**B** to **E**). The twisting QRS pattern was more evident in lead aVF during the second half of the VT episode. The transition in QRS axis (between V7 and V10) correlated with the bifurcation of a predominantly single rotating wavefront (scroll) into two separate simultaneous wavefronts rotating around the left ventricular and right ventricular cavities. The final transition in QRS axis (between V10 and V11) correlated with the termination of the right ventricular circuit and the reestablishment of a single left ventricular circulating wave front. P indicates P waves. Modified from Reference 25, with permission.

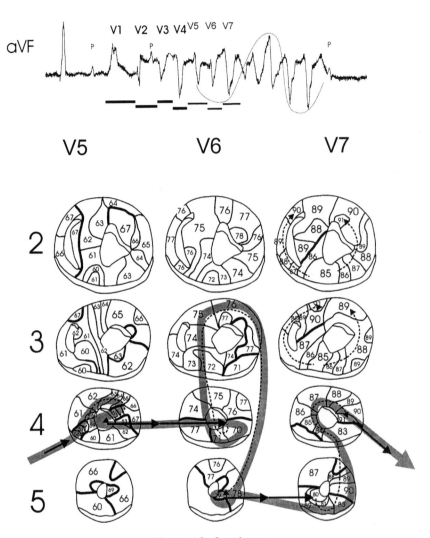

Figure 3C. Continues.

posterior border of the septum. In other instances, the right ventricular circulating wavefront was extinguished through collision with an opposing wavefront in the interventricular septum. The right ventricular circulating wavefront usually did not exhibit a localized zone of slow conduction. This may suggest that the conduction block that develops at the border between the thin right ventricular free wall and the much thicker interventricular septum may be, at least in part, secondary to an impedance-mismatch mechanism.[29] On the other hand, left ventricular circuits frequently encompassed a varying zone of slow conduction, and conduction block usually developed in this slow zone probably secondary to

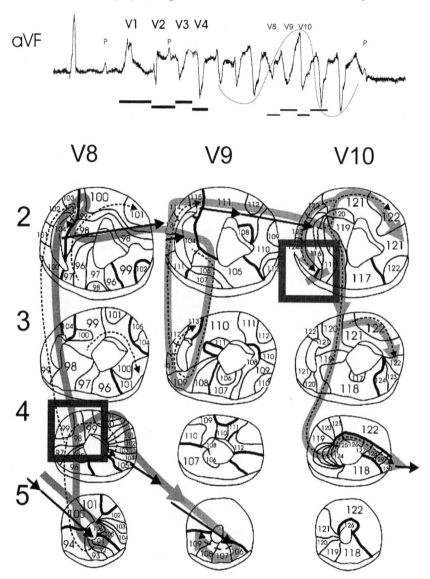

Figure 3D. Continues.

decremental conduction. Although it was more difficult to correlate accurately, there was evidence that a period of transitional complexes covering more than one cycle was associated with gradual dominance of one of the two circulating wavefronts before termination of the other wavefront (see the transitional QRS complexes labeled V8 and V9 in Fig. 3). Although the AP-A model seems to represent many of the phenotypic features of

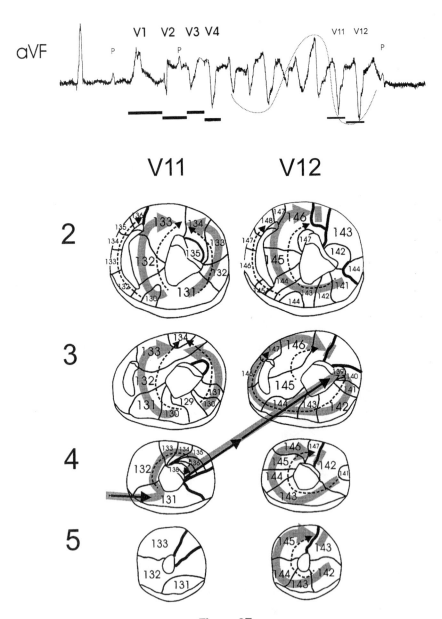

Figure 3E.

LQTS, it should be obvious that "sanitized" surrogate experimental models do not reflect the complex pathophysiology that is present in the clinical LQTS where multiple factors tend to modulate the phenotypic expression of the disease.

Short-Long Cardiac Sequence and the Onset of TdP

One or more short-long cardiac cycles, usually the result of a ventricular bigeminal rhythm, frequently precede the onset of malignant ventricular tachyarrhythmias. This is seen in patients with organic heart disease and apparently normal QT intervals[30] as well as in patients with either the congenital[31] or acquired[32,33] LQTS. The electrophysiological mechanisms that underlie this relationship have not been fully explored. This was recently investigated in the canine AP-A model, a surrogate of LQT3.[34] The bigeminal beats consistently arose from a subendocardial focal activity (SFA) from the same or different sites while TdP was due to encroachment of the SFA on a substrate of dispersion of repolarization to induce reentrant arrhythmias. In the presence of a multifocal bigeminal rhythm, TdP followed the SFA that had both a critical site of origin and local coupling interval in relation to the underlying pattern of dispersion of repolarization that promoted reentry. In the presence of a unifocal bigeminal rhythm, the following mechanisms for the onset of TdP were observed: 1) a second SFA from a different site infringed on the dispersion of repolarization of the first SFA to initiate reentry; 2) a slight lengthening of the preceding CL(s) resulted in increased dispersion of repolarization at key sites due to differential increase of local repolarization at midmyocardial zones compared with epicardial zones. This resulted in de novo arcs of functional conduction block and slowed conduction to initiate reentry (Figs. 4 through 6). Thus, the transition of a bigeminal rhythm to TdP was due to well-defined electrophysiological changes with predictable consequences that promoted reentrant excitation.

QT/T Wave Alternans and TdP

It has long been known that tachycardia-dependent T wave alternans occurs in patients with the congenital or idiopathic form of the LQTS and may presage the onset of polymorphic VT known as TdP.[35,36]

In a recent analysis of 1103 LQTS patients with rate-corrected QT (QTc) interval greater than 0.44 s from the International LQTS Registry, T wave alternans was recorded in 30 patients.[37] The frequency of occurrence of T wave alternans was directly proportional to the length of the QTc interval on the enrollment ECG. T wave alternans occurred in one

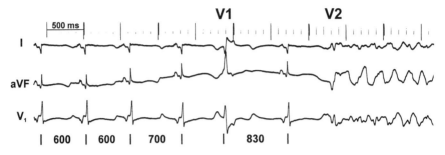

Figure 4. Electrocardiographic recordings from a canine anthopleurin-A (AP-A) surrogate model of LQT3 in which ventricular tachyarrhythmia was initiated by the ventricular premature beat (V2) that followed the first short-long cardiac sequence. The latter was due to the occurrence of a ventricular premature beat (V1, the short cycle) followed after a compensatory pause by a sinus beat (the long cycle). Note that V1 followed a sudden lengthening of the sinus cycle length. The numbers represent cardiac cycle length in ms. Reproduced from Reference 34, with permission.

or more occasions during an average 4-year follow-up in 21% of the patients with QTc greater than 0.60 s, but in less than 0.2% of the patients with QTc less than 0.50 s. Patients with advanced forms of T wave alternans (those with bidirectional beat-to-beat changes in T wave polarity; n=21) were younger, had longer QTc values, had a higher incidence of complex ventricular tachyarrhythmias, and were more likely to experience a cardiac event (syncope or cardiac arrest) than those with less advanced forms of T wave alternans (those without bidirectional beat-to-beat changes in T wave polarity; n=9).

Alternation of the duration and/or configuration of the repolarization wave of the body surface ECG, usually referred to as QT or T wave alternans, is seen under diverse experimental and clinical conditions.[38,39] Interest in repolarization alternans is attributed to the hypothesis that it may reflect an underlying dispersion of repolarization in the heart. Although overt T wave alternans in the ECG is not common, in recent years digital signal processing techniques have made it possible to detect subtle degrees of T wave alternans. This suggests that the phenomenon may be more prevalent than previously recognized and may represent an important marker of vulnerability to ventricular tachyarrhythmias in general.[40]

The electrophysiological basis of arrhythmogenicity of QT/T alternans in LQTS was recently investigated in the AP-A model of LQT3.[41] The arrhythmogenicity of QT/T alternans was primarily due to the greater degree of spatial dispersion of repolarization during alternans than during slower rates not associated with alternans (Fig. 7). The dispersion of repolarization was most marked between midmyocardial and epicardial zones in the left ventricular free wall. In the presence of a critical degree

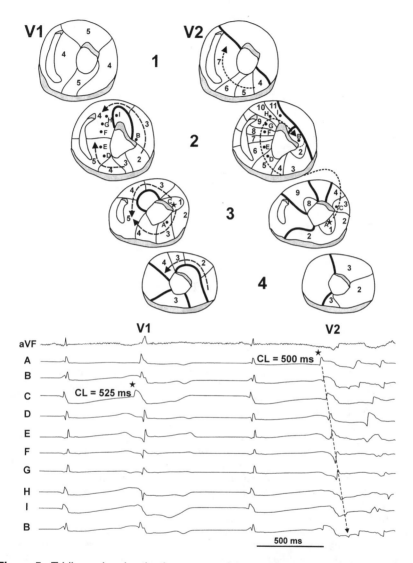

Figure 5. Tridimensional activation pattern of the two ventricular premature beats, V1 and V2, shown in Figure 4, as well as selected electrograms along the reentrant pathway initiated by the V2 beat. The two V beats arose from two different sites (marked by stars in section 3 of the maps and by electrograms C and A for V1 and V2 beats, respectively). The V2 beat had a shorter "local" coupling interval compared with V1. The V1 beat resulted in multiple zones of functional conduction block, but there was no significant area of slow conduction, and the total ventricular activation time was 100 ms. By contrast, the V2 beat resulted in more extensive zones of functional conduction block and a slow circulating wavefront in section 2 to initiate the first reentrant cycle ms. Reproduced from Reference 34, with permission.

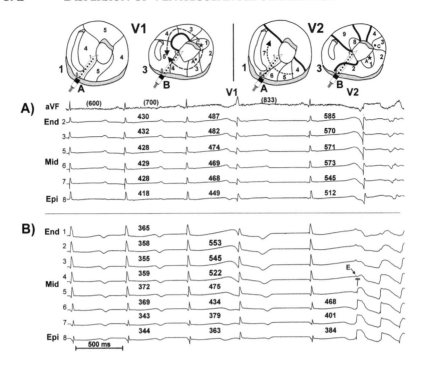

Figure 6. Unipolar electrograms recorded from two plunge needle electrodes (in sections 1 and 3, respectively) from the experiment shown in Figures 4 and 5. Recordings from electrode sites #1 and #4 in needle A are not shown. The recordings illustrate the alterations in the repolarization pattern and dispersion of repolarization that followed the lengthening of preceding cycle length (CL) and that created the substrate for reentrant excitation. The members in the figure represent the local activation-recovery intervals (ARIs), and the numbers in parentheses are the cardiac CLs. Needle A shows that the increase of the sinus CL preceding V1 resulted in lengthening of ARI of all epicardial (Epi), midmyocardial (Mid), and endocardial (End) sites compared with preceding sinus beats with shorter and relatively constant CLs. The longer compensatory CL after V1 resulted in further lengthening of ARIs of the next sinus beat. Critical analysis revealed that the degree of lengthening of ARI at Epi sites was less compared with subEpi, Mid, and End sites, resulting in greater dispersion between these sites. For needle A, the dispersion of ARIs between Epi site #8 and "adjacent" subEpi site #7, separated by 1 mm, was 10 ms during the stable sinus rhythm at a CL of 600 ms, and increased to 19 ms after the lengthening of the last sinus cycle before V1 to 700 ms. The dispersion of ARI then increased to 37 ms after the longer CL of 833 ms of the S-L sequence. Needle B showed similar directional increases of local ARIs after the lengthening of the preceding CL, but the degree of lengthening was more pronounced. Still, the lengthening of ARI at Epi sites was less marked compared with Mid and End sites. The lengthening of the sinus CL from 600 ms to 700 ms resulted in 19-ms and 38-ms increase of the ARI at the two most Epi sites #8 and #7, respectively, compared with Mid/End sites (ranging from 65 ms at site #6 to 195 ms at site #2). The most illustrative consequence of differential changes in ARI in response to lengthening of preceding CL is seen in the sinus beat

of dispersion of repolarization, propagation of the activation wavefront could be blocked between these zones to initiate reentrant excitation and polymorphic VT. Two factors contributed to the modulation of repolarization during QT/T alternans, resulting in greater magnitude of dispersion of repolarization between midmyocardial and epicardial zones at critical short CLs: 1) differences in restitution kinetics at midmyocardial sites, characterized by larger ΔARI and a slower time constant (τ) compared with epicardial sites, and 2) differences in the diastolic interval that would result in different input to the restitution curve at the same constant CL. The longer ARI of midmyocardial sites resulted in shorter diastolic interval during the first short cycle and thus a greater degree of ARI shortening.

An important observation was that marked repolarization alternans could be present in local electrograms without manifest alternation of the QT/T segment in the surface ECG. The latter was seen at critically short CLs associated with reversal of the gradient of repolarization between epicardial and midmyocardial sites, with a consequent reversal of polarity of the intramyocardial QT wave in alternate cycles. This observation provides the rationale for the recent digital signal processing techniques that attempt to detect subtle degrees of T wave alternans.[40]

The Autonomic Nervous System and LQTS

Sympathetic imbalance has been invoked to explain an arrhythmogenic substrate of the LQTS.[42] The concept proposed that reduced right cardiac sympathetic innervation, presumably of a congenital basis, results in reflex elevation of left cardiac sympathetic activity. The hypothesis was originally based on earlier studies in dogs showing that left stellate ganglion stimulation and right stellate ganglion interruption prolong QT interval.[43] The data were obtained from measurement of the QT interval in only one ECG lead. Later studies showed that neuronal or intravenous adrenergic stimulation can transiently prolong the QT interval, followed by shortening.[44] Studies in the in vivo model of cesium-induced LQTS suggest that the left stellate ganglion exerts a "quantitatively" greater adrenergic influence on the ventricles than the right stellate ganglion.[45] The larger EAD amplitude in monophasic AP recordings from the left

←————————————————————————————————

Figure 6 *(continued)*. after the S-L sequence in needle B. Conduction block occurred between Mid sites #5 and #4. The ARIs could only be estimated at sites #6 to #8 and showed further lengthening compared with the sinus beat before V1. The ARI could not be accurately estimated at sites #1 to #5 because of superimposition of the local activation potential (site #5) or electrotonic potentials (sites #1 to #4) on the depolarization wave. However, it is clear that the dispersion of local ARI between sites #5 and #4 was the substrate for the resulting functional conduction block ms. Reproduced from Reference 34, with permission.

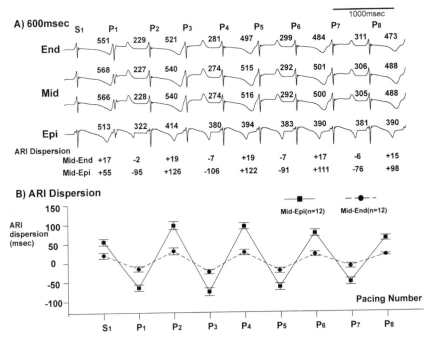

Figure 7. Transmural recording from a plunge needle electrode in the left ventricular free wall from a dog during infusion of anthopleurin-A (AP-A). The recording illustrates unipolar electrograms from endocardial (End), midmyocardial (Mid), and epicardial (Epi) sites. QT alternans was induced by abrupt decrease of the cardiac cycle length (CL) from 1000 ms (S1) to 600 ms (P1, P2, P3, etc.). The numbers represent the activation-recovery interval (ARI) in ms. Note that even though the overall QT interval is shorter at 600 ms compared with 1000 ms, the degree of ARI dispersion between Epi and Mid sites was greater at 600 ms. Also note the reversal of the gradient of ARI between Epi and Mid sites, with a consequent reversal of polarity of the intramyocardial QT wave in alternate cycles. **B.** Graphic illustration of mean ± SEM of ARI dispersion between Mid and Epi sites and between Mid and End sites during successive short CLs of 600 ms from 12 different sites from the left ventricular free wall from the same experiment. Reproduced from Reference 41, with permission.

ventricle observed with left or bilateral ansae subclaviae stimulation, compared with right ansae subclaviae stimulation, may simply reflect more epinephrine release or a greater mass of affected myocardium. The potential role of α_1-adrenoreceptors in the LQTS was highlighted by studies that showed that α_1-adrenoreceptor stimulation increased and α_1-adrenoreceptor blockade decreased EAD amplitude and incidence of VT in the canine cesium model of LQTS and TdP.[46] In a rabbit model of LQTS and TdP, induced by Class III antiarrhythmic agents, the α_1-adrenoreceptor agonist methoxamine significantly lengthened the QT interval and increased the incidence of TdP.[47] However, the effects of α_1-adrenoreceptor agonists can be complex. In another study,[48] using measurements of ARI in the rabbit, α_1-agonist effect resulted in prolongation of ARIs but a decrease of the dispersion of ARIs on the epicardial surface. The latter effect was explained by the α_1-agonist improving cellular coupling via enhanced gap junctional conductance.[49] It remains unknown, however, whether α_1-agonists could affect dispersion of refractoriness in the tridimensional ventricle.

Recent preliminary clinical observations suggest that the onset of TdP in LQT3 patients with a mutant Na channel may occur at rest or during sleep rather than during exercise, possibly in association with relative bradycardia.[50] On the other hand, patients with mutant K channels, especially LQT1, usually have syncope or cardiac arrest under stressful conditions possibly because of an arrhythmogenic effect of catecholamine and/or differences in the rate and degree of accommodation of the QT interval to CL shortening.[50]

A recent study investigated the differential effects of β-adrenergic stimulation on the frequency-dependent electrophysiological actions of three different Class III agents, dofetilide, a pure I_{kr} blocker, ambasilide, a nonselective I_k blocker, and chromanol 293B, a selective I_{ks} blocker.[51] The AP prolonging effect of dofetilide was significantly reduced by isoproterenol while that of ambasilide was much less reduced. In contrast, the AP prolonging effect of chromanol 293B was increased in the presence of isoproterenol. This observation is of interest, since the most significant correlation of autonomic stimulation and the onset of TdP is seen in LQT1 patients in whom the I_{ks} channel is mutated. Possible mechanisms for such a reversed effect of isoproterenol in the presence of chromanol remain speculative.

From an electrophysiologically mechanistic point of view, autonomic manipulations can be arrhythmogenic in the LQTS by means of two interrelated mechanisms: 1) by enhancing or suppressing the generation of EADs and their conduction in the heart, and 2) by enhancing or suppressing the dispersion of repolarization. The latter mechanism is essential for the occurrence of reentrant excitation. It is possible that in patients with LQT1, due to depressed I_{ks}, autonomic stimulation results in differential effect on APD in epicardial versus midmyocardial and endocardial zones, with consequent increase of dispersion of repolarization and onset of reentrant excitation. Given this framework, it becomes obvious that a major limitation in this area is the lack of quantitative data on the effects of autonomic manipulations on the tridimensional spatial dispersion of repolarization in vivo in a surrogate model of LQT1.

Conclusion

The electrophysiological mechanism(s) of LQTS and TdP continue to unravel. It is a prime example of how molecular biology, ion channel, cellular, and organ physiology coupled with clinical observations is the future paradigm for advancement of medical knowledge.

References

1. El-Sherif N, Craelius W, Boutjdir M, et al. Early afterdepolarizations and arrhythmogenesis. *J Cardiovasc Electrophysiol* 1990;1:145-160.
2. Antzelevich C, Sicouri S. Clinical relevance of cardiac arrhythmias generated by afterdepolarizations: Role of M cells in the generation of U waves, triggered activity and torsade de pointes. *J Am Coll Cardiol* 1994;23:259-277.
3. El-Sherif N, Caref EB, Yin H, et al. The electrophysiological mechanism of ventricular tachyarrhythmias in the long QT syndrome: Tridimensional mapping of activation and recovery patterns. *Circ Res* 1996;79:474-492.
4. Dessertenne F. La tachycardie ventriculaire a deux foyers opposes variables. *Arch Mal Coeur* 1996;59:263-272.
5. Roden DM, Lazzara R, Rosen M, et al. Multiple mechanisms in the long QT syndrome. Current knowledge, gaps, and future directions. *Circulation* 1996;94:1996-2012.
6. Jackman WM, Clark M, Friday KJ, et al. Ventricular tachyarrhythmias in the long QT syndrome. *Med Clin North Am* 1984;68:1079-1104.
7. Leenhardt A, Glaser E, Burguera M, et al. Short-coupled variant of torsade de pointes. A new electrocardiographic entity in the spectrum of idiopathic ventricular tachyarrhythmias. *Circulation* 1994;89:206-215.
8. El-Sherif N. Proarrhythmic consequences of pharmacologically prolonged repolarization: Experimental considerations. In Singh BN, Wellens HJJ, Hiraoka M (eds): *Pharmacological Control of Cardiac Arrhythmias. To Delay Conduction or to Prolong Refractoriness?* Mount Kisco: Futura Publishing Co.; 1994:335-356.
9. Vincent GM. The molecular basis of the long QT syndrome: Genes causing fainting and sudden death. *Annu Rev Med* 1998;49:263-274.
10. Wang Q, Curran ME, Splawski I, et al. Positional cloning of a novel potassium channel gene: KVLQT1 mutations cause cardiac arrhythmias. *Nat Genet* 1996;12:17-23.
11. Barhanin J, Lesage F, Guillemare E, et al. KvLQT1 and IsK (minK) proteins associate to form the I_ks cardiac potassium current. *Nature* 1996;384:78-80.
12. Sanguinetti MC, Curran ME, Zou A, et al. Coassembly of KVLQT1 and minK (IsK) proteins to form cardiac I_ks potassium channel. *Nature* 1996;384:80-83.
13. Curran ME, Splawski I, Timothy KW, et al. A molecular basis for cardiac arrhythmia: HERG mutations cause long QT syndrome. *Cell* 1995;80:795-803.
14. Wang Q, Shen J, Splawski I, et al. SCN5A mutations associated with an inherited cardiac arrhythmia, long QT syndrome. *Cell* 1995; 80:805-811.
15. Sanguinetti MC, Jiang C, Curran ME, et al. A mechanistic link between an inherited and an acquired cardiac arrhythmia: HERG encodes the Ikr potassium channel. *Cell* 1995;81:299-307.
16. Schott JJ, Charpentier F, Peltier S, et al. Mapping of a gene for long QT syndrome to chromosome 4q25-27. *Am J Hum Genet* 1995;57:1114-1122.
17. Neyroud N, Tesson F, Denjoy I, et al. A novel mutation in the potassium channel gene KVLQT1 causes the Jervell and Lange-Nielsen cardioauditory syndrome. *Nat Genet* 1997;15:186-189.
18. Rubie C, Hordt M, Towbin JA, et al. KCNE1 mutations cause Jervell and Lange-Nielsen syndrome. *Nat Genet* 1997;17:267-268.

19. Canadian Adverse Drug Reaction Newsletter: Drugs causing prolongation of QT interval and torsade de pointes. *Can Med Assoc J* 1998;158:103-104.
20. El-Sherif N, Zeiler RH, Craelius W, et al. QTU prolongation and polymorphic ventricular tachyarrhythmias due to bradycardia-dependent early afterdepolarizations. *Circ Res* 1988;63:286-305.
21. Boutjdir M, El-Sherif N. Pharmacological evaluation of early afterdepolarisations induced by sea anemone toxin (ATXII) in dog heart. *Cardiovasc Res* 1991;25:815-819.
22. El-Sherif N, Fozzard HA, Hanck DA. Dose-dependent modulation of the cardiac sodium channel by the sea anemone toxin ATXII. *Circ Res* 1992;70:285-301.
23. Boutjdir M, Restivo M, Wei Y, et al. Early afterdepolarization formation in cardiac myocytes: Analysis of phase plane patterns, action potential, and membrane currents. *J Cardiovasc Electrophysiol* 1994;5:609-620.
24. Bennett PB, Yazawa K, Makita N, et al. Molecular mechanism for an inherited cardiac arrhythmia. *Nature* 1995;376:683-685.
25. El-Sherif N, Chinushi M, Caref EB, et al. Electrophysiological mechanism of the characteristic electrocardiographic morphology of torsade de pointes tachyarrhythmias in the long QT syndrome. Detailed analysis of ventricular tridimensional activation patterns. *Circulation* 1997;96:4392-4399.
26. Haws CW, Lux RL. Correlation between in vivo transmembrane action potential durations and activation recovery intervals from electrograms: Effects of interventions that alter repolarization time. *Circulation* 1991;81:281-288.
27. Antzelevitch C, Sicouri S, Litovsky SH, et al. Heterogeneity within the ventricular wall: Electrophysiology and pharmacology of epicardial, endocardial, and M cells. *Circ Res* 1991;69:1427-1449.
28. Sicouri S, Antzelevitch C. Electrophysiologic characteristics of M cells in the canine left ventricular free wall. *J Cardiovasc Electrophysiol* 1995;6:591-603.
29. Fast VG, Kleber AG. Block of impulse propagation at an abrupt tissue expansion: Evaluation of the critical strand diameter in a 2- and 3-dimensional computer models. *Cardiovasc Res* 1995;30:449-459.
30. Leclerq JF, Maison-Blanche P, Cauchemez B, et al. Respective role of sympathetic tone and cardiac pauses in the genesis of 62 cases of ventricular fibrillation recorded during Holter monitoring. *Eur Heart J* 1988;9:1276-1283.
31. Viskin S, Alla SR, Barron HV, et al. Mode of onset of torsades de pointes in congenital long QT syndrome. *J Am Coll Cardiol* 1996;28:1262-1268.
32. Roden DM, Woosley RL, Primm RK. Incidence and clinical features of the quinidine associated long QT syndrome: Implications for patient care. *Am Heart J* 1986;111:1088-1093.
33. Kay GN, Plumb VJ, Arciniegas JG, et al. Torsades de pointes: The long-short initiating sequence and other clinical features; observations in 32 patients. *J Am Coll Cardiol* 1990;2:806-817.
34. El-Sherif N, Caref EB, Chinushi M, et al. Mechanism of arrhythmogenicity of short-long cardiac sequence that precedes ventricular tachyarrhythmias in the long QT syndrome. *J Am Coll Cardiol* 1999;33:1415-1423.
35. Schwartz PJ, Malliani A. Electrical alternation of the T-wave: Clinical and experimental evidence of its relationship with the sympathetic nervous system and with the long Q-T syndrome. *Am Heart J* 1975;89:45-50.
36. Habbab MA, El-Sherif N. TU alternans, long QTU, and torsade de pointes: Clinical and experimental observations. *PACE* 1992;15:916-931.

37. Moss AJ. Long QT syndrome. In Podrid PJ, Kowey PR (eds): *Cardiac Arrhythmias. Mechanisms, Diagnosis, and Management.* Baltimore: Williams & Wilkins; 1995:1110-1120.
38. Surawicz B, Fisch C. Cardiac alternans: Diverse mechanisms and clinical manifestations. *J Am Coll Cardiol* 1992;20:483-499.
39. Verrier RL, Nearing BD. Electrophysiologic basis for T wave alternans as an index of vulnerability to ventricular fibrillation. *J Cardiovasc Electrophysiol* 1994;5:445-461.
40. Rosenbaum DS, Jackson LE, Smith GM, et al. Electrical alternans and vulnerability to ventricular arrhythmias. *N Engl J Med* 1994;330:235-241.
41. Chinushi M, Restivo M, Caref EB, et al. Electrophysiological basis of the arrhythmogenicity of QT/T alternans in the long QT syndrome. Tridimensional analysis of the kinetics of cardiac repolarization. *Circ Res* 1998; 83:614-628.
42. Schwartz PJ, Locati E, Priori SG, et al. The long QT syndrome. In Zipes DP, Jalife J (eds): *Cardiac Electrophysiology: From Cell to Bedside.* Philadelphia: W.B. Saunders Co.; 1990:589-605.
43. Yanowitz R, Preston JB, Abildskov JA. Functional distribution of right and left stellate innervation to the ventricles: Production of neurogenic electrocardiographic changes by unilateral alteration of sympathetic tone. *Circ Res* 1966;18:416-428.
44. Abildskov JA. Adrenergic effects on the QT interval of the electrocardiogram. *Am Heart J* 1976;92:210-216.
45. Ben David J, Zipes DP. Differential response to right and left ansae subclaviae stimulation of early afterdepolarizations and ventricular tachycardia induced by cesium in dogs. *Circulation* 1988;78:1241-1250.
46. Ben David J, Zipes DP. Alpha adrenoceptor stimulation and blockade modulates cesium-induced early afterdepolarizations and ventricular tachyarrhythmias in dogs. *Circulation* 1990;82:225-233.
47. Carlsson L, Almgren O, Duker G. QTU-prolongation and torsade de pointes induced by putative class III antiarrhythmic agents in the rabbit: Etiology and interventions. *J Cardiovasc Pharmacol* 1990;16:276-285.
48. Dhein S, Gerwin R, Ziskoven V, et al. Propranolol unmasks class III like electrophysiological properties of norepinephrine. *Arch Pharmacol* 1993; 348:643-649.
49. Kolb HA, Somogyi R. Biochemical and biophysical analysis of cell-to-cell channels and regulation of gap junctional permeability. *Rev Physiol Biochem Pharmacol* 1991;118:1-48.
50. Schwartz PJ, Priori SG, Locati EH, et al. Long QT syndrome patients with mutations of the SCN5A and HERG genes have differential responses to Na^+ channel blockade and to increases in heart rate. Implications for gene-specific therapy. *Circulation* 1995;92:3381-3386.
51. Schreieck J, Wang Y, Gjini V, et al. Differential effect of beta-adrenergic stimulation on the frequency-dependent electrophysiologic actions of the new class III antiarrhythmics dofetilide, ambasilide, and chromanol 293B. *J Cardiovasc Electrophysiol* 1997;8:1420-1430.

12

Spatial Dispersion of Ventricular Repolarization in the Long QT Syndrome

Carlo Napolitano, Silvia G. Priori, and Peter J. Schwartz

Introduction

The long QT syndrome (LQTS) is a genetically transmitted life-threatening disease characterized by prolongation of the QT interval on the electrocardiogram (ECG) and by frequent syncope or cardiac arrest occurring usually in conditions of psychological or physical stress. These syncopal episodes are due to ventricular tachycardia "torsade de pointes" (TdP) that often degenerates in ventricular fibrillation and eventually results in the sudden death of most of the affected patients. This disease manifests itself in young age and most patients are diagnosed when they are children or teenagers. Mortality among untreated, or incorrectly treated, patients is extremely high, as 21% of patients die within 1 year from the first episode and 60% die within 10 years.[1,2]

The evidence of a familial pattern of inheritance (as an autosomal dominant trait in most families) in the LQTS opened the way to the identification of the disease-related loci by linkage studies and thereafter to the demonstration of the LQTS genes. It has been recognized that the LQTS phenotype is caused by mutations in some of the genes encoding for ion channel proteins regulating cardiac electrical activity. Mutations in four different genes have been demonstrated: *KCNQ1, HERG, SCN5A,* and *KCNE1*.[3] Expression studies also showed that the abnormal function of these ion channel proteins affects cardiac repolarization and it is likely to create a vulnerable substrate that can lead to the development of repetitive

From Olsson SB, Amlie JP, Yuan S (eds): *Dispersion of Ventricular Repolarization: State of the Art.* ©Futura Publishing Company, Inc., Armonk, NY, 2000.

ventricular arrhythmias, often triggered by an acute adrenergic activation (exercise or emotions).[2]

Despite the very rapid increase in the knowledge of the pathophysiological determinants of LQTS observed in recent years, the electrophysiological mechanisms leading to arrhythmias are less clearly understood. This chapter summarizes the experimental and clinical evidence supporting the role of dispersion of ventricular repolarization as one of the determinants of the onset of ventricular arrhythmias in the LQTS, and reviews the current possibilities for the detection of this arrhythmogenic substrate in the clinical setting.

Mechanism(s) for Arrhythmias in the Inherited LQTS

Despite the fact that the clinical manifestation and the basic molecular defects underlying LQTS are well characterized, the mechanisms responsible for the onset of arrhythmias are less clear. TdP, a polymorphic ventricular tachycardia with peculiar "twisting" of the QRS axis, is the typical LQTS-related arrhythmia.[4] Reentry and abnormal automaticity have both been hypothesized as arrhythmogenic mechanisms in LQTS, the first being facilitated by the presence of dispersion of ventricular repolarization, and the latter due to the onset of early afterdepolarization and triggered activity.[1,2] Evidence in favor of both mechanisms has been provided and a unifying hypothesis has been proposed, with focal activity being the first initiating event of the arrhythmias, which thereafter become sustained with a reentrant mechanism favored by the presence of heterogeneity of ventricular repolarization.[2]

Recently, El-Sherif and coworkers provided experimental evidence in favor of this unifying hypothesis.[5] In their study high-resolution tridimensional mapping was performed in pharmacologically induced LQTS, demonstrating that the initial beat of polymorphic ventricular tachycardia consistently arose as focal activity, whereas subsequent beats were due to successive subendocardial focal activity and reentrant excitation.

Evidence for a Spatial Dispersion of Repolarization in the LQTS

One of the landmark features of the LQTS is the abnormal repolarization pattern. QT interval prolongation is often associated with morphological alterations of the T wave that may be notched, diphasic, and with a prominent late "second" component.[2,6] However, a QT interval prolongation per se does not demonstrate that the process of repolarization is heterogeneous, since uniform prolongation action potential duration and refractory periods throughout the myocardium may indeed stabilize the electrical activity of the myocardium producing an antiarrhythmic effect.[7]

As outlined above, the primary defect of LQTS is a genetically determined abnormal function of some of the ion channel proteins regulating cardiac electrical activity. Thus, we have to postulate that in order to cause heterogeneity of cardiac action potentials these abnormalities affect cardiac myocytes differentially. After the identification of the LQTS-related genes,[3] attempts have been made to reproduce in experimental controlled settings the electrophysiological consequences of the LQTS-related genetic defects.[8,9] In a cellular model mimicking the electrophysiological consequences of LQTS mutations, we have demonstrated that these alterations are indeed able to create a vulnerable substrate with prolonged action potential duration, where early afterdepolarizations and triggered activity may arise in presence of β-adrenergic stimulation.[8] These observations were subsequently extended in two studies by Antzelevitch's group that showed that the transmural differences of action potential recovery time are critical in determining the heterogeneity of repolarization in the heart[10] and that when this dispersion is worsened by simultaneous presence of altered I_{Ks} current (as it happens for the LQT1 subtype of LQTS) and β-adrenergic stimulation, TdP develops.[9] This latter evidence also supports the role for the dispersion of repolarization as the substrate of arrhythmias and confirms the importance of the sympathetic nervous system as a trigger for events in LQTS.

The evidence of the presence of a significant degree of dispersion of repolarization in LQTS raises the intriguing possibility that some of the protein structures involved in the pathophysiology of LQTS might be differently expressed in the myocardium, thus representing a molecular substrate of the dispersion. Interestingly, recent preliminary findings, showing transmural differences in the pattern of expression of the *KCNQ1* protein support this concept and provide a possible "molecular" justification for the transmural dispersion of repolarization.[11]

Spatial Dispersion of Repolarization in LQTS: Clinical Evidence

Monophasic action potential (MAP) recordings, which provide a measure of the duration of the cardiac action potential,[12,13] were used in the earlier studies as a direct measure of the dispersion of ventricular repolarization in humans. Bonatti and coworkers,[14] using MAPs recorded from different myocardial sites of the right ventricle, showed dispersion up to 40 ms in normal subjects. Significantly higher values, from 100 to 270 ms, were found in patients with LQTS. These data were subsequently extended demonstrating, in LQTS patients, the presence of dispersion of left ventricle recovery times as well as refractoriness.[15]

Despite the fact that the MAP recordings provide a direct quantification of the dispersion of repolarization, the usefulness of this technique as a risk stratifier is limited by the need for an invasive approach. Therefore, noninvasive markers of dispersion have been proposed in order to overcome these limitations and to allow the evaluation of larger patient groups, including the many children affected by LQTS.

QT Dispersion

The QT interval is the marker of the electrical activity of the ventricles at the surface level. It is generally accepted that the duration of this interval reflects the time from the earliest cardiac activation to the latest repolarization in the myocardium.[16]

In 1988 Cowan et al[17] proposed that even a standard 12-lead ECG recording may provide information on the heterogeneity of ventricular repolarization by estimating the QT interlead variability or "QT dispersion." Day and colleagues[18,19] provided data that further supported the role of this index in the correct identification of the spatial dishomogeneity of repolarization. Based on the concept that each specific lead may reflect the regional duration of ventricular repolarization they defined QT dispersion as the difference between the longest and the shortest QT interval within the 12 standard leads.

Evidence for an abnormally increased QT dispersion in LQTS patients has been provided by Day et al,[18] who also showed a direct correlation of the degree of QT dispersion with cardiac events.

These results were subsequently confirmed and extended by Priori et al.[20] In this study, a clinically important correlation between reduction of QT dispersion and efficacy of therapeutic interventions was observed. Indeed, the LQTS patients, destined to remain free of syncope or cardiac arrest while being treated with β-blockers, had a QT dispersion not different from that of healthy controls. By contrast, those patients who, despite β-blockade, continued to have life-threatening arrhythmias had a greatly increased QT dispersion. Moreover, the LQTS patients who continued to remain highly symptomatic despite β-blockade and who underwent successful left cardiac sympathetic denervation (i.e., without recurrences at follow-up) had a reduction of QT dispersion to a level not different from that of healthy controls.[20]

Statistical analysis showed 80% sensitivity, 82% specificity, and an 80% positive and 77% negative predictive value for a cutoff value of 100 ms for QT dispersion in predicting patients' responsiveness to β-blockade. Finally, no correlation was observed between QT interval duration and the degree of QT dispersion, suggesting that the electrophysiological background of electrical heterogeneity is different from that of QT prolongation.

Thus, an increased QT dispersion is often detectable in LQTS patients, and its reduction appears to correlate with a positive response to therapy. However, the clinical value of QT dispersion has been criticized recently, mainly based on the evidences of its overall poor intra- and interobserver reproducibility,[21,22] stimulating the search for other noninvasive and reliable tools capable of detecting and quantifying the dispersion of ventricular repolarization at the clinical level.

Principal Component Analysis

Principal component analysis (PCA) is a mathematical procedure that can identify the spatial characteristics of a waveform, providing a quantification of the different components (vectors) that concur with the definition of the waveform itself.[23,24] The analysis of the cardiac repolarization based on PCA is usually referred to as T wave complexity analysis.[24] The most important advantage of PCA applied to the quantification of the ST-T segment spatial heterogeneity is represented by the fact that, at variance of QT dispersion, it avoids the need for a precise definition of the individual points such as the T wave offset. Indeed, the isoelectric segments following the T wave offset, if included in the measure, do not contribute to the definition of the spatial vectors. Therefore, PCA by definition is highly reproducible and observer-independent.

In the PCA analysis the T wave is first decomposed in one set of values (eigenvalues), which numerically describe the waveform by means of appropriate multiplication factors.[23] PCA of the T wave can be grossly visualized as the short and long axis of T wave loop of the vectorcardiogram, where a "thin" loop represents a relatively "smooth" repolarization (i.e., only one prominent vector describes T wave), while a "fat" or irregular loop corresponds to a complex repolarization pattern (i.e., other minor, yet quantitatively significant, vectors are present).

PCA *in* LQTS

The initial attempts for clinical application of PCA to study the cardiac repolarization took advantage of the body surface mapping technique.[25]

The earliest evaluation by our group of PCA analysis in a group of LQTS patients showed abnormally higher eigenvalues, corresponding to an increased complexity of repolarization with respect to healthy controls.[26] These observations were subsequently confirmed in a more extensive study, in which the diagnostic power of PCA applied to body surface mapping was also evaluated, showing a 87% sensitivity and a 96% specificity in the diagnosis of LQTS.[27]

Based on the encouraging experience of PCA applied to body surface mapping, we tried to develop a new strategy in order to overcome the technical limitations of body surface mapping and increase the practical feasibility of PCA in the clinical setting. We developed a new algorithm for the calculation of PCA from 12-lead Holter recordings.[23] We identified a set of eight values (eigenvectors) representing the magnitude of the different components of the entire repolarization process. The quantification of the relative contribution of these components provided an estimate of the complexity of repolarization.

Using this technique we evaluated a population of LQTS patients and compared it to healthy controls. The complexity of repolarization (CR), calculated every hour during Holter recordings and averaged (CR_{24h}), was found to be significantly higher in the LQTS group[23] (Fig. 1). In this study CR_{24h} showed a 88% sensitivity and 91% negative predictive value for the identification of LQTS patients. We also took advantage of the possibility of a dynamic assessment of complexity of repolarization allowed by the use of the Holter technique. Interestingly, among LQTS patients not only was CR_{24h} higher but its variability was significantly increased (Fig. 1). Indeed, the 24 hours trend of CR in LQTS patients presented some "downslopes" where the values were close to those observed in healthy controls. In agreement with this observation we demonstrated that the diagnostic power of PCA is reduced when it is applied

Complexity of Repolarization in the Long QT Syndrome

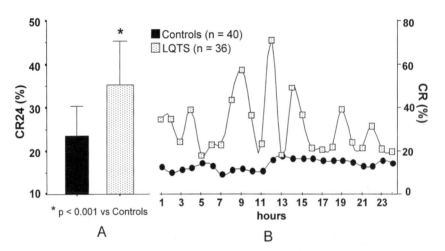

Figure 1. Complexity of repolarization (CR) in long QT syndrome (LQTS) patients quantified by principal component analysis during Holter recordings. **A.** Bar graph showing the mean 24-hour complexity (CR_{24h}) in healthy controls and LQTS patients. **B.** Example of hourly sampled measures of CR during Holter recordings in a LQTS patient (squares) and in a healthy subject (circles).

to a single ECG,[23] suggesting that, in LQTS patients, the assessment of repolarization should include multiple samples within a 24-hour period.

These data support the concept that PCA may represent a useful diagnostic tool in LQTS, constituting a novel and highly reproducible noninvasive technology to detect the degree of spatial dispersion of repolarization in LQTS as well as in other arrhythmogenic conditions. Along this line, the preliminary results obtained in a still limited patient population (Napolitano C, unpublished observation), show that the CR is significantly different in LQTS patient subgroups that carry mutations of different genes, being higher in patients with mutations in the *SCN5A* and *HERG* genes. Based on the multicenter report with data from the LQTS international registry demonstrating that the malignancy of cardiac events in LQTS is higher in patients with *SCN5A* mutations,[28] it is tempting to propose that PCA may help in the risk stratification of LQTS patients.

Conclusions

Overall, the results of the genetic studies and the evidence provided by the experimental models allow us to hypothesize that the pathophysiology of LQTS is characterized by a genetically determined alteration of cardiac repolarization producing an arrhythmogenic substrate that favors the onset of repetitive arrhythmias. One of the major consequences of the altered function of cardiac ion channel proteins is indeed the generation of a heterogeneous pattern of ventricular repolarization.

However, while these pathophysiological features are quite well characterized, our ability to precisely quantify this substrate in the clinical setting remains much less efficient. MAP recordings, body surface mapping, QT dispersion, and, lately, PCA have been proposed as clinical tools targeted to such an endpoint. So far, although all these techniques have been proven valuable in the identification of the abnormal pattern of repolarization in LQTS patients, they are still inadequate for the risk stratification of major arrhythmic events. PCA applied to 12-lead Holter recordings is a promising approach, being able to overcome at least some of the limitations inherent to the other techniques. However, only the availability of large prospective studies will definitively prove or dismiss the strength of this tool to predict arrhythmias in LQTS patients. The time has come for a large comparative study of the different noninvasive methodologies.

References

1. Schwartz PJ. Idiopathic long QT syndrome: Progress and questions. *Am Heart J* 1985;109:399-411.

2. Schwartz PJ, Priori SG, Napolitano C. Long QT syndrome. In Zipes DP, Jalife J (eds): *Cardiac Electrophysiology: From Cell to Bedside.* 3rd ed. Philadelphia: W.B. Saunders Co.; 2000:597-615.

3. Priori SG, Barhanin J, Hauer RN, et al. Genetic and molecular basis of cardiac arrhythmias: Impact on clinical management parts I and II. *Circulation* 1999;99:518-28.

4. Napolitano C, Priori SG, Schwartz PJ. Torsades de pointes: Mechanisms and management. *Drugs* 1994;47:51-65.

5. El-Sherif N, Caref EB, Yin H, Restivo M. The electrophysiological mechanism of ventricular arrhythmias in the long QT syndrome. Tridimensional mapping of activation and recovery patterns. *Circ Res* 1996;79:474-492.

6. Malfatto G, Beria G, Sala S, et al. Quantitative analysis of T wave abnormalities and their prognostic implications in the idiopathic long QT syndrome. *J Am Coll Cardiol* 1994;23:296-301.

7. Singh BN. *Control of Cardiac Arrhythmias by Lengthening Repolarization.* Mount Kisco; Futura Publishing Co.; 1988.

8. Priori SG, Napolitano C, Cantù F, et al. Differential response to Na+ channel blockade, β-adrenergic stimulation, and rapid pacing in a cellular model mimicking the SCN5A and HERG defects present in the long QT syndrome. *Circ Res* 1996;78:1009-1015.

9. Shimizu W, Antzelevitch C. Cellular basis for the ECG features of the LQT1 form of the long-QT syndrome: Effects of β-adrenergic agonists and antagonists and sodium channel blockers on transmural dispersion of repolarization and torsade de pointes. *Circulation* 1998;98:2314-2322.

10. Yan GX, Antzelevitch C. Cellular basis for the normal T wave and the electrocardiographic manifestations of the long-QT syndrome. *Circulation* 1998;3(98):1928-1936.

11. Dumaine R, Sheng WU, Antzelevich C. KvLQT1 but not minK mRNA parallels the distribution of IKs in the canine heart. *PACE* 1999;22(Pt. II):856. Abstract.

12. Edvardsson N, Hirsch I, Olsson SB. Right ventricular monophasic action potentials in healthy young men. *PACE* 1984;7:813-821.

13. Olsson SB, Brorson L, Edvardsson N, Varnauskas E. Estimation of ventricular repolarization in man by monophasic action potential recording technique. *Eur Heart J* 1985;6(suppl D):71-79.

14. Bonatti V, Rolli A, Botti G. Monophasic action potential studies in human subjects with prolonged ventricular repolarization and long QT syndromes. *Eur Heart J* 1985;6(suppl D):131-143.

15. Vassallo JA, Cassidy DM, Kindwall KE, et al. Nonuniform recovery of excitability in the left ventricle. *Circulation* 1988;78:1365-1372.

16. Surawicz B. Mechanisms of QT prolongation and arrhythmias. In Butrous GG, Schwartz PJ (eds): *Clinical Aspects of Ventricular Repolarization.* London: Farrand Press; 1989:225-242.

17. Cowan CJ, Yusoff K, Moore M, et al. Importance of lead selection in QT interval measurement. *Am J Cardiol* 1988;61:83-87.

18. Day CP, McComb JM, Campbell RWF. QT dispersion: An indication of arrhythmia risk in patients with long QT intervals. *Br Heart J* 1990;63:342-344.

19. Day CP, McComb JM, Campbell RWF. QT dispersion in sinus beats and ventricular extrasystoles in normal hearts. *Br Heart J* 1991;64:39-41.

20. Priori SG, Napolitano C, Diehl L, Schwartz PJ. Dispersion of the QT interval. A marker of therapeutic efficacy in the idiopathic long QT syndrome. *Circulation* 1994;89:1681-1689.

21. Fei L, Statters DJ, Camm AJ. QT-interval dispersion on 12 lead electrocardiogram in normal subjects: Its reproducibility and relation to the T wave. *Am Heart J* 1994;127:1654-1655.
22. Kautzner J, Yi G, Camm AJ, Malik M. Short- and long-term reproducibility of QT, QTc, and QT dispersion measurement in healthy subjects. *PACE* 1994;17:928-937.
23. Priori SG, Mortara DW, Napolitano C, et al. Evaluation of the spatial aspects of T-wave complexity in the long-QT syndrome. *Circulation* 1997;96:3006-3012.
24. Lux RL, Evans AK, Burgess MJ, et al. Redundancy reduction for improved display and analysis of body surface potential maps. I. Spatial compression. *Circ Res* 1981;49:186-196.
25. Mirvis DM. Spatial variation of QT intervals in normal persons and patients with acute myocardial infarction. *J Am Coll Cardiol* 1985;5:625-631.
26. De Ambroggi L, Bertoni T, Locati E, et al. Mapping of body surface potentials in patients with idiopathic long QT syndrome. *Circulation* 1986;74:1334-1345.
27. De Ambroggi L, Negroni MS, Monza E, et al. Dispersion of ventricular repolarization in the long QT syndrome. *Am J Cardiol* 1991;68:614-620.
28. Zareba W, Moss AJ, Schwartz PJ, et al. Influence of genotype on the clinical course of the long-QT syndrome. International Long-QT Syndrome Registry Research Group. *N Engl J Med* 1998;339:960-965.

Dispersion of Ventricular Repolarization and Cardiac Disorders

13

Role of Ischemia on Dispersion of Repolarization

Peter Taggart and Peter Sutton

Introduction

Acute ischemia is accompanied by a series of electrophysiological changes that alter the timing of repolarization.[1,2] Within the first few minutes of ischemia the action potential plateau is abbreviated and repolarization occurs earlier. However, more or less simultaneously, conduction slowing occurs resulting in delayed activation. The delayed onset of the action potential may therefore offset the earlier repolarization of the cells due to action potential duration (APD) shortening. The overall effect of ischemia on repolarization is therefore a complex function of the balance between action potential shortening on the one hand and conduction slowing on the other.

In this chapter we first consider some aspects of methodology in the assessment of dispersion of repolarization. Next we illustrate some of the effects of ischemia on APD and conduction, which combine to determine the time of local repolarization and hence dispersion of repolarization. We then review the effects of acute ischemia on QT dispersion. Finally we consider the possible relevance of changes in repolarization and dispersion of repolarization induced by ischemia.

Methodology in the Assessment of Dispersion of Repolarization

Several techniques have been used to assess dispersion of repolarization, none of which are without some degree of limitation. A major difficulty relates to the nature of the ischemic process itself. Regional ischemia

From Olsson SB, Amlie JP, Yuan S (eds): *Dispersion of Ventricular Repolarization: State of the Art.* ©Futura Publishing Company, Inc., Armonk, NY, 2000.

is characteristically inhomogeneous not only between ischemic and non-ischemic areas but also within ischemic areas.[1,3] For example, in one study action potentials recorded with floating microelectrodes in intact pig hearts often showed good responses from cells only a few millimeters away from cells that are nearly unresponsive[1] (Fig. 1). Ideally, some form of high-intensity mapping would therefore be preferred. The use of voltage-sensitive dyes provides a means of obtaining a satisfactory measure of repolarization simultaneously at a large number of closely spaced sites.[4] However, technical requirements, movement artifact, and toxicity pose limitations for the application of the method, and preclude its use in humans. Consequently, much of our insight on dispersion of repolarization relies on information obtained using floating microelectrodes or monophasic action potentials (MAPs) obtained from a limited number of sites or even a single site, or extrapolation from in vitro recordings. MAPs have been recorded simultaneously from several sites using either pressure contact or suction electrodes in several animal models of ischemia.[5-7] MAP recordings have also been obtained from a single site during ischemia in humans from endocardium in patients during cardiac catheterization[8-10] and from epicardium in patients during cardiac surgery.[11] Extrapolation from single cell experiments requires caution. Although

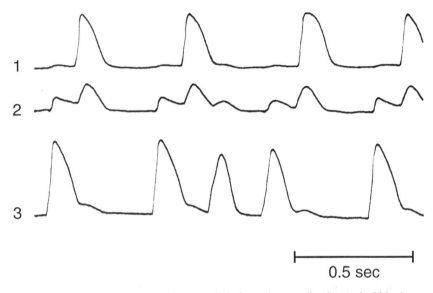

0.5 sec

Figure 1. Transmembrane action potentials from three cells situated within 1 mm of each other in the intact porcine heart. Stimulation of cell 3 results in a good action potential which is conducted to cell 1 with a delay of about 100 ms. A premature stimulus initiated a large action potential in cell 3 but did not conduct to cell 1. The double potentials in cell 2 probably represent electrotonic current from cells 1 and 3 and indicate lack of response of cell 2. From Reference 1.

marked differences in the effect of ischemic conditions on the time course of repolarization have been demonstrated in cells isolated from different locations within the ventricular wall,[12] the extent to which these differences occur in vivo when cells are electrically and mechanically coupled is an unresolved and somewhat controversial issue.[13] Recently activation-recovery intervals, measured as the interval between the activation moment of the local electrogram and the maximum derivative of the T wave, have been validated as a surrogate marker for APD during ischemia.[14] This now provides a means of obtaining multiple simultaneous measurements of repolarization, i.e., high-intensity repolarization mapping. QT dispersion, i.e., the difference between the shortest and longest QT interval, in the clinical electrocardiogram (ECG) is being increasingly used as a measure of dispersion of repolarization. Although several studies addressing the relationship between the QT interval and the underlying electrophysiology support the concept that QT interval does reflect dispersion of repolarization, definitive proof is still awaited (see other chapters for discussion). Nevertheless, the technique has the advantage of being noninvasive and simple to use in the clinical situation.

Effect of Ischemia on Action Potential Repolarization

The effects of ischemia on the action potential have been studied in a number of in vitro and in vivo experimental models (for extensive reviews see References 2 and 15). In brief, the early effects of ischemia are loss of resting membrane potential accompanied by slowing of upstroke velocity, loss of plateau amplitude, and shortening of APD. If ischemia continues these changes progress until loss of excitability occurs. Studies in patients using MAPs show qualitatively similar results[8-11] with a trend to a more rapid evolution in humans.[16] To illustrate the effects of regional ischemia on action potential repolarization, a record obtained from a patient undergoing angioplasty for a proximal left anterior descending coronary artery stenosis is shown in Figure 2. The angioplasty procedure involves the positioning of a balloon catheter within the lumen of the coronary artery at the site of a narrowing responsible for symptoms of angina. The balloon is then inflated for a period of between 1 and 3 minutes in order to stretch open the narrowed segment. During this time the artery is occluded and the myocardium served by the vessel is rendered ischemic. In this patient a MAP catheter electrode was positioned on the right ventricular anterior septal wall, i.e., in the area rendered ischemic during occlusion of the artery. During ischemia APD shortens progressively with loss of amplitude. At 2½ minutes the MAP shows marked shortening of APD and the cells generating these signals are probably close to the point of inexcitability. Immediately following defla-

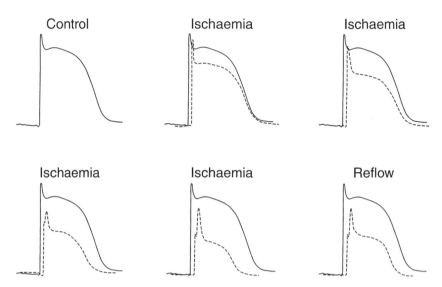

Figure 2. Monophasic action potential (MAP) from the endocardium in an area rendered ischemic during angioplasty of the left anterior descending coronary artery (see text). The control MAP (solid lines) and MAP during 1, 1½, 2, and 2½ minutes of ischemia and reflow (dotted lines) are superimposed, illustrating the progressive development of dispersion of repolarization between the normal and ischemic myocardium during the first minutes of ischemia.

tion of the balloon the MAP duration increases although the APD remains short. In this example comparison of the control MAPs with MAPs at 2½ minutes of ischemia shows reduction in APD at 90% repolarization from 270 ms to 180 ms. As there is no reason to suppose that APD in the nonischemic regions altered appreciably during ischemia, this would imply an APD difference of 90 ms between the ischemic and nonischemic territory. In the presence of alternans APD differences between ischemic and nonischemic regions alternate from beat to beat.[2,17] An example after 7 minutes of ischemia in an isolated perfused pig heart is shown in Figure 3. During ischemia (middle panel) the first action potential is small and the electrogram is monophasic, indicating the absence of local electrical activity. The second electrogram shows T wave inversion, indicating delayed local repolarization.

Influence of Local Conduction on the Timing of Action Potential Repolarization

As emphasized earlier and illustrated in Figure 3, the timing of repolarization at a given site is determined not only by the duration of the action potential but also by the time required for local activation.[18] Conduction slowing develops early during ischemia, initially mainly due to loss

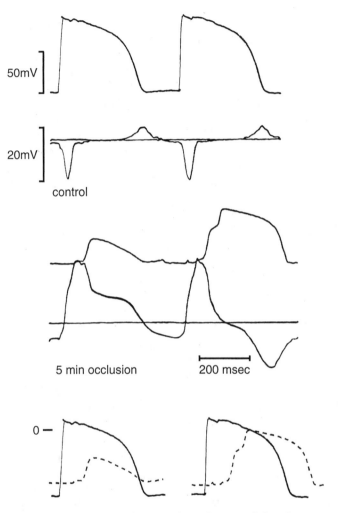

Figure 3. Transmembrane action potentials and extracellular electrograms from intact porcine heart under control conditions (**top**) and during ischemia (**middle**). Ischemia results in electrical alternans with alternating short and long action potentials. In the **bottom panel** the normal and ischemic action potentials are superimposed. The alternating action potential duration together with the activation delay during ischemia result in an alternation in the potential gradient during repolarization between normal and ischemic myocardium. Redrawn from Kléber AG et al; *Circ Res* 1978;42(5):603-613.

of inward current secondary to reduction in resting membrane potential and later, after approximately 10 to 15 minutes, also as a consequence of cell uncoupling (for review and discussion see References 2 and 15). Conduction delay is particularly marked on epicardium where activation is delayed relative to endocardium.[19-22] This has been attributed to either enhanced sensitivity of epicardium to ischemia or relative preservation of endocardium due to oxygenation from intracavity blood or electrotonic coupling to Purkinje fibers, which are more resistant to ischemia.[23] Studies in canines have shown that delay occurs mainly in the mid wall.[24] Recent work in humans confirms this finding and demonstrates an inhomogeneity that would be consistent with a role of anisotropy in the conduction delay.[25] A study was performed in humans in order to obtain some quantitative measure of the combined effects of conduction slowing across the ventricular wall and APD shortening on repolarization during the first few minutes of ischemia.[26] A MAP was recorded from the left ventricular epicardium in patients undergoing coronary artery surgery. During atrial pacing (normal endocardial to epicardial conduction and activation) transmural time was measured between an adjacent subendocardial plunge electrode and the MAP electrode. Conduction time was calculated as the interval between the dv/dtmin of the subendocardial electrogram and the dv/dtmax of the MAP upstroke. Once on cardiopulmonary bypass a 3-minute period of global ischemia was created using the procedure of cross-clamping the aorta between the input from the pump oxygenator and the coronary arteries routinely employed during the procedure to create a bloodless operating field. During ischemia the MAP showed the expected APD shortening (Fig. 4, top panel). Conduction time increased (Fig. 4, middle panel) thereby offsetting the effect of APD shortening on repolarization at the MAP electrode site (Fig. 4, bottom panel). These data relate only to the first 3 minutes of ischemia. More prolonged ischemia would be expected to be associated with further action potential and conduction changes occurring in a markedly inhomogeneous fashion.

Repolarization Gradients—Lateral or Transmural

In normal myocardium where cells are electrically and mechanically well coupled, steep repolarization gradients usually do not occur. Local electrotonic current flow exerts an averaging effect that tends to lengthen the shorter action potentials and shorten the longer action potentials.[27,28] It is nevertheless well known that during early ischemia, while cells remain well coupled, marked differences in APD develop. An example is shown in Figure 5 from a study that used floating microelectrodes on the epicardium in porcine hearts during regional ischemia and showed a range of action potentials from normal to very short.[1] Thus, the effects of ischemia clearly outweigh any electrotonic averaging effect, and substantial differences in APD develop both within the ischemic area and between the ischemic area surrounding normal myocardium. The situation within the ventricular wall is less clear. Cells isolated from subepicardial regions show a greater sensitivity to ischemic conditions than do subendocardial cells (Fig. 6).[12] However, the extent to which these differ-

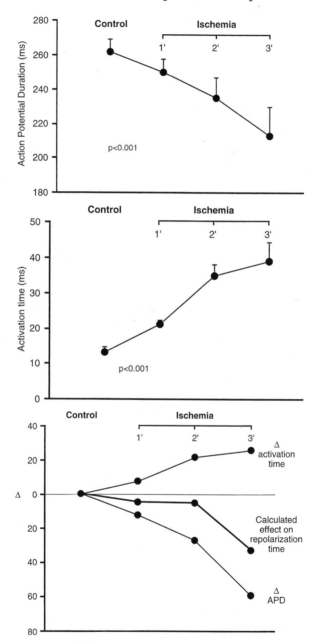

Figure 4. Epicardial monophasic action potential (MAP) recordings and transmural activation time from the left ventricular free wall in a patient during cardiac surgery. During a 3-minute period of global ischemia epicardial MAP duration shortens and transmural activation time increases. The activation delay offsets the effect of ischemia on the time of epicardial repolarization. From Reference 26.

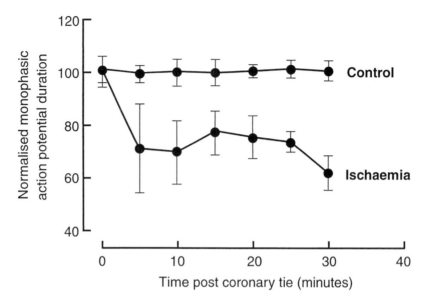

Figure 5. Changes in epicardial monophasic action potential (MAP) duration from an area of isolated ischemia and surrounding normal myocardium (control) in in situ porcine heart. MAP duration shortens in the ischemic area resulting in a repolarization gradient between the ischemic and surrounding myocardium. This gradient develops within the first few minutes of ischemia while intercellular coupling is maintained. From Murphy CF, Horner SM, Dick DJ, et al. Electrical alternans and the onset of rate-induced pulsus alternans during acute regional ischaemia in the anaesthetised pig heart. *Cardiovasc Res* 1996;32:138-147.

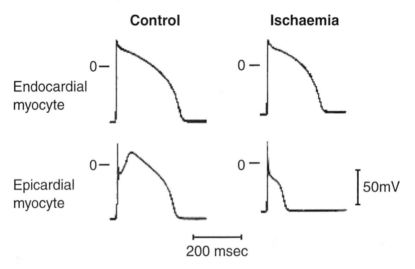

Figure 6. The effect of simulated ischemia on isolated myocytes from canine ventricle. The effect of ischemic conditions is much more profound on epicardial compared with endocardial myocytes. Redrawn from Reference 12.

ences become manifest in vivo may be influenced not only by electrotonic interaction but by several other factors.[13,29,30] During regional ischemia myocardial blood flow is redistributed in favor of the more epicardial regions.[31,32] The lower subendocardial perfusion, together with the greater intramyocardial tension within the subendocardial muscle layers, intensifies the ischemic burden in the subendocardium and reduces it subepicardially. In vivo studies during ischemia have yielded mixed results. One study on isolated cat ventricular wall showed greater APD shortening on epicardium compared with endocardium.[33] Electrograms obtained from plunge electrode recordings in porcine hearts showed similar changes and different intramyocardial depths in resting membrane potential and ST amplitude during regional ischemia.[34] It is a well-known clinical observation that acute episodes of regional ischemia for example during exercise are most commonly accompanied by ST depression in the ECG. On the basis of solid angle theory,[35] this is conventionally interpreted as indicating subendocardial ischemia and the ECG manifestation the result of electrophysiological gradients between the more ischemic subendocardial regions and the less or nonischemic subepicardial regions. This would imply that despite a greater sensitivity of the subepicardium to ischemia the effect in vivo is for dominant subendocardial electrophysiological changes. However, evidence has recently been presented indicating that the electrophysiological gradients giving rise to ST depression in regional ischemia are not parallel to the epicardium, as solid angle theory would predict, but occur at the lateral margins of the ischemic area.[36]

These findings question the interpretation of ST changes as indicating subendocardial ischemia and the existence of a transmural electrophysiological gradient in these patients. Thus, at present the orientation of electrophysiological gradients and dispersion of repolarization within the ventricular wall during ischemia is unclear.

QT Dispersion during Ischemia

QT dispersion provides a global measure of dispersion of repolarization. Several studies have used the approach to evaluate arrhythmia risk in patients with ischemic heart disease and in post myocardial infarction patients[37] (see sections in book). A recent study demonstrated the ability of QT dispersion to provide a dynamic measure of dispersion of repolarization, i.e., to register progressive changes in QT dispersion during the development of acute ischemia.[38] Patients with coronary disease were studied during an incremental pacing protocol. Following routine cardiac catheterization atrial pacing was established at just above the patient's intrinsic heart rate. Every 2 minutes the basic rate was increased by 10 beats per minute until either the onset of the patient's usual angina or the attainment of 110 beats per minute. QT dispersion was measured in the ECG with simultaneous 12-lead acquisition. Initial QT dispersion was 44 ms (39 to 49 95% CI), which was similar to QT dispersion in other reported patient studies under basal conditions (Fig. 7). During ischemia QT interval increased progressively to 82 ms (73 to 92 95% CI) at maximum. Patients undergoing cardiac catheterization for atypical chest pain in whom coronary artery anatomy and left ventricular function were shown to be normal constituted a control group. In this group QT dispersion did not change significantly during a similar pacing protocol. The increase in QT dispersion during pacing was related to the extent of the coronary artery disease. As shown in Figure 8, the extent of inducible QT dispersion during the incremental pacing was greater in patients with three vessel disease compared with patients with single vessel disease.

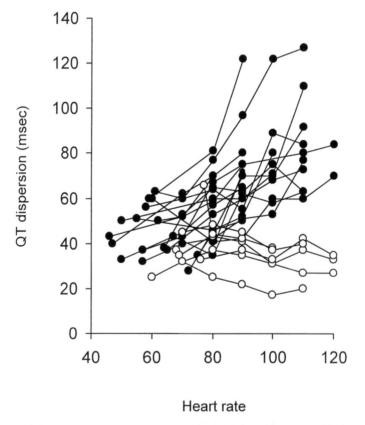

Figure 7. QT dispersion during an incremental atrial pacing protocol in individual patients with coronary artery disease (solid circles) and a control group (open circles). An increase in heart rate was accompanied by clinical evidence of ischemia and an increase in QT dispersion in the coronary artery disease group but no increase in QT dispersion in the control subjects. From Reference 38.

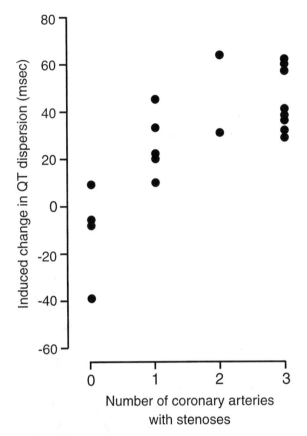

Figure 8. A greater increase in QT dispersion during an incremental atrial pacing protocol was seen in patients with three vessel coronary artery disease compared with patients with single vessel disease. From Reference 38.

Other studies of QT dispersion during acute ischemia in patients include patients undergoing coronary artery angioplasty. QT dispersion increased from control values 25±11 ms before balloon occlusion of the artery to 52±14 ms immediately following a 1-minute occlusion and from 43±20 ms to 61±19 ms at the end of a 2-minute occlusion of the artery.[39] The increase in QT dispersion was lessened progressively during repeated occlusions, a result arguably attributable to preconditioning.[40] Exercise on an ergometer increased QT dispersion from 61.5±5.2 ms to 94.5±7.8 ms in patients with coronary artery disease compared with a nonsignificant increase in a control group of patients from 45.2±5.0 ms to 50.7±4.5 ms.[41] A similar overall effect was obtained by Rankema et al[42] in patients during treadmill exercise. These authors demonstrated a blunting effect of beta blockade on the increase in QT dispersion during exercise in patients with coronary artery disease.[42] In the study by Lee et al,[41] dobutamine infusion increased QT dispersion in the patients with coronary artery disease from 57.2±4.9 ms to 109.4±10.1 ms compared with 58.0±4.3ms to 55.2±7.3 ms in a control group.

QT dispersion has recently been used to assess the effects of mental stress in patients with coronary artery disease.[43] Patients undergoing coronary angiography for chest pain were studied using a structured psychological stress protocol. The mental stress resulted in an increase in QT dispersion in patients with coronary artery disease that did not occur in patients with atypical chest pain and normal coronary artery anatomy (Fig. 9). Of particular interest is that no patient developed angina or ST segment evidence of ischemia in the ECG. This raises the question as to

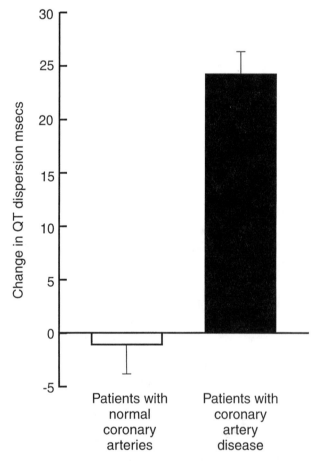

Figure 9. Mental stress induced by a structured interview resulted in an increase in QT dispersion in patients with coronary artery disease but not in persons with normal angiographic coronary anatomy and normal ventricular function. From Reference 43.

whether mental stress induced subclinical ischemia,[44] which was then sufficient to cause enhanced QT dispersion, or whether in these patients with ischemic heart disease the substrate is present that alters the electrophysiological response to mental stress.

Dispersion of Repolarization during Ischemia as a Measure of Dispersion of Refractoriness

Much of the importance attached to dispersion of repolarization centers on the relationship between repolarization and refractoriness in normal ventricular myocardium. In normal conditions recovery of excitability following excitation is largely voltage-dependent and is regained as the action potential repolarizes toward threshold voltage.[45] Refractoriness therefore approximates to the time of repolarization. As increased dispersion of refractoriness is well known to increase susceptibility to ventricular arrhythmias, therefore increased dispersion of repolarization provides a marker of enhanced susceptibility to arrhythmia.[46,47] However, as ischemia progresses, recovery of excitability becomes delayed beyond the time when repolarization is complete, due to the phenomenon of postrepolarization refractoriness.[1,48] Although studies of ischemia consistently show action potential shortening, the behavior of refractoriness is less clear. Some studies have reported that during ischemia refractory period shortens,[49-54] others that it lengthens,[55-57] and others that it shows a biphasic response.[57-59] It is likely that these differing results relate at least partly to the models of ischemia employed and to methodological problems inherent in measuring refractory periods in ischemia (see Reference 55 for discussion). Recent work in humans suggests that during global ischemia that might be expected to correspond to the center of an area of regional ischemia,[3] refractoriness prolongs and outlasts action potential repolarization as early as 1 to 2 minutes after the onset of ischemia.[26] In border zones refractory periods shorten, probably due to the diffusion of extracellular potassium and other metabolic products of ischemia.[55] Thus, although it is difficult to draw definite conclusions from the available data, it seems likely that the center of an ischemic zone or in global ischemia refractory periods prolong, and do so early in humans, whereas in the border zones refractory periods may shorten, possibly maintaining the relationship with APD. It is, however, evident that the interpretation of dispersion of refractoriness on the basis of measurements of repolarization during ischemia in quantitative terms may be inappropriate and is likely to be misleading. It may be that under ischemic conditions indices of repolarization such as QT dispersion nevertheless reflect dispersion of refractoriness. Further work is needed to clarify the relation between APD and refractoriness in the dynamic context of early ischemia.

References

1. Downar E, Janse MJ, Durrer D. The effect of acute coronary artery occlusion on subepicardial transmembrane potentials in the intact porcine heart. *Circulation* 1977:56:217-224.
2. Janse MJ, Wit AL. Electrophysiological mechanisms of ventricular arrhythmias resulting from myocardial ischaemia and infarction. *Physiol Rev* 1989: 69:1049-1169.
3. Coronel R, Fiolet JWT, Wilms-Schopman FJG, et al. Distribution of extracellular potassium and its relation to electrophysiologic changes during acute myocardial ischemia in the isolated perfused porcine heart. *Circulation* 1988;77: 1125-1138.
4. Rosenbaum DS, Kaplan DT, Kanai A, et al. Repolarization abnormalities in ventricular myocardium change dynamically with abrupt cycle length shortening. *Circulation* 1991;84:1333-1345.
5. Kingaby RO, Lab MJ, Cole AW, Palmer TN. Relation between monophasic action potential duration, ST segment elevation and regional myocardial blood flow after coronary occlusion in the pig. *Cardiovasc Res* 1986;20:740-751.
6. Taggart P, Sutton PMI, Spear DW, et al. Simultaneous endocardial and epicardial monophasic action potential recordings during brief periods of coronary artery ligation in the dog: Influence of adrenaline, beta blockade and alpha blockade. *Cardiovasc Res* 1988;12:900-909
7. Franz MR, Flaherty JT, Platia EV, et al. Localization of regional myocardial ischemia by recording monophasic action potentials. *Circulation* 1984;69: 593-604.
8. Taggart P, Sutton PMI, John R, et al. The epicardial electrogram: A quantitative assessment during balloon angioplasty incorporating monophasic action potential recordings. *Br Heart J* 1989;62:342-352.
9. John RM, Taggart PI, Sutton PM, et al. Direct effect of dobutamine on action potential duration in ischemic compared to normal areas in the human ventricle. *J Am Coll Cardiol* 1992;20:896-903.
10. Taggart P, Sutton PMI, Boyett MR, et al. Human ventricular action potential duration during short and long cycles. Rapid modulation by ischaemia. *Circulation* 1996;94:2526-2534.
11. Taggart P, Sutton P, Runnalls M, et al. Use of monophasic action potential recordings during routine coronary artery bypass surgery as an index of localised myocardial ischaemia. *Lancet* 1986;1:1462-1464.
12. Lucas A, Antzelevitch C. Differences in the electrophysiological response of canine ventricular epicardium and endocardium to ischemia: Role of the transient outward current. *Circulation* 1993;88:2903-2915.
13. Nabauer M. Electrical heterogeneity in the ventricular wall—and the M cell. *Cardiovasc Res* 1998;40:248-250.
14. Ejima J, Martin D, Engle C, et al. Ability of activation recovery intervals to assess action potential duration during no flow ischemia in the in situ porcine heart. *J Cardiovasc Electrophysiol* 1998;9:832-844.
15. Gettes LS, Cascio WE. Effect of acute ischaemia on cardiac electrophysiology. In Fozzard HA, Harber E, Jennings RB, et al (eds): *The Heart and Cardiovascular System.* 2nd ed. New York: Raven Press; 1992:2021-2054.
16. Coronel R, Opthof T, Taggart P, et al. Differential electrophysiology of repolarisation from clone to clinic. *Cardiovasc Res* 1997;33:503-517.

17. Dilly SG, Lab MJ. Electrophysiological alternans and restitution during acute regional ischaemia in myocardium of anaesthetised pig. *J Physiol (Lond)* 1988;402:315-333.
18. Kuo CS, Amlie JP, Munakata K, et al. Dispersion of monophasic action potential durations and activation times during atrial pacing, ventricular pacing and ventricular stimulation in canine ventricles. *Cardiovasc Res* 1983;17:152-161.
19. Cox JL, Daniel TM, Boineau JP. The electrophysiologic time course of acute myocardial ischemia and the effects of early coronary artery reperfusion. *Circulation* 1973;48:971-983.
20. Williams DO, Scherlag BJ, Hope RR, et al. The pathophysiology of malignant ventricular arrhythmias during acute myocardial ischemia. *Circulation* 1974;50:1163-1172.
21. Elharrar V, Gaum WE, Zipes DP. Effect of drugs on conduction delay and incidence of ventricular arrhythmias induced by acute coronary occlusion in dogs. *Am J Cardiol* 1977;39:544-549.
22. Ruffy R, Lovelace DE, Mueller TM, et al. Relationship between changes in left ventricular bipolar electrograms and regional myocardial blood flow during acute coronary occlusion in the dog. *Circ Res* 1979;45:764-770.
23. Antzelevitch C, Litofsky SH, Lukas A. Epicardium versus endocardium: Electrophysiology and pharmacology. In Zipes DP, Jalife J (eds): *Cardiac Electrophysiology: From Cell to Bedside*. Philadelphia: W.B. Saunders Co.; 1990:386-395.
24. Arenal A, Villemaire C, Nattel S. Mechanism of selective epicardial activation delay during acute myocardial ischemia in dogs. *Circulation* 1993;88(Pt. 1):2381-2388.
25. Taggart P, Sutton PMI, Opthof T, et al. Early onset of stepwise transmural activation delay in patients with coronary heart disease during ischemia. *Circulation* 1998;98(suppl):I817.
26. Sutton PMI, Taggart P, Opthof T, et al. Ischaemia delays epicardial activation on human epicardium: Is this pro-arrhythmic or anti-arrhythmic? *J Physiol (Lond)* 1999;518P:16P.
27. Hoffman BF. Electrotonic modulation of the T wave. *Am J Cardiol* 1982;50:361-362.
28. Moe GK. Oscillating concepts in arrhythmia research. A personal account. *Int J Cardiol* 1984;5:109-113.
29. Anyukhovsky EP, Sosunov EA, Gainullin RZ, Rosen MR. The controversial M cell. *J Cardiovasc Electrophysiol* 1999;10:244-260.
30. Antzelevitch C, Shimizu W, Yan G-X, et al. The M cell: Its contribution to the ECG and to normal electrical function of the heart. *J Cardiovasc Electrophysiol* 1999;10:1124-1152.
31. Griggs DM, Nakamura Y. Effect of coronary constriction on myocardial distribution of iodantipyrine-I[131]. *Am J Physiol* 1968;215:1082-1086.
32. Bache RJ, McHale PA, Greenfield JC Jr. Transmural myocardial perfusion during restricted coronary inflow in the awake dog. *Am J Physiol* 1977;332:H645-H651.
33. Kimura S, Bassett AL, Kohya T, et al. Simultaneous recording of action potentials from endocardium and epicardium during ischemia in the isolated cat ventricle: Relation of temporal electrophysiologic heterogeneities to arrhythmias. *Circulation* 1986;74:401-409.
34. Janse MJ, Cinca J, Morena H, et al. The '"border zone"' in myocardial ischemia. An electrophysiological, metabolic and histochemical correlation in the pig heart. *Circ Res* 1978;44:576-588.

35. Holland RP, Arnsdorf MF. Solid angle theory and the electrocardiogram: Physiologic and quantitative interpretations. *Prog Cardiovasc Dis* 1977;19:431-455.
36. Li D, Li CY, Yong AC, Kilpatrick D. Source of electrocardiographic ST changes in subendocardial ischemia. *Circ Res* 1998;82:957-970.
37. Higham PD, Furniss SS, Campbell RWF. QT dispersion and components of the QT interval in ischaemia and infarction. *Br Heart J* 1995;73:32-36.
38. Sporton SC, Taggart P, Sutton PM, et al. Acute ischaemia: A dynamic influence on QT dispersion. *Lancet* 1997;349:306-309.
39. Tarabey R, Sukenik D, Molnar J, Somberg J. Effect of intracoronary balloon inflation at percutaneous transluminal coronary angioplasty on QT dispersion. *Am Heart J* 1998;135:519-522.
40. Okishige K, Yamashita K, Yoshinaga H, et al. Electrophysiologic effects of ischemic preconditioning on QT dispersion during coronary angioplasty. *J Am Coll Cardiol* 1996;28:70-73.
41. Lee HS, Cross SJ, Rowles J, Jennings KP. QT dispersion in patients with coronary artery disease—effect of exercise, dobutamine and dipyridamole myocardial stress. *Br Heart J* 1994;71(suppl 5):98.
42. Rankema G, Singh JP, Meijs M, et al. Effect of exercise-induced ischemia on QT interval dispersion. *Am Heart J* 1998;135:88-92.
43. James R, Taggart P, Jeeves R, et al. Acute psychological stress and the propensity to ventricular arrhythmias: Evidence for a linking mechanism. *Eur Heart J* 2000;21:1023-1028.
44. Deanfield JE, Shea M, Kennett M, et al. Silent myocardial ischaemia due to mental stress. *Lancet* 1984;2:1001-1005.
45. Hoffman BF, Cranefield PF. *Electrophysiology of the Heart.* New York: McGraw Hill; 1960.
46. Han J, Moe GK. Nonuniform recovery of excitability of ventricular muscle. *Circ Res* 1964;14:44-60.
47. Kuo CS, Manakata K, Reddy CP, Surawicz B. Characteristics and possible mechanism of ventricular arrhythmia dependent on the dispersion of action potential duration. *Circulation* 1983;67:1356-1367.
48. El-Sherif N, Scherlag BJ, Lazzara R, Samet P. Pathophysiology of tachycardia- and bradycardia-dependent block in the canine proximal His-Purkinje system after acute myocardial ischemia. *Am J Cardiol* 1974;33:529-540.
49. Elharrar V, Foster PR, Jirak TL, et al. Alterations in canine myocardial excitability during ischemia. *Circ Res* 1977;40:98-105.
50. Kuppersmith J, Antman EM, Hoffman BF. In vivo electrophysiological effects of lidocaine in canine acute myocardial infarction. *Circ Res* 1975;36:84-91.
51. Ramanathan KB, Bodenheimer M, Banka VS, Helfant RH. Electrophysiological effects of partial coronary occlusions and reperfusion. *Am J Cardiol* 1977;40:50-54.
52. Batsford WPD, Cannon DS, Zaret BI. Relationship between ventricular refractoriness and regional myocardial blood flow after acute coronary occlusion. *Am J Cardiol* 1978;41:1083-1088.
53. Stewart JR, Burmeister WE, Burmeister J, Luccest BR. Electrophysiologic and antiarrhythmic effects of phentolamine in experimental coronary artery occlusion and reperfusion in the dog. *J Cardiovasc Pharmacol* 1980;2:77-81.
54. Wolk R, Cobbe SM, Hicks MN, Kane KA. Effects of lignocaine on dispersion of repolarisation and refractoriness in a working rabbit heart model of regional myocardial ischaemia. *J Cardiovasc Pharmacol* 1998;31:253-261.

55. Janse MJ, Capucci A, Coronel R, Fabius MAW. Variability in recovery of excitability in the normal canine and the ischemic porcine heart. *Eur Heart J* 1985;6(suppl D):41-52.
56. Horacek T, Neumann M, Van Mutius S, Meesmann W. Nonhomogeneous electrophysiological changes and the bimodal distribution of early ventricular arrhythmias during acute coronary occlusion. *Basic Res Cardiol* 1984;79:649-667.
57. Russell DG, Oliver MF. Ventricular refractoriness during acute myocardial ischaemia and its relationship to ventricular fibrillation. *Cardiovasc Res* 1978;12:221-227.
58. Penny WJ. The deleterious effects of myocardial catecholamines on cellular electrophysiology and arrhythmias during ischaemia and reperfusion. *Eur Heart J* 1984;55:960-973.
59. Gilmour RF, Zipes DP. Different electrophysiological responses of canine endocardium and epicardium to combined hyperkalemia, hypoxia and acidosis. *Circ Res* 1980;46:814-825.

14

Dispersion of Repolarization in Patients with Dilated Cardiomyopathy

Wolfram Grimm, Katrin Leuchtenberger, and Bernhard Maisch

The prognosis of patients with idiopathic dilated cardiomyopathy (IDC) is poor despite the introduction of vasodilator drugs. Reported annual mortality rates range between 5% and 45% depending on patient selection and severity of the disease.[1-3] In up to 50% of patients with IDC, death is sudden, presumably caused by rapid ventricular tachycardia (VT), ventricular fibrillation (VF), primary bradyarrhythmias, or electromechanical dissociation.[1-7] Implantable cardioverter-defibrillator (ICD) therapy has recently been shown to be superior to antiarrhythmic drugs for increasing overall survival in patients with VF or symptomatic VT.[8] Furthermore, prophylactic ICD therapy has been demonstrated to improve survival in selected postinfarct patients with a left ventricular (LV) ejection fraction ≤35%, nonsustained VT on Holter, and inducible, nonsuppressible VT on electrophysiological study.[9] In contrast to postinfarct patients, no consensus exists on how to select asymptomatic patients with dilated cardiomyopathy for prophylactic ICD implantation. A recent study at our institution did not show VT or VF inducibility during electrophysiological study to be helpful for arrhythmia prediction in IDC.[10] To date, a variety of noninvasive methods have been proposed for arrhythmia risk stratification in IDC including the degree of LV dysfunction, ventricular arrhythmias on Holter, abnormal findings by signal-averaged ECG, changes in autonomic tone as indexed by heart rate variability and baroreflex sensitivity, microvolt T wave alternans, and dispersion of ventricu-

This work was supported in part by a grant from the German Science Foundation.

From Olsson SB, Amlie JP, Yuan S (eds): *Dispersion of Ventricular Repolarization: State of the Art.* ©Futura Publishing Company, Inc., Armonk, NY, 2000.

lar repolarization. Increased QT dispersion, measured as interlead variability of QT intervals in the 12-lead surface ECG, has been evaluated as a noninvasive tool to predict life-threatening ventricular arrhythmias and sudden death in a variety of clinical settings including idiopathic long QT syndrome, remote myocardial infarction, hypertension, mixed patient populations with heart failure, as well as patients with amiodarone therapy or ICD therapy.[11-17] To date, however, only very limited data are available about the clinical significance of an increased dispersion of repolarization in patients with dilated cardiomyopathy.

Design and Results of the Marburg Cardiomyopathy Pilot Study from 1992 to 1995

Patient Characteristics and Control Group

From December 1992 until August 1995, 107 patients with IDC (26 women) were prospectively enrolled in this study at our institution.[18] The mean age was 50 ± 12 years and the mean LV ejection fraction was $31 \pm 15\%$. All patients with IDC met the following inclusion criteria: 1) LV ejection fraction $\leq 50\%$ without greater than 50% stenosis of any major coronary branch during cardiac catheterization; 2) LV enlargement by angiography and echocardiography; and 3) absence of valvular heart disease, systemic hypertension, or other conditions known to cause cardiomyopathy.[19] Patients were excluded if they had atrial fibrillation or pacemaker dependency, electrolyte imbalance, Class I or Class III antiarrhythmic drug treatment, New York Heart Association (NYHA) Class IV, cancer, or renal failure requiring hemodialysis. The control group consisted of 100 subjects (33 women, 67 men, age: 50 ± 13 years) without structural heart disease to provide information on QT dispersion in normal individuals with an age and sex comparable to that of the IDC population.

Analysis of QT and QTc Dispersion Using a High-Resolution Digitizer

In the Marburg Cardiomyopathy Pilot Study,[18] QT intervals and R-R intervals in all leads of the standard 12-lead electrocardiogram (ECG), which was recorded at a paper speed of 50 mm/s were measured routinely in three consecutive beats by one observer using a high-resolution digitizer (SummaSketch III, Summagraphics, London, Great Britain) connected to a 486 personal computer. Rate-corrected QT (QTc) was then automatically calculated using Bazett's formula. The investigator was blinded with respect to the patient to which the ECG under analysis belonged. QT intervals were measured from the beginning of the Q wave to the return of the T wave to the isoelectric line in each lead, in which the end of the T wave could be discerned. In the presence of a U wave, the end of the T wave was defined as the intersection of the tangent to the repolarization slope with the isoelectric line (Fig. 1). QT intervals could be measured in a mean of 10 ± 2 leads per 12-lead standard ECG in this study (range: 5 to 12 leads). Repeated measurement of QT dispersion of 50 randomly chosen 12-lead ECGs from patients with IDC showed a nonsignificant intraobserver variability of QT dispersion of 8 ± 7 ms (range 1 to 31 ms).

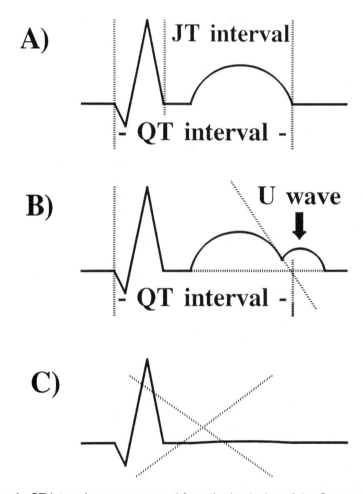

Figure 1. QT intervals were measured from the beginning of the Q wave to the return of the T wave to the isoelectric line in each lead, in which the end of the T wave could be discerned (**A**). In the presence of a U wave, the end of the T wave was defined as the intersection of the tangent to the repolarization slope with the isoelectric line (**B**). If the end of the T wave could not be determined properly, this lead was excluded from analysis (**C**).

QT Dispersion in IDC without Bundle Branch Block Compared with Controls

The results of QT dispersion measurements in patients with IDC without bundle branch block versus healthy controls are summarized in Table 1. As a result, heart rate, QTc intervals, QT dispersion, QTc dispersion, and adjusted QTc dispersion were all found to be significantly increased in patients with IDC compared with healthy controls.

Relation between QT Dispersion and Major Arrhythmic Events during Follow-up

During 13±7 months of follow-up, major arrhythmic events occurred in 12 of 107 study patients with IDC (11%) including sudden deaths in 5 patients, sustained VT in 1 patient, and appropriate ICD shocks for VT or VF in 6 patients, in whom prophylactic ICD implantation had been performed at study entry. The relation between QT dispersion measurements at study entry and major arrhythmic events during follow-up is summarized in Table 2. QT dispersion was increased in patients with arrhythmic events compared with patients without arrhythmic events during follow-up (76±17 versus 60±26 ms; P=0.03). QTc dispersion and adjusted QTc dispersion, however, were not significantly different between patients with and without major arrhythmic events during follow-up (Table 2). The considerable overlap of QT dispersion and QTc dispersion in patients with and without major arrhythmic events is shown in Figure 2. Of note, patients with major arrhythmic events also had a lower LV ejection fraction compared with patients without arrhythmic events (25±8 versus 32±10%; P<0.05). There was no significant difference in the remaining clinical variables including age, gender, and treatment for heart failure between patients with and without arrhythmic events during follow-up.[18]

Table 1
QT Dispersion in Dilated Cardiomyopathy Compared with Controls

	Dilated Cardiomyopathy	Controls	P Value
Patients (n)	76*	100	
RR interval (ms)	715±163	867±150	<0.01
Mean QT interval (ms)	382±49	396±32	0.03
Mean QTc interval (ms)	455±35	427±21	<0.01
QT dispersion (ms)	57±25	41±11	<0.01
QTc dispersion (ms)	71±34	46±11	<0.01
Adjusted QTc dispersion (ms)	24±11	14±3	<0.01

*After exclusion of patients with bundle branch block (QRS≥120 ms).

Table 2
Relation Between QT Dispersion and Arrhythmic Events during Follow-Up

	Arrhythmic Events	Arrhythmia-Free	P Value
All 107 study pateints (n)	**12**	**95**	
R-R interval (ms)	698±96	725±160	ns
QT dispersion (ms)	76±17	60±26	0.03
QTc dispersion (ms)	86±22	75±35	0.18
Adjusted QTc dispersion (ms)	27±6	24±10	ns
Patients without BB block (n)	**8**	**68**	
R-R interval (ms)	680±69	719±171	ns
QT dispersion (ms)	78±17	55±25	0.01
QTc dispersion (ms)	84±24	71±35	0.19
Adjusted QTc dispersion (ms)	27±6	24±11	ns

BB block = bundle branch block.

Interpretation of the Results of the Marburg Cardiomyopathy Pilot Study[18]

Similar to previous studies in patients with any form of cardiac disease, we were not surprised to find a significant increase in QT dispersion, QTc dispersion, and adjusted QTc dispersion in patients with IDC compared with 100 age- and sex-matched healthy control subjects. QT dispersion was increased in patients with arrhythmic events compared with patients without arrhythmic events during follow-up. Measures of QTc dispersion and adjusted QTc dispersion between patients with IDC with and without arrhythmic events, however, failed to reach statistical significance in this study. Thus, although QT dispersion was increased in patients with IDC and arrhythmic events during follow-up, its clinical usefulness for risk stratification appears to be very limited due to the large overlap of QT dispersion between patients with and without arrhythmic events (Fig. 2). Of note, QT dispersion analysis in the Marburg Cardiomyopathy Pilot Study had several important limitations. Similar to previous studies, the 12-lead ECGs in this study were recorded with a Siemens Mingograph, which was able to record only six leads simultaneously, usually the six limb leads followed by the six chest leads. Ideally, one would like to have an ECG with all 12 standard leads recorded simultaneously for QT dispersion analysis. In addition, QT and R-R intervals in the present study were measured using a digitizer connected to a personal computer. Although QT dispersion measurement with a high-resolution digitizer board had an acceptable nonsignificant intraobserver variability of 8±7 ms in our study, this method is very time consuming and probably less accurate than newer methods that are based on computerized measurements of scanned and enlarged 12-lead ECGs. Although great care was taken to use consistent criteria to define the end of the QT

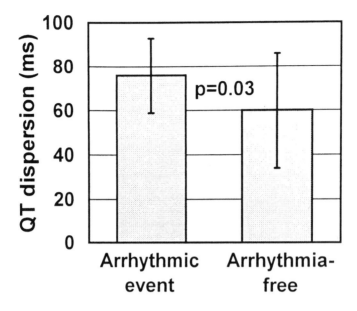

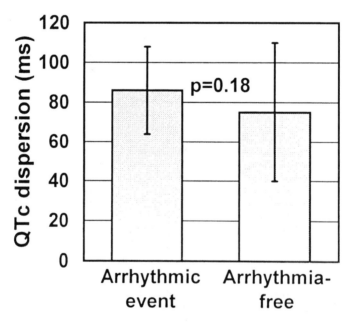

Figure 2. QT and QTc dispersion in patients with idiopathic dilated cardiomyopathy with and without arrhythmic events during 13±7 months prospective follow-up.

interval by a single experienced observer as described above, the lack of a uniformly accepted definition of the end of the QT interval remains a limitation of any study dealing with QT dispersion measurements. It is of note, however, that this study has been conducted prospectively and that all measurements have been performed by a single observer who was blinded with respect to the patient to which the ECG under analysis belonged.

Design and First Results of the Marburg Cardiomyopathy Study[20]

The Marburg Cardiomyopathy Study (MACAS) is a prospective observational study that was started in 1996, supported by a grant from the German Science Foundation. The purpose of MACAS is to determine the value of the following potential noninvasive arrhythmia risk predictors in at least 200 patients with IDC with a mean follow-up of 5 years: NYHA functional class, LV ejection fraction, LV end-diastolic diameter determined by echocardiography, left bundle branch block and atrial fibrillation on ECG, rate-corrected QT/JT dispersion on 12-lead ECG, signal-averaged ECG, ventricular arrhythmias and heart rate variability on 24-hour digital Holter ECG recordings, baroreflex sensitivity, and microvolt T wave alternans. Of note, MACAS will also comprise a control group of 100 age- and sex-matched healthy volunteers in order to be able to determine how many "false positive results" can be expected when performing such a comprehensive noninvasive arrhythmia risk stratification. Primary endpoints in MACAS are total mortality and major arrhythmic events defined as sustained VT or VF or sudden cardiac death. Until January 1999, a total of 156 patients with dilated cardiomyopathy and sinus rhythm were enrolled in MACAS (Fig. 3). Forty-four patients were women (28%) with a mean age of 47 ± 12 years and a LV ejection fraction of $31\pm10\%$.

Analysis of Ventricular Repolarization in MACAS

In contrast to the Marburg Cardiomyopathy Pilot Study described above, all QTc and JTc dispersion measurements were performed using high-quality laser-printed ECGs (600 dpi) with all standard 12-leads recorded simultaneously with the Cambridge Heart system CH 2000 at a paper speed of 50 mm/s. Instead of using a high-resolution digitizer board as in the MACAS Pilot Study, all ECG recordings in MACAS were scanned directly with a resolution of 1200×1200 dpi into commercially available graphics software (Corel Photo Paint for Windows 95) using an IBM personal computer with a Pentium II processor. Then, the scanned 12-lead ECG was displayed on a 21-inch high-resolution computer screen

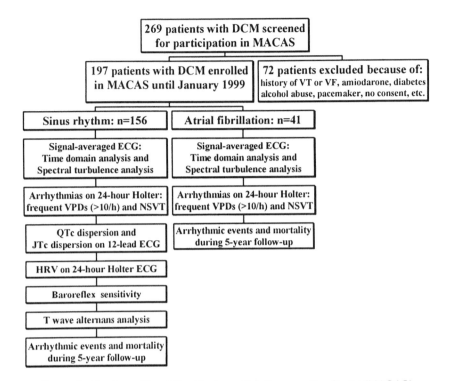

Figure 3. Study profile of the Marburg Cardiomyopathy Study (MACAS).

in order to perform computer-assisted repolarization measurements with manual correction by two experienced observers who were completely unaware of the clinical characteristics of the patients. By using this software, the size of any chosen QRS complex and T wave beat could be magnified as much as needed on the 21-inch screen in order to facilitate determination of the shortest and longest QT interval as well as JT interval in any of the 12 leads, in which the end of the T wave could be discerned as shown in Figure 1. Preliminary results of QT and JT dispersion analysis in MACAS are summarized in Table 3.

Clinical Implications of the Results of MACAS

The prognostic significance of the findings in MACAS will be determined by multivariate Cox analysis at the end of 5-year follow-up (toward the end of the year 2003).[20] The results of MACAS will have important implications for the design of future trials to evaluate the role of prophylactic ICD therapy in asymptomatic patients with idiopathic dilated cardiomyopathy.

Table 3
QT Dispersion in the Marburg Cardiomyopathy Study (MACAS)

	All patients	BB block	No BB block
Patients (n)	156	58	98
R-R interval (ms)	700±145	664±123	721±153*
Uncorrected QT values (ms)			
Minimum QT interval	354±42	371±39	344±41*
Maximum QT interval	399±45	419±40	388±44*
QT dispersion	45±18	47±17	44±17
Uncorrected JT values (ms)			
Minimum JT interval	234±37	217±31	243±37*
Maximum JT interval	279±39	265±32	287±41*
JT dispersion	46±17	48±18	44±17
Rate corrected QT values[#] (ms)			
Minimum QTc interval	426±42	458±38	407±32*
Maximum QTc interval	481±43	517±36	460±30*
QTc dispersion	55±21	59±22	52±19
Rate corrected JT values[#] (ms)			
Minimum JTc interval	280±32	268±30	288±31*
Maximum Jc interval	335±39	327±28	340±29*
JTc dispersion	55±20	59±21	53±19

*$P<0.05$ for patients with versus patients without bundle branch block (BB block).
[#]According to Bazett's formula.

References

1. Fuster V, Gersh BJ, Guilani ER, et al. The natural history of idiopathic dilated cardiomyopathy. *Am J Cardiol* 1981;47:525-531.
2. Anderson KP, Freedman RA, Mason JW. Sudden death in idiopathic dilated cardiomyopathy. *Ann Intern Med* 1987;107:104-106.
3. Stevenson LW, Fowler MB, Schroeder JS, et al. Poor survival of patients considered too well for transplantation. *Am J Med* 1987;83:871-876.
4. Tamburro P, Wilber D. Sudden death in idiopathic dilated cardiomyopathy. *Am Heart J* 1992;124:1035-1045.
5. Sugrue DD, Rodeheffer RJ, Codd MB, et al. The clinical course of idiopathic dilated cardiomyopathy. *Ann Intern Med* 1992;117:117-123.
6. Redfield MM, Gersh BJ, Bailey KR, et al. Natural history of idiopathic dilated cardiomyopathy: Effect of referral bias and secular trend. *J Am Coll Cardiol* 1993;22:1921-1926.
7. Luu M, Stevenson WG, Stevenson LW, et al. Diverse mechanisms of unexpected cardiac arrest in advanced heart failure. *Circulation* 1989;80:1675-1680.
8. The Antiarrhythmics Versus Implantable Defibrillators (AVID) Investigators. A comparison of antiarrhythmic-drug therapy with implantable defibrillators in patients resuscitated from near-fatal ventricular arrhythmias. *N Engl J Med* 1997;337:1576-1583.
9. Moss AJ, Hall J, Cannom DS, et al for the Multicenter Automatic Defibrillator Implantation Trial Investigators. Improved survival with an implanted defibrillator in patients with coronary disease at high risk for ventricular arrhythmia. *N Engl J Med* 1996;335:1933-1940.

10. Grimm W, Hoffmann J, Menz V, et al. Programmed ventricular stimulation for arrhythmia risk prediction in patients with idiopathic dilated cardiomyopathy and nonsustained ventricular tachycardia. *J Am Coll Cardiol* 1998;32:739-745.
11. Priori SG, Napolitano C, Diehl L, Schwartz PJ. Dispersion of the QT interval: A marker of therapeutic efficacy in the idiopathic long QT syndrome. *Circulation* 1994;89:1681-1689.
12. Barr CS, Naas A, Freemann M, et al. QT dispersion and sudden unexpected death in chronic heart failure. *Lancet* 1994;343:327-329.
13. Glancy JM, Garratt CJ, Woods KL, deBono DP. QT dispersion and mortality after myocardial infarction. *Lancet* 1995;354:945-948.
14. Perkiömäki JS, Koistinen J, Yli-Mayry S, Huikuri HV. Dispersion of QT interval in patients with and without susceptibility to ventricular tachyarrhythmias after previous myocardial infarction. *J Am Coll Cardiol* 1995;26:174-179.
15. Grimm W, Steder U, Menz V, Maisch B. Predictive value of QT dispersion for ventricular tachyarrhythmias in patients with implantable cardioverter-defibrillator. *Ann Noninvas Electrocardiol* 1996;1:419-422.
16. Grimm W, Steder U, Menz V, et al. Effect of amiodarone on QT dispersion in the 12-lead standard electrocardiogram and its significance for subsequent arrhythmic events. *Clin Cardiol* 1997;20:107-110.
17. Zabel M, Klingenheben T, Franz MR, Hohnloser SH. Assessment of QT dispersion for prediction of mortality or arrhythmic events after myocardial infarction. *Circulation* 1998;97:2543-2550.
18. Grimm W, Steder U, Menz V, et al. QT dispersion and arrhythmic events in idiopathic dilated cardiomyopathy. *Am J Cardiol* 1996;78:458-461.
19. Richardson P, McKenna W, Bristow M, et al. Report of the 1995 World Health Organization/International Society and Federation of Cardiology Task Force on the Definition and Classification of Cardiomyopathies. *Circulation* 1996;93:841-842.
20. Grimm W, Glaveris C, Hoffmann J, et al. Noninvasive arrhythmia risk stratification in idiopathic dilated cardiomyopathy—Design and first results of the Marburg Cardiomyopathy Study. *PACE* 1998;21(Pt. II):2551-2556.

15

Dispersion of Repolarization in Patients with Hypertension

Juha S. Perkiömäki

Introduction

Hypertension is a very common disease. The reported prevalence rates vary depending on the definitions used and the populations studied. Hypertension affects approximately 20% to 25% of the adult population.[1,2] It may alter the dispersion of cardiac repolarization in many ways. Elevated blood pressure per se may increase the signs of inhomogeneity of repolarization.[3,4] Left ventricular hypertrophy (LVH) has been detected echocardiographically in 12% to 20%,[5,6] 50%,[7] and almost 90%[8] of patients with hypertension, depending on the severity of the disease and the population studied, and it is a major determinant of the dispersion of ventricular repolarization in hypertension. Furthermore, long-standing hypertension may potentiate atherosclerosis[9-11] and thereby aggravate coronary artery disease or lead to heart failure[12,13] and stroke,[14] which may all contribute to the heterogeneity of repolarization in patients with hypertensive disease.[15-22]

It has been suggested that ventricular arrhythmias play an important role in the occurrence of sudden death in hypertensive patients with LVH,[23] but there has been some controversy about this.[24,25] Increased dispersion of repolarization favors the genesis of ventricular arrhythmias,[26-29] which may be one mechanism of sudden death in hypertensive patients with LVH.

Dispersion of Repolarization and Refractoriness

Cellular repolarization is a complex cascade of different ion currents, of which the various voltage-dependent potassium currents are the most

From Olsson SB, Amlie JP, Yuan S (eds): *Dispersion of Ventricular Repolarization: State of the Art.* ©Futura Publishing Company, Inc., Armonk, NY, 2000.

important. One of them, the transient outward potassium current (I_{to}), plays a crucial role in the early phases of repolarization (phase 1 of the action potential) and in setting the voltage of the plateau phase. After its beginning, repolarization is interrupted by an inward calcium current and a persisting inward sodium current, resulting in the plateau phase of the action potential. McDonald and Trautwein[30,31] described the kinetics of the delayed rectifier K current (I_K) in cat papillary muscles, and their results were supplemented by Kleiman and Houser,[32] who found a negative-slope region in the current-voltage relationship of the inward rectifier K current (I_{K1}) in feline myocytes. I_{K1} contributes to the terminal phase of repolarization and the resting membrane potential. The action of the ionic pumps makes the whole process self-regenerating.[33]

The dispersion of refractoriness parallels the dispersion of repolarization in a normal myocardium, but not in a diseased or pharmacologically altered myocardium, where it lags behind the end of repolarization; this is known as postrepolarization refractoriness.[34] The risk of cardiac arrhythmias increases when the dispersion of repolarization in the myocardium increases.[26-29] Ventricular tachyarrhythmias caused by a reentrant mechanism require the presence of nonhomogenous conduction, nonhomogenous refractoriness, or both.[29] The role of increased dispersion of repolarization in the genesis of torsade de pointes ventricular tachycardia and ventricular fibrillation has been well recognized. Furthermore, the data suggest that increased dispersion of repolarization is an important factor in the genesis of monomorphic ventricular tachycardia.[35]

The current methods of measuring the recovery time dispersion (i.e., the epicardial or endocardial monophasic action potentials) and body surface mapping are useful in research work but are not very practicable in routine clinical use. Increased evidence supports the assumption that QT dispersion reflects local differences in repolarization and the recovery time of the myocardium.[36-40]

Dispersion of Repolarization in Hypertension and Myocardial Hypertrophy

Data on the dispersion of repolarization in patients with hypertension before the development of hypertrophy are very sparse. It is known that changes in blood pressure and fast-developing hypertension are arrhythmogenic factors.[41-43] Animal tests have mainly been done to evaluate the influence of myocardial hypertrophy, induced by renal hypertension or some other condition, on the dispersion of repolarization by comparing hypertrophied hearts with normotensive hearts. Such studies have given a lot of valuable information on the changes of the repolarization process in hypertensive hypertrophied hearts, but only scant information on the influence of hypertension per se without hypertrophy on the dispersion of repolarization. However, it should be borne in mind that cardiac hypertrophy is a continuous process, which begins in hypertensive disease long before the criteria of hypertrophy are fulfilled. For example, asymmetric left ventricular remodeling due to isolated relative septal thickening has been found to be common in untreated hypertensive subjects with normal left ventricular mass.[44] The findings on hypertensive patients suggest that electrical changes in the left ventricular myocardium (as determined by QT dispersion measurement) may precede structural and morphological abnormalities.[3] However, much more is known of the dispersion of repolarization in myocardial hypertrophy.

Experimental Data

Myocardial hypertrophy causes abnormalities in ion channels and currents. The precise importance of the changes of different ion currents relative to each other in disturbing repolarization has not, however, been fully established.[45] At any rate, it is clear that these changes in ion channels and currents are among the basic factors contributing to the altered repolarization in LVH. In general, action potential is prolonged in a hypertrophied myocardium.[45] This prolongation may be inhomogeneous in different areas, resulting in heterogeneity of repolarization.

In hypertrophied rat hearts, a decrease in I_{to} appears to be one cause of prolongation of the action potential.[46,47] In an experiment with cats, LVH was shown to have a pronounced effect on the dispersion of refractoriness and repolarization and to favor vulnerability to ventricular fibrillation. Blockade of the voltage-dependent potassium channel, but not the slow inward calcium channel, narrowed the dispersion of recovery of excitability and protected against ventricular fibrillation.[48] Interestingly, in feline myocytes isolated from a hypertrophied right ventricle, the magnitude of the I_K was found to be decreased, which may contribute to the prolongation of the action potential duration. In addition, the magnitude of the I_{K1} was found to be increased, suggesting that the prolongation of the action potential duration cannot be explained by changes in this component of the cell current.[32] In accordance with these data, the peak amplitude of I_{K1} was observed to be increased in cells from cat papillary muscles obtained from hypertrophied right ventricles.[49] On the contrary, the results of the study on the electrophysiological characteristics of left ventricular myocytes isolated from spontaneously hypertensive rats suggested that the reduced I_{K1} density leads to a lower outward repolarizing current via the inward rectifier and to an observable prolongation of the action potential. Furthermore, there was no detectable difference in the transient outward potassium current, the delayed rectifier potassium current, or the magnitude of the L-type calcium current.[50] However, in a work with cats, regional electrophysiological disparities induced by LVH in the anterior papillary muscle were subsequently reduced by vera-pamil.[51] In congruence with this finding, it has been suggested that abnormalities of the slow inward Ca current may contribute to the prolongation of the action potential duration in cardiac hypertrophy.[52] There is some evidence that the sodium-calcium exchange activity is altered in sarcolemmal vesicles from hypertrophied rat hearts,[53] and changes in the currents generated by sodium-calcium exchange may play an important role in alterations of the action potential duration in cardiac hypertrophy.

Generally speaking, ischemia abbreviates the refractory period in the affected area of the myocardium[26] and may thus cause inhomogeneity of repolarization. Furthermore, cardiac hypertrophy favors ischemia. Although hypertrophy prolongs the action potential duration, it enhances shortening of the action potential duration during global ischemia, which could increase the dispersion of repolarization during regional ischemia.[54] In addition, ischemia may contribute to electrical cell-to-cell uncoupling and an increase of extracellular resistance.[55] These changes decrease conduction velocity and may unmask intrinsic heterogeneities in repolarization, which both favor reentrant arrhythmias.[56] However, the results of an experiment on preparations of rat hearts suggested that alterations in electrotonic coupling between cells are unlikely to account for the action potential prolongation in hypertrophied myocardium. The results also showed that the latter half of repolarization is prolonged selectively in epicardial cells in contrast to the overall lengthening of repolarization in endocardial and papillary muscle fibers, indicating that the action potential prolongation that accompanies hypertrophy is not uniform.[57] On the other hand, the normal endocardial/epicardial gradient in the early phase of the action potential duration was reduced and the gradient in the plateau phase of the action potential duration reversed in myocytes isolated from rat hearts with isoproterenol-induced hypertrophy, which could explain the observed T wave inversion. Interestingly, in subendocardial myocytes hypertrophy was associated with a significant reduction in the plateau phase of the action potential duration.[58] However, the previous observations did not show consistent correlation between surface T wave configuration and regional (endocardial/epicardial) differences in intracellular action potential duration in hypertrophied rat hearts.[59]

Low K has been shown to produce increased shortening of the action potential in hypertrophied left ventricular myocytes isolated from spontaneously hypertensive rats. This may cause shortening of the wavelength of excitation and increase the inhomogeneity of repolarization, favoring reentrant ventricular tachyarrhythmias.[60] This finding has some interest in view of the previous controversial observation concerning the increased coronary heart disease mortality of hypertensive men with electrocardiogram (ECG) abnormalities, including LVH, who are treated with diuretics.[61]

Cardiac hypertrophy is associated with many histologic alterations.[62,63] In LVH, interstitial fibrosis may distort the electrical properties of different areas and change impulse propagation.[64-66] Interfibrillar collagen tissue may increase nonuniform anisotropy of the myocardium.[67] This facilitates reentrant arrhythmias.[68] It may be speculated that, in LVH, increased anisotropy may also cause increased dispersion of repolarization, as may also the stretching of myocardial fibers. In animal studies using isolated cells from hypertrophied myocardium, the effects of such features as myocardial fibrosis, myocyte loss, and ischemic foci, etc., are lost. However, these may all contribute substantively to the increased inhomogeneity of repolarization in hypertrophied hearts in hypertension.

The autonomic nervous system is known to regulate ventricular repolarization and refractoriness. In experiments on mongrel dogs, various means of sympathetic stimulation, both sympathetic nervous and humorous adrenergic, have been found to shorten the refractory period.[26] On the other hand, vagus stimulation has been shown to prolong ventricular refractoriness.[69] Thus, the possible changes in the autonomic control of the heart in hypertension and hypertrophy are also potential factors, which may alter the dispersion of repolarization.

Data from Human Studies

Data from the endocardial and epicardial monophasic action potential recordings in patients with LVH due to long-standing aortic valve disease suggest that hypertrophy increases the dispersion of repolarization and that the inverse relationship between the activation time and action potential duration is lost in hypertrophy, probably due to diminished electrotonic interaction, which may explain the observed increased dispersion of repolarization.[70] Mechanical changes in the heart cause electrophysiological changes, a phenomenon called mechanoelectric coupling. An increase in the afterload shortens the action potential duration,[71,72] and this may contribute to the increased heterogeneity of repolarization in hypertension.

The information on the dispersion of repolarization from human studies of patients with hypertension and myocardial hypertrophy is based mainly on indirect methods, such as QT dispersion measurement, which only reflect the dispersion of repolarization. The data suggest that QT dispersion is increased in hypertensive compared to nonhypertensive individuals and that the increase may occur before the development of echocardiographic LVH.[3] QT dispersion has been found to be increased in essential hypertensive patients with severe disease (i.e., the ones with the greatest left ventricular mass index and blood pressure).[4]

Accumulating evidence supports the notion that QT dispersion is prolonged in hypertensive patients with echocardiographic LVH[73-78] and that QT dispersion is associated with the left ventricular mass.[74,75] Particularly the dispersion QT apex interval (the interval from the beginning of the QRS complex to the apex of the T wave) has been shown to be increased in hypertensive patients with LVH, suggesting that LVH results in more marked inhomogeneity of the plateau phase than the downslope phase of repolarization.[73] The finding concurs with the experimental observations, which have demonstrated that myocardial hypertrophy may alter the ion channels that are operative during this phase of repolarization.[32,52] Interestingly, the prolongation of QT dispersion in hypertensive patients has been attributed particularly to concentric LVH,[76] which has been found to be associated with the highest incidence of adverse outcomes.[79,80] Furthermore, it has been shown that QT dispersion is increased in nondipper hypertensives compared with nocturnal dippers.[77] This finding can be partly explained by the observations that nondippers have more severe LVH than dippers.[77,81]

Increased QT dispersion reflects inhomogeneity of repolarization, and it may make the hypertrophied myocardium vulnerable to ventricular arrhythmias. However, this assumption is not supported by the data from 24-hour Holter studies. Although the presence of LVH correlated positively with increased QT dispersion in patients with essential arterial hypertension, prolonged QT dispersion was not found to be an adjunctive risk factor for complex ventricular arrhythmias in a 24-hour Holter monitoring.[78] In congruence with this observation, the previous data on mixed patient populations with LVH suggest that there is no relation between the degree of change in QT dispersion and the incidence of ventricular arrhythmias in 24-hour Holter monitoring.[19]

Other noninvasive methods have also been used to study abnormalities in repolarization in patients with hypertension. It has been proposed that the increasing repolarization abnormalities along with the progress of hypertension could be better detected by using magnetocardiograms than ECGs.[82] In addition, data from the body surface potential maps in patients with essential hypertension have shown that severe LVH causes alterations in the intrinsic repolarization properties.[83]

Analyses of heart rate variability have yielded variable results in patients with hypertension.[73,84-87] However, there are suggestions of disturbances in sympathovagal balance.[85,87,88] Changes in autonomic cardiac regulation may alter ventricular repolarization, a notion supported by animal studies, and thus potentially favor heterogeneity of repolarization in hypertensive patients.

A simplified schematic presentation of the factors that may increase the dispersion of repolarization in patients with hypertension is given in Figure 1.

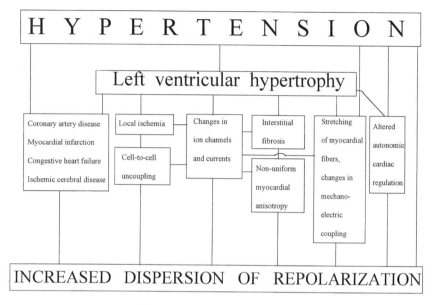

Figure 1. Simplified schematic presentation of the factors that may increase the dispersion of repolarization in patients with hypertension.

Influence of Antihypertensive Medication on the Dispersion of Repolarization

Data on the influence of antihypertensive medication on the dispersion of repolarization are scant and are mainly based on assessments of the effects of antihypertensive therapy on QT dispersion. It has been shown in hypertensive patients with an elevated left ventricular mass index that antihypertensive treatment with ramipril, an angiotensin-converting enzyme inhibitor, and felodipine, a calcium antagonist, could reduce QT dispersion. QT dispersion did not increase after drug washout, suggesting that the improvement in this parameter might be mediated by a concomitant reduction in the left ventricular mass index rather than by a direct antiarrhythmic effect.[74] Consistent with these findings, the left ventricular mass index regressed and the QT dispersion decreased in hypertensive patients with LVH during long-term enalapril treatment[89] and in mildly hypertensive patients with concentric hypertrophy after treatment with various antihypertensive medications.[76]

Thus, it seems obvious that changes in QT dispersion may reflect progression and regression of LVH. However, the changes that determine the QT dispersion reduction during antihypertensive therapy and LVH regression are not fully established. Furthermore, it is not known if there are any differences between the different antihypertensive medications in their ability to decrease QT dispersion. Some observations have suggested that not all antihypertensive agents are equally effective in reducing left ventricular mass,[90-93] but this matter is not completely settled. Particularly the data on diuretics in this respect have been contradictory.[90,92,94] Evidence from a meta-analysis supports the assumption that angiotensin-converting enzyme inhibitors may be the most effective antihypertensive drugs in causing regression of LVH.[95] However, the information on the effectiveness of different antihypertensive medications in regressing LVH cannot be directly extrapolated to the effectiveness in decreasing QT dispersion.

Speculatively, it may be assumed that the reduction in the dispersion of repolarization (suggested by the decrease in QT dispersion) by antihypertensive medication may be one of the fundamental mechanisms to explain why the regression of cardiac hypertrophy in hypertensive patients is associated with a reduction in the risk of cardiovascular events.[96]

Dispersion of Repolarization in Diseases Associated with Hypertension

Hypertension is an important risk factor in coronary vascular disease, and LVH on ECG is associated with a threefold to fivefold increase in the risk of coronary cardiopathy.[2] LVH accelerates the rate of myocardial infarction progression.[97] Furthermore, hypertension is a common cause of congestive heart failure.[12,13] These conditions may contribute substantively to the heterogeneity of repolarization in patients with hypertension,[15,16,18,19,36,98-101] as may possibly also ischemic cerebral disease and stroke,[20-22] for which hypertension is a well-known risk factor[14] (Fig. 1).

Conclusions

Dispersion of repolarization may increase in patients with hypertension even before the development of myocardial hypertrophy. However, ventricular hypertrophy is the major determinant of increased dispersion of repolarization in hypertension. Changes in the different ion channels and currents, interstitial fibrosis, local ischemia, electrical cell-to-cell uncoupling, nonuniform myocardial anisotropy, stretching of myocardial fibers, changes in mechanoelectric coupling, disturbances in autonomic cardiac regulation (and particularly heterogeneous distributions of these changes), and hypertension-associated diseases (coronary artery disease, myocardial infarction, congestive heart failure, and possibly cerebral ischemic disease) may all contribute to the inhomogeneity of repolarization in patients with hypertension and LVH. Increased dispersion of repolarization favors reentry and perhaps triggered activity and thereby the genesis of life-threatening ventricular arrhythmias. The mechanisms by which LVH predisposes hypertensive patients to sudden death are not fully established. Increased dispersion of repolarization may be an important factor, which may make these patients vulnerable to arrhythmic events. The markers of heterogeneity of repolarization can be decreased by regressing LVH with antihypertensive medication. This reduction may be notably involved with the concomitant regression of hypertrophy, but its involvement with other factors, such as the possible direct antiarrhythmic effects of antihypertensive drugs, is not well understood. Furthermore, it is not known if all the antihypertensive agents that can cause LVH regression are also effective in reducing dispersion of repolarization. Previous data suggest that the regression of LVH by antihypertensive therapy reduces the risk of cardiovascular events. The proof for this notion awaits the results of the ongoing multicenter studies, which will hopefully also answer the question of whether this possible reversal of the risk is independent of the decrease of blood pressure and the antiarrhythmic and other actions of antihypertensive drugs. However, the significance and possible benefits of reducing the dispersion of repolarization by antihypertensive medication in patients with hypertension and LVH remain to be proved.

References

1. Hypertension prevalence and the status of awareness, treatment and control in the United States. Final report of the Sub-committee on Definition and Prevalence of the 1984 Joint National Committee. *Hypertension* 1985;7:457-468.
2. Kannel WB. Left ventricular hypertrophy as a risk factor in arterial hypertension. *Eur Heart J* 1992;13(suppl D):82-88.
3. Vilas-Boas F, Lima AA, Torreao J, et al. Temporal QT dispersion in patients with systemic blood hypertension. *Arquivos Brasileiros de Cardiologia* 1997;68:343-346.
4. Clarkson PBM, Naas AAO, McMahon A, et al. QT dispersion in essential hypertension. *Q J Med* 1995;88:327-332.
5. Hammond IW, Devereux RB, Alderman MH, et al. The prevalence and correlates of echocardiographic left ventricular hypertrophy among employed patients with uncomplicated hypertension. *J Am Coll Cardiol* 1986;7:639-650.
6. Savage DD, Garrison RJ, Kannel WB, et al. The spectrum of left ventricular hypertrophy in a general population sample: The Framingham Study. *Circulation* 1987;75(suppl I):I26-I33.
7. Savage DD, Drayer JI, Henry WL, et al. Echocardiographic assessment of cardiac anatomy and function in hypertensive subjects. *Circulation* 1979;59:623-632.
8. Devereux RB, Casale PN, Hammond IW, et al. Echocardiographic detection of pressure-overload left ventricular hypertrophy: Effect of criteria and patient population. *J Clin Hypertens* 1987;3:66-78.
9. Hollander W, Madoff I, Paddock J, et al. Aggravation of atherosclerosis by hypertension in a subhuman primate model with coarctation of the aorta. *Circ Res* 1976;38(suppl 2):63-72.

10. Hollander W, Prusty S, Kirkpatrick B, et al. Role of hypertension in ischemic heart disease and cerebral vascular disease in the cynomolgus monkey with coarctation of the aorta. *Circ Res* 1977;40(suppl I):I70-I83.

11. Pick R, Johnson PJ, Glick G. Deleterious effects of hypertension on the development of aortic and coronary atherosclerosis in stumptail macaques (Macaca speciosa) on an atherogenic diet. *Circ Res* 1974;35:472-482.

12. McKee PA, Castelli SP, McNamara PM, et al. The natural history of congestive heart failure: The Framingham Heart Study. *N Engl J Med* 1971;285:1441-1446.

13. Kannel WB, Castelli WP, McNamara PM, et al. Role of blood pressure in the development of congestive heart failure: The Framingham Heart Study. *N Engl J Med* 1972;287:781-787.

14. Sacco RL. Identifying patient populations at high risk for stroke. *Neurology* 1998;51(suppl 3):S27-S30.

15. Sporton SC, Taggart P, Sutton PM, et al. Acute ischaemia: A dynamic influence on QT dispersion. *Lancet* 1997;349:306-309.

16. Stoletniy LN, Pai RG. Value of QT dispersion in the interpretation of exercise stress test in women. *Circulation* 1997;96:904-910.

17. Struthers AD, Davidson NC, Naas A, et al. QT dispersion and triple-vessel coronary disease. *Lancet* 1997;349:1174-1175.

18. Nabauer M, Kaab S. Potassium channel down-regulation in heart failure. *Cardiovasc Res* 1998;37:324-334.

19. Davey PP, Bateman J, Mulligan IP, et al. QT interval dispersion in chronic heart failure and left ventricular hypertrophy: Relation to autonomic nervous system and Holter tape abnormalities. *Br Heart J* 1994;71:268-273.

20. Davis TP, Alexander J, Lesch M. Electrocardiographic changes associated with acute cerebrovascular disease: A clinical review. *Prog Cardiovasc Dis* 1993;36:245-260.

21. Abmann I, Müller E. Prognostic significance of different QT-intervals in the body surface ECG in patients with acute myocardial infarction and in patients with acute or chronic cerebral processes. *Acta Cardiol* 1990;XLV:501-504.

22. Perkiömäki JS, Sourander LB, Levomäki L, et al. Electrocardiographic QT interval dispersion and left ventricular hypertrophy as predictors of stroke mortality in the elderly. Submitted for publication.

23. McLenachan JM, Henderson E, Morris KI, et al. Ventricular arrhythmias in patients with hypertensive left ventricular hypertrophy. *N Engl J Med* 1987;317:787-792.

24. Dunn FG, Pringle SD. Sudden cardiac death, ventricular arrhythmias and hypertensive left ventricular hypertrophy. *J Hypertens* 1993;11:1003-1010.

25. Aronow WS, Epstein S, Koenigsberg M, et al. Usefulness of echocardiographic LVH, ventricular tachycardia and complex ventricular arrhythmias in predicting ventricular fibrillation or sudden cardiac death in elderly patients. *Am J Cardiol* 1988;62:1124-1125.

26. Han J, Moe GK. Nonuniform recovery of excitability in ventricular muscle. *Circ Res* 1964;XIV:44-60.

27. Merx W, Yoon MS, Han J. The role of local disparity in conduction and recovery time on ventricular vulnerability to fibrillation. *Am Heart J* 1977;94:603-610.

28. Kuo CS, Munakata K, Reddy CP. Characteristics and possible mechanisms of ventricular arrhythmia dependent on the dispersion of action potential durations. *Circulation* 1983;67:1356-1367.

29. Kuo CS, Reddy CP, Munakata K, et al. Mechanism of ventricular arrhythmias caused by increased dispersion of repolarization. *Eur Heart J* 1985;6(suppl D):63-70.

30. McDonald TF, Trautwein W. Membrane currents in cat myocardium: Separation of inward and outward components. *J Physiol (Lond)* 1978;274:193-216.

31. McDonald TF, Trautwein W. The potassium current underlying delayed rectification in cat ventricular muscle. *J Physiol (Lond)* 1978;274:217-246.

32. Kleiman RB, Houser SR. Outward currents in normal and hypertrophied feline ventricular myocytes. *Am J Physiol* 1989;256:H1450-H1461.

33. Rosen MR. Mechanisms of cardiac impulse initiation and propagation. In Saksena S, Goldschlager N (eds): *Electrical Therapy for Cardiac Arrhythmias: Pacing, Antitachycardia Devices, Catheter Ablation.* Philadelphia: W.B. Saunders Co.; 1990:3-8.

34. Surawicz B. Will QT dispersion play a role in clinical decision-making? *J Cardiovasc Electrophysiol* 1996;7:777-784.

35. Yuan S, Wohlfart B, Olsson SB, et al. The dispersion of repolarization in patients with ventricular tachycardia. A study using simultaneous monophasic action potential recordings from two sites in the right ventricle. *Eur Heart J* 1995;16:68-76.

36. Cowan JC, Yusoff K, Moore M, et al. Importance of lead selection in QT interval measurement. *Am J Cardiol* 1988;61:83-87.

37. Day CP, McComb CM, Campbell RWF. QT dispersion: An indicator of arrhythmia risk in patients with long QT intervals. *Br Heart J* 1990;63:342-344.

38. Day CP, McComb JM, Matthews J, et al. Reduction in QT dispersion by sotalol following myocardial infarction. *Eur Heart J* 1991;12:423-427.

39. Dritsas A, Gilligan D, Nichoyannopoulos P, et al. Amiodarone reduces QT dispersion in patients with hypertrophic cardiomyopathy. *Int J Cardiol* 1992;36:345-349.

40. Zabel M, Portnoy S, Franz MR. Electrocardiographic indexes of dispersion of ventricular repolarization: An isolated heart validation study. *J Am Coll Cardiol* 1995;25:746-752.

41. Sideris DA, Toumanidis ST, Kostis EB, et al. Arrhythmogenic effect of high blood pressure: Some observations on its mechanisms. *Cardiovasc Res* 1989;23:983-992.

42. Sideris DA, Kontoyannis DA, Michalis C, et al. Acute changes in blood pressure as a cause of cardiac arrhythmias. *Eur Heart J* 1987;8:45-52.

43. James MA, Jones JV. Systolic wall stress and ventricular arrhythmia: The role of acute change in blood pressure in the isolated working rat heart. *Clin Sci* 1990;79:499-504.

44. Verdecchia P, Porcellati C, Zampi I, et al. Asymmetric left ventricular remodeling due to isolated septal thickening in patients with systemic hypertension and normal left ventricular masses. *Am J Cardiol* 1994;73:247-252.

45. Hart G. Cellular electrophysiology in cardiac hypertrophy and failure. *Cardiovasc Res* 1994;28:933-946.

46. Benitah JP, Gomez AM, Bailly P, et al. Heterogeneity of the early outward current in ventricular cells isolated from normal and hypertrophied rat hearts. *J Physiol* 1993;469:111-138.

47. Cerbai E, Barbieri M, Li Q, et al. Ionic basis of action potential prolongation of hypertrophied cardiac myocytes isolated from hypertensive rats of different ages. *Cardiovasc Res* 1994;28:1180-1187.

48. Kowey PR, Friehling TD, Sewter J, et al. Electrophysiological effects of left ventricular hypertrophy. Effect of calcium and potassium channel blockade. *Circulation* 1991;83:2067-2075.
49. Barrington PL, Harvey RD, Mogul DJ, et al. Na current (I_{Na}) and inward rectifying K current (I_{K1}) in cardiocytes from normal and hypertrophic right ventricles of cat. *Biophys J* 1988;53:426a. Abstract.
50. Brooksby P, Levi AJ, Jones JV. The electrophysiological characteristics of hypertrophied ventricular myocytes from the spontaneously hypertensive rat. *J Hypertens* 1993;11:611-622.
51. Cameron JS, Miller LS, Kimura S, et al. Systemic hypertension induces disparate localized left ventricular action potential lengthening and altered sensitivity to verapamil in left ventricular myocardium. *J Mol Cell Cardiol* 1986;18:169-175.
52. Kleiman RB, Houser SR. Calcium currents in normal and hypertrophied isolated feline ventricular myocytes. *Am J Physiol* 1988;255:H1434-H1442.
53. Hanf R, Drubaix I, Marotte F, et al. Rat cardiac hypertrophy. Altered sodium-calcium exchange activity in sarcolemmal vesicles. *FEBS Lett* 1990;236:145-149.
54. Hicks MN, McIntosh MA, Kane KA, et al. The electrophysiology of rabbit hearts with left ventricular hypertrophy under normal and ischaemic conditions. *Cardiovasc Res* 1995;30:181-186.
55. Kléber AG, Riegger CB, Janse MJ. Electrical uncoupling and increase of extracellular resistance after induction of ischemia in isolated, arterially perfused rabbit papillary muscle. *Circ Res* 1987;61:271-279.
56. Priori SG, Barhanin J, Hauer RNW, et al. Genetic and molecular basis of cardiac arrhythmias: Impact on clinical management. Part III. *Circulation* 1999;99:674-681.
57. Keung ECH, Aronson RS. Non-uniform electrophysiological properties and electrotonic interaction in hypertrophied rat myocardium. *Circ Res* 1981;49:150-158.
58. Shipsey SJ, Bryant SM, Hart G. Effects of hypertrophy on regional action potential characteristics in the rat left ventricle. A cellular basis for T-wave inversion? *Circulation* 1997;96:2061-2068.
59. Keung EC, Aronson RS. Transmembrane action potentials and the electrocardiogram in rats with renal hypertension. *Cardiovasc Res* 1981;15:611-614.
60. Evans SJ, Jones JV, Levi AJ. Reduction in external K causes increased action potential shortening in ventricular myocytes from the spontaneously hypertensive rat. *J Hypertens* 1997;15:659-666.
61. Multiple Risk Factor Intervention Trial Research Group. Multiple Risk Factor Intervention Trial. Risk factor changes and mortality results. *JAMA* 1982;248:1465-1477.
62. Wendt-Gallitelli MF, Jacob R. Time course of electron microscopic alterations in the hypertrophied myocardium of Goldblatt rats. *Basic Res Cardiol* 1977;72:209-213.
63. Maron BJ, Ferrans VJ, Roberts WC. Ultrastructural features of degenerated cardiac muscle cells in patients with cardiac hypertrophy. *Am J Pathol* 1975;79:387-434.
64. Weber KT, Brilla CG. Pathological hypertrophy and cardiac interstitium-fibrosis and renin-angiotensin-aldosterone systems. *Circulation* 1991;83:1849-1865.
65. Messerli FH, Kaesser UR, Josem CJ. Effects of antihypertensive therapy on hypertensive heart disease. *Circulation* 1989;80(suppl IV):145-150.

66. Toyoshima H, Park YD, Ishikawa Y, et al. Effects of ventricular hypertrophy on conduction velocity of action front in the ventricular myocardium. *Am J Cardiol* 1982;49:1938-1945.
67. Aguilar JC, Martinez AH, Conejos FA: Mechanisms of ventricular arrhythmias in the presence of pathological hypertrophy. *Eur Heart J* 1993;14(suppl J):65-70.
68. Spach MS, Miller WT, Geselowitz DB, et al. The discontinuous nature of propagation in normal canine cardiac muscle. Evidence for recurrent discontinuity of intracellular resistance that affect the membrane currents. *Circ Res* 1981;48:39-54.
69. Martins JB, Zipes DP. Effects of sympathetic and vagal nerves on recovery properties of the endocardium and epicardium of the canine left ventricle. *Circ Res* 1980;46:100-110.
70. Franz MR, Bargheer K, Lichtlen PR, et al. Myocardial repolarization in normal and hypertrophied human left ventricles. In Butrous GS, Schwartz PJ (eds): *Clinical Aspects of Ventricular Repolarization.* London: Farrand Press; 1989:219-226.
71. Taggart P, Sutton PM, Treasure T, et al. Contraction-excitation feedback in man? *Br Heart J* 1988;59:109.
72. Taggart P, Sutton PM, Treasure T, et al. Monophasic action potentials at discontinuation of cardiopulmonary bypass: Evidence for contraction-excitation feedback in man. *Circulation* 1988;77:1266-1275.
73. Perkiömäki JS, Ikäheimo MJ, Pikkujämsä SM, et al. Dispersion of the QT interval and autonomic modulation of heart rate in hypertensive men with and without left ventricular hypertrophy. *Hypertension* 1996;28:16-21.
74. Mayet J, Shahi M, McGrath K, et al. Left ventricular hypertrophy and QT dispersion in hypertension. *Hypertension* 1996;28:791-796.
75. Ichkhan K, Molnar J, Somberg J. Relation of left ventricular mass and QT dispersion in patients with systematic hypertension. *Am J Cardiol* 1997;79:508-511.
76. Tomiyama H, Doba N, Fu Y, et al. Left ventricular geometric patterns and QT dispersion in borderline and mild hypertension: Their evolution and regression. *Am J Hypertens* 1998;11:286-292.
77. Kohno I, Takusagawa M, Yin D, et al. QT dispersion in dipper- and nondipper-type hypertension. *Am J Hypertens* 1998;11:280-285.
78. Cavallini B, Perri V, Sali M. Dispersion of QT interval in arterial hypertension with left ventricular hypertrophy. *Minerva Cardioangiol* 1996;44:45-48.
79. Koren MJ, Devereux RB, Casale PN, et al. Relation of left ventricular mass and geometry to morbidity and mortality in uncomplicated essential hypertension. *Ann Intern Med* 1991;114:345-352.
80. Krumholz HM, Larson M, Levy D. Prognosis of left ventricular geometric patterns in the Framingham Heart Study. *J Am Coll Cardiol* 1995;25:879-884.
81. Verdecchia P, Schillaci G, Guerrieri M, et al. Circadian blood pressure changes and left ventricular hypertrophy in essential hypertension. *Circulation* 1990;81:528-536.
82. Nomura M, Fujino K, Katayama M, et al. Analysis of the T wave of the magnetocardiogram in patients with essential hypertension by means of isomagnetic and vector arrow maps. *J Electrocardiol* 1988;21:174-182.
83. Igarashi H, Kubota I, Ikeda K, et al. Body surface mapping for the assessment of left ventricular hypertrophy in patients with essential hypertension. *Jpn Circ J* 1987;51:284-292.

84. Furlan R, Guzzetti S, Crivellaro W, et al. Continuous 24-hour assessment of the neural regulation of systemic arterial pressure and RR variabilities in ambulant subjects. *Circulation* 1990;81:537-547.

85. Guzzetti S, Piccaluga E, Casati R, et al. Sympathetic predominance in essential hypertension: A study employing spectral analysis of heart rate variability. *J Hypertens* 1988;6:711-717.

86. Dassi S, Balsama M, Guzzetti S, et al. Twenty-four hour power spectral analysis of heart rate variability and of arterial pressure values in normotensive and hypertensive subjects. *J Hypertens* 1991;9(suppl 6):S72-S73.

87. Chakko S, Mulintapang RF, Huikuri HV, et al. Alterations in heart rate variability and its circadian rhythm in hypertensive patients with left ventricular hypertrophy free of coronary artery disease. *Am Heart J* 1993;126:1364-1372.

88. Langewitz W, Rüddel H, Schächinger H. Reduced parasympathetic cardiac control in patients with hypertension at rest and under mental stress. *Am Heart J* 1994;127:122-128.

89. González-Juanatey JR, Garcia-Acuña JM, Pose A, et al. Reduction of QT and QTc dispersion during long-term treatment of systemic hypertension with enalapril. *Am J Cardiol* 1998;81:170-174.

90. Liebson PR. Clinical studies of drug reversal of hypertensive left ventricular hypertrophy. *Am J Hypertens* 1990;3:512-517.

91. Schulman S, Weiss J, Becker L, et al. The effects of antihypertensive therapy on left ventricular mass in elderly patients. *N Engl J Med* 1990;322:1350-1356.

92. Dahlöf B, Pennert K, Hansson L. Reversal of left ventricular hypertrophy in hypertensive patients: A metaanalysis of 109 treatment studies. *Am J Hypertens* 1992;5:95-110.

93. Thürmann PA, Kenedi P, Schmidt A, et al. Influence of the angiotensin II antagonist valsartan on left ventricular hypertrophy in patients with essential hypertension. *Circulation* 1998;98:2037-2042.

94. Gottdiener JS, Reda DJ, Massie BM, et al. Effects of single-drug therapy on reduction of left ventricular mass in mild to moderate hypertension. Comparison of six antihypertensive agents. The Department of Veterans Affairs Cooperative Study Group on Antihypertensive Agents. *Circulation* 1997;95:2007-2014.

95. Schmieder RE, Martus P, Klingbeil A. Reversal of left ventricular hypertrophy in essential hypertension: Meta-analysis of randomized double-blind studies. *JAMA* 1996;275:1507-1513.

96. Muiesan ML, Salvetti M, Rizzoni D, et al. Association of change in left ventricular mass with prognosis during long-term antihypertensive treatment. *J Hypertens* 1995;13:1091-1095.

97. Polese A, De Cesare N, Montorsi P, et al. Upward shift of the lower range of coronary flow autoregulation in hypertensive patients with hypertrophy of the left ventricle. *Circulation* 1991;83:845-853.

98. Kurz RW, Ren XL, Franz MR. Dispersion and delay of electrical restitution in the globally ischaemic heart. *Eur Heart J* 1994;15:547-554.

99. Glancy JM, Garratt CJ, Woods KL, et al. QT dispersion and mortality after myocardial infarction. *Lancet* 1995;345:945-948.

100. Higham PD, Campbell RWF. QT dispersion. *Br Heart J* 1994;71:508-510.

101. van de Loo A, Arendts W, Hohnloser SH. Variability of QT dispersion measurements in the surface electrocardiogram in patients with acute myocardial infarction and in normal subjects. *Am J Cardiol* 1994;74:1113-1118.

16

QT Dispersion in Patients with Congestive Heart Failure and Ventricular Arrhythmias

*Michel Galinier, Atul Pathak, Bruno Dongay,
Daniel Curnier, Joelle Fourcade, Serge Boveda,
and Jean-Paul Bounhoure*

Introduction

Identification of patients with congestive heart failure who are at risk for sudden cardiac death remains problematic. QT dispersion has been demonstrated to provide an indirect measurement of the inhomogeneity of myocardial repolarization,[1] and increased QT dispersion may predispose to arrhythmic events.[2-5] To date, only little information is available on the prognostic significance of QT dispersion in congestive heart failure, and results of previous studies remain controversial. Most have shown that patients with congestive heart failure,[6,7] secondary to ischemic heart disease[8] or to idiopathic dilated cardiomyopathy,[9] who presented with arrhythmic events during follow-up had significantly greater QT dispersion than those without arrhythmic events. But some recent studies failed to demonstrate a predictive value of QT dispersion for arrhythmic events in patients with congestive heart failure.[10,11] In a large patient cohort with congestive heart failure, we sought to examine the correlations between QT interval dispersion and the other arrhythmogenic markers, ventricular premature beats on Holter monitoring and ventricular late potentials on

From Olsson SB, Amlie JP, Yuan S (eds): *Dispersion of Ventricular Repolarization: State of the Art.* ©Futura Publishing Company, Inc., Armonk, NY, 2000.

signal-averaged electrocardiograms (ECGs), to evaluate the prognostic value of QT interval dispersion.

Methods

Patients

From January 1990 until December 1995, 205 patients with congestive heart failure in sinus rhythm, mean age 58±11 years, 170 men and 35 women, were prospectively enrolled in this study at Rangueil University Hospital (Toulouse, France). Inclusion criteria were 1) New York Heart Association (NYHA) Class II to IV; 2) left ventricular ejection fraction less than 45%; 3) left ventricular enlargement; and 4) absence of valvular heart disease. Exclusion criteria were 1) atrial fibrillation; 2) permanent pacing; 3) electrolyte disturbance; 4) medical regimen consisted of Class I antiarrhythmic; and 5) recent myocardial infarction or unstable angina. Patients with bundle branch block were included but considered separately. Clinical investigations included 12-lead ECG, chest radiography, two-dimensional Doppler echocardiography, cardiac catheterization with coronary angiography, and left ventricular angiography. Holter ECG recording for 24 hours and signal-averaged ECG were also realized.

The etiologies of congestive heart failure were ischemic heart disease in 86 patients, idiopathic dilated cardiomyopathy in 101 patients, and hypertensive dilated cardiomyopathy in 18 patients. The diagnosis of dilated cardiomyopathy was made according to usual criteria,[12] in the presence of a depressed left ventricular ejection fraction and in the absence of significant coronary artery disease and other specific heart muscle diseases. In comparison to patients with dilated cardiomyopathy (n=119), those with ischemic heart disease (n=86) were older (60±10 versus 57±13 years; P<0.05) and had less bundle branch block on ECG recording (30% versus 47%; P<0.05). No differences were stated between these two groups concerning sex, NYHA status (51% versus 49% in grades III to IV), cardiothoracic ratio (57±6% versus 57±6%), ejection fraction (28±8% versus 29±9%), and left ventricular end-diastolic dimension (65±8 versus 67±9 mm). For the medical regimen at inclusion, there was no difference between the two groups for angiotensin-converting enzyme inhibitor (90% and 96%) and amiodarone (46% versus 43%). The percentages of patients taking diuretics (79% versus 90%; P<0.05) and digoxin (41% versus 58%; P<0.05) were slightly different.

Arrhythmogenic Markers

Evaluation of QT interval dispersion was realized in the whole cohort of patients (n=205). All measurements were made on standard ECGs with simultaneous 12-lead acquisition, recorded at a speed of 25 mm/s. The

QT interval, defined as the interval between the beginning of QRS complex and the end of the T wave (i.e., return to the TP baseline), was measured in all 12 leads in two consecutive cycles by a physician who was unaware of clinical conditions at the time of QT measurements. When U waves were present, the end of the T wave was defined as the intersection of the isoelectric line and the tangent of the maximal slope on the downward limb of the T wave.[13] QT interval dispersion was calculated as the difference between the maximum and the minimum QT intervals in any of the 12 leads.

Holter ECG recordings for 24 hours were obtained from 187 patients, using a Marquette Electronics 8000 system. Premature ventricular beats, polymorphism, ventricular doublets, and nonsustained ventricular tachycardia (Lown Class IVb) were noted and classified according to the Lown criteria.

Signal-averaged ECGs were recorded in 194 patients, on a Marquette MAC 15 machine, using about 300 QRS cycles and a high-pass digital filter of 40 Hz; a noise level of less than 0.4 μV was considered as acceptable. Ventricular late potentials were considered to be present if at least two of the following criteria existed: 1) in the absence of bundle branch block: filtered QRS duration greater than 120 ms; root-mean square voltage in the last 40 ms less than 20 μV; low-amplitude signals less than 40 μV greater than 40 ms; and 2) in the presence of bundle branch block: filtered QRS duration greater than 145 ms; root-mean square voltage in the last 40 ms less than 17 μV; low-amplitude signals less than 40 μV greater than 55 ms.

Follow-up

Survival data were obtained by direct patient examination or from general practitioners who took care of the enrolled patients. Cause of patients' death was determined by direct communication whether with the patients' families, or with their general practitioners; if information was still not available, hospital charts were reviewed. Every effort was made to differentiate sudden death from pump failure death. Arrhythmic events during follow-up were defined as: 1) sudden cardiac death, i.e., death within 1 hour after the onset of symptoms in a previously medically stable patient, death during sleep, or unwitnessed death (that occurred within 1 hour of the patients last being seen alive); 2) spontaneous symptomatic sustained ventricular tachycardia or ventricular fibrillation. Patients who underwent cardiac transplantation during follow-up were considered alive at the date of intervention and were excluded for further analysis.

Statistical Analysis

Quantitative values are reported as mean ± SD. Continuous variables (QT interval dispersion, ventricular premature beats, left ventricular ejection fraction...) were treated by linear regression and the correlation coefficient was calculated. Mean QT interval dispersion for every Lown class was tested by analysis of variance. When significant data emerged, the mean values were treated in pairs by Fischer's PLSD test. The Student t test for independent series was used to compare the mean QT interval dispersion values depending on the presence or the absence of nonsustained ventricular tachycardia on Holter or ventricular late potentials. The results of these tests are considered significant if a P value of less than 0.05 is obtained.

Survival Analysis

Survival time estimates calculated by the method of Kaplan Meier and statistical comparisons between survival curves were done using the log-rank test. The significance of each categorical variable was determined by a P≤0.05. The following continuous variables were transformed into dichotomized variables: cardiothoracic ratio ≤60 or greater than 60%; left ventricular ejection fraction ≥25 or less than 25%; QT interval dispersion ≤80 or greater than 80 ms, as the value superior to the 75th percentile of the QT interval dispersion distribution measured in our population. The relative risk and the significance for each categorical variable were assessed using a discrete Cox model. Multivariate survival analysis was performed with the Cox proportional hazards model to determine which factors were significantly associated with global, cardiac, or sudden death and arrhythmic events after adjustment for the other variables. Variables selected to be tested in multivariate analysis were those with a P less than 0.10 in the univariate model. A stepwise selection was done using a P to remove from and a P to enter into the model ≤0.05 with both prior backward selection after inclusion of all selected variables (saturated model) and then forward selection. The P value refers to the likelihood ratio test of the hypothesis that the regression coefficient was zero. Results are expressed as relative risk with confidence intervals (CI 95%). A significant increase of risk is obtained if CI 95% excludes 1 and P of Wald test ≤0.05 (computed with STATVIEW package).

Results

QT interval dispersion was normally distributed, and the mean QT interval dispersion was 65.4±27.9 ms and varied between 10 and 160 ms. There was no significant difference in QT interval dispersion between patients with ischemic heart disease or dilated cardiomyopathy (65.8±28.8 versus 65.0±27.4 ms; P=0.846). QT interval dispersion was significantly greater in patients with bundle branch block (71.7 ± 29.3 versus 61.1 ± 26.2 ms; P=0.008). In this cohort 38 patients (18.5%) had a QT interval dispersion greater than 80 ms.

Correlation of QT Interval Dispersion and Other Arrhythmogenic Markers

QT interval dispersion was not significantly related to serum potassium level, ventricular premature complex frequency, or Lown classes. There was no significant difference in QT interval dispersion between patients with or without nonsustained ventricular tachycardia (60.0 ± 24.3 ms versus 65.5 ± 26.7 ms; P=0.16) and between patients with and without ventricular late potentials (66.7 ± 26.9 ms versus 65.0 ± 28.7 ms; P=0.66). QT interval dispersion was not significantly related to age, sex, NYHA classification, cardiothoracic ratio, left ventricular ejection fraction, and left ventricular end-diastolic dimension. The same lack of correlation between the QT interval dispersion and the other arrhythmogenic markers was found in patients with or without ischemic heart disease.

QT Interval Dispersion and Treatments

QT interval dispersion was not significantly different in patients treated with or without amiodarone (67.0 ± 28.8 ms versus 64.0 ± 27.2 ms; P=0.446). In contrast, QT interval dispersion was significantly lower in patients treated with digoxin compared with those not treated with this drug (61.2 ± 28.1 ms versus 69.6 ± 27.2 ms; P<0.05). QT interval dispersion was not significantly related to angiotensin-converting enzyme inhibitors or treatment with diuretics.

Predictive Value of QT Interval Dispersion

During 24 ± 16 months of follow-up in the 205 patients with congestive heart failure, 66 patients died; 56 of them died of cardiac causes, including 22 from sudden death. Seven patients presented with spontaneous symptomatic sustained ventricular tachycardia. Ten patients underwent heart transplantation. For five patients no follow-up data could be obtained and they were excluded from the survival analysis and considered lost from study.

The 4-year mortality rate was 47%. Baseline QT interval dispersion was significantly greater in patients who died than in survivors (70.9 ± 30.3 ms versus 62.4 ± 26.8 ms; P<0.05), in patients who died suddenly (80.0 ± 30.4 ms versus 63.4 ± 27.4 ms; P<0.01), and in patients with arrhythmic events (80.3 ± 27.4 ms versus 62.6 ± 27.6 ms; P=0.002). A same significant difference (P<0.05) for QT interval dispersion between patients with and without arrhythmic events was found for patients without (75.7±24.1 ms versus 59.1±26.1 ms) and with bundle branch block (84.7±29.4 ms versus 68.6±28.0 ms).

Univariate Survival Analysis

In the 200 patients with congestive heart failure (Table 1), a QT interval dispersion longer than 80 ms tended to be related with all cause and cardiac mortality but the P values were not inferior to 0.05. The 4-year mortality rates in patients with a QT interval dispersion greater than 80 ms compared with those with a QT interval dispersion ≤80 ms were 56.6±8.8% versus 41.9±6.1% for all cause death and 50.8±9.6% versus 39.1±6.3% for cardiac death. The presence of an ischemic heart disease, a NYHA Class III to IV, a cardiothoracic ratio greater than 60%, a left ventricular ejection fraction less than 25%, and the use of amiodarone were closely related with all cause and cardiac mortality. A QT interval dispersion greater than 80 ms tended to be related to sudden death, but the P value was not inferior to 0.05 and was the sole studied parameter significantly related to arrhythmic events (P<0.05).

Multivariate Analysis

After testing the appropriateness of Cox regression model for the different mortality classes and arrhythmic events, we selected for multivariate survival analysis different parameters that showed a significant relation with mortality or arrhythmic events in univariate analysis: etiologies of congestive heart failure, NYHA classes, cardiothoracic ratio, left ventricular ejection fraction, and amiodarone treatment. We also included all of the parameters that in univariate analysis displayed a P value less than 0.1, for which prognostic influence was considered possible: QT interval dispersion and Lown Class IVb.

For all cause mortality, the presence of an ischemic heart disease, a NYHA Class III to IV, and a cardiothoracic ratio greater than 60% were retained as independent predictors of death. For cardiac mortality, these three parameters but also a QT interval dispersion greater than 80 ms were retained as independent predictors of cardiac death. For sudden death, only the QT interval dispersion was retained as an independent predictor of sudden death. A QT interval dispersion greater than 80 ms increased the sudden death risk 2.53-fold (95% CI 1.04 to 6.17; P<0.05). For arrhythmic events, only a QT interval dispersion greater than 80 ms was retained as an independent predictor of arrhythmic events (RR: 2.66; 95% CI 1.22 to 5.84; P<0.02). The same results were obtained in the subgroup of patients without bundle branch block.

Table 1
Relative Risk and Confidence Intervals of 95% in Univariate Survival Analysis for All-Cause, Cardiac and Sudden Death, and Arrhythmic Events in 200 Patients with Congestive Heart Failure

	All Cause Mortality			Cardiac Mortality			Sudden Death		Arrhythmic Events		
	R-R	95% CI	P	R-R	95% CI	P	R-R	95% CI	R-R	95% CI	P
QTd>80 ms	1.59	0.92-2.76	0.096	1.68	0.93-3.04	0.082	2.17	0.89-5.33	2.22	1.01-4.89	0.042
Lown IVb	1.49	0.90-2.47	0.116	1.64	0.95-2.82	0.073	1.72	0.73-4.05	0.78	0.58-2.84	0.540
VLP	1.08	0.65-1.75	0.781	0.80	0.46-1.39	0.427	0.97	0.40-2.38	1.41	0.67-3.03	0.363
NYHA III-IV	2.09	1.26-3.46	0.003	2.54	1.44-4.46	0.008	0.58	0.25-1.36	0.80	0.38-1.65	0.539
EF<25%	1.64	1.00-2.67	0.046	1.82	1.08-3.09	0.024	1.75	0.75-4.07	2.01	0.96-4.19	0.057
CTR>60%	2.77	1.65-466	0.0001	2.87	1.63-5.04	0.0001	2.6	1.04-6.51	2.03	0.89-4.64	0.085
BBB	1.27	0.78-2.04	0.344	1.32	0.78-2.22	0.290	1.69	0.74-4.00	1.49	0.72-3.12	0.272
Amiodarone	1.75	1.09-2.86	0.021	2.00	1.17-3.44	0.009	1.54	0.66-3.57	1.19	0.57-2.44	0.647
Digoxin	1.12	0.69-1.82	0.637	1.19	0.70-2.04	0.506	0.68	0.28-1.61	0.70	0.33-1.49	0.359
Age	1.01	0.99-1.03	0.187	1.01	0.99-1.03	0.354	1.00	0.96-1.03	1.00	0.97-1.03	0.980
IHD	1.96	1.21-3.20	0.006	1.89	1.12-3.21	0.016	1.85	0.80-4.29	1.97	0.94-4.09	0.066

BBB = bundle branch block; CI = confidence interval; CTR = cardiothoracic ratio; EF = ejection fraction; IHD = ischemic heart disease; NYHA = New York Heart Association; QTd = QT interval dispersion; RR = relative risk; VLP = ventricular late potentials.

Discussion

Measure of QT Interval Dispersion in Patients with Congestive Heart Failure

Our data confirmed that QT interval dispersion is greater in patients with congestive heart failure than in normal subjects, in whom it was usually found between 20 and 50 ms.[14,15] Even though the reproducibility of the measurement of QT interval dispersion in healthy volunteers is known to be relatively poor,[13] the mean QT interval dispersion in the present study (65.4±27.9 ms) is very similar to the value reported recently by Fei et al[16] in a group of 60 patients with congestive heart failure secondary to idiopathic dilated cardiomyopathy: 66±16 ms. Furthermore, the mean QT interval dispersion in our study found in patients with or without bundle branch block (71.7±29.3 ms and 61.1±26.2 ms) was very similar to the values reported recently by Grimm et al[15] in a group of 107 patients with idiopathic dilated cardiomyopathy: 71±27 and 57±25 ms, respectively, in patients with and without bundle branch block. Similar to previous studies in patients with coronary artery disease with congestive heart failure[8] or following myocardial infarction[5] in whom QT interval dispersion was reported between 60 and 80 ms, the mean QT interval dispersion in our patients with ischemic heart disease was 65.8±28.8 ms.

Since we measured QT interval on standard ECGs with simultaneous 12-lead acquisition, we did not correct the QT interval for heart rate. In fact, it was recently reported by Zaidi et al,[17] in a group of 54 patients with dilated cardiomyopathy, with or without bundle branch block, compared with 53 normal subjects, that the uncorrected QT interval values were lower than the corrected values but in the same proportions. Furthermore, it is now well accepted that correction of the QT interval for heart rate is potentially misleading under certain circumstances.[18] Hysteresis in the QT interval adaptation to the change of heart rate within a period of few beats makes the correction for heart rate less important. Dispersion of repolarization does not increase to the same extent with longer cycle length as does the duration of repolarization.[19] This viewpoint is supported by the studies of Fei et al,[16] who demonstrated that there were no significant beat-to-beat variations in QT dispersion measured on simultaneously recorded 12-lead ECGs and that there was no significant relationship between QT dispersion and R-R intervals.

Correlations of QT Interval Dispersion in Patients with Congestive Heart Failure

A significant correlation between QT interval dispersion and frequency of ventricular extrasystoles or the presence of nonsustained ventricular tachycardia on Holter monitoring was not demonstrated by us in this study, or by Davey et al[6] in patients with chronic heart failure, or by Fei et al[16] in patients with idiopathic dilated cardiomyopathy. A lack of correlation was also found in the present study between abnormal QT interval dispersion and the presence of ventricular late potentials. Differences in the mechanism generating these two electric phenomena may be responsible for this lack of correlation: an inhomogeneity of myocardial repolarization for QT interval dispersion[1,2] and a fragmentation of final depolarization for late potentials.

Prognostic Value of QT Interval Dispersion in Heart Failure

In our population of patients with congestive heart failure, only an abnormal QT interval dispersion was retained in multivariate analysis as an independent predictor of arrhythmic events and sudden death. In contrast, nonsustained ventricular tachycardia on Holter ECG and ventricular late potentials had no prognostic value.

In patients with dilated cardiomyopathy, we have previously demonstrated the value of QT interval dispersion as a predictive marker for arrhythmias.[20] An abnormal QT interval dispersion was an independent predictor of arrhythmic events and sudden death, increasing arrhythmic risk approximately fivefold. In the same way, Pye et al[9] demonstrated increased QT interval dispersion in nine patients with dilated cardiomyopathy with a documented history of ventricular arrhythmias (84 ms) compared with eight patients with ventricular arrhythmias and good left ventricular function (58 ms). Davey et al[21] reported increased QT interval dispersion in patients with left ventricular failure who later died suddenly but not in those dying from progressive pump failure compared with survivors. Recently, Grimm et al,[15] in a prospective study of 107 patients with idiopathic dilated cardiomyopathy followed up 13 ± 7 months in whom 12 (11%) arrhythmic events occurred (five sudden deaths), reported a significant increased QT interval dispersion in patients with versus without arrhythmic events during follow-up, as well as in all patients (76 ± 17 versus 60 ± 26) and in patients without bundle branch block (78 ± 17 versus 55 ± 25). In this study, when the QT interval dispersion was corrected for heart rate, no significant difference between patients with versus without arrhythmic events during follow-up was found. Recently, in a retrospective study of 163 patients with congestive heart failure, secondary to idiopathic dilated cardiomyopathy or ischemic heart disease, Fu et al[7] found a larger QT interval dispersion in patients who died suddenly or experienced spontaneous ventricular tachycardia (95 ± 19 ms) than in survivors (54 ± 21 ms) or in patients who died of other cardiac causes (47 ± 15 ms). In contrast, in a prospective study of 60 patients with congestive heart failure secondary to idiopathic dilated cardiomyopathy, Fei et al[16] found no significant difference in QT interval dispersion between the eight patients who died and the survivors during 34 ± 23 months of follow-up. However, this study was unable to state a conclusion regarding the difference in QT interval dispersion between patients who died suddenly and survivors, due to a small number (n=2) of patients who died suddenly. Recently, Strunk-Mueller et al,[22] in a retrospective study of 223 patients with dilated cardiomyopathy, also found no significant difference in QT interval dispersion corrected for heart rate between the 20 patients who died suddenly and the survivors, but this study included patients in atrial fibrillation. Nevertheless, the usefulness of QT interval dispersion for arrhythmia risk prediction was limited by the large overlap of QT dispersion between patients with and without arrhythmic events.

In patients with ischemic heart disease, the value of QT interval dispersion for arrhythmia prediction remains controversial. Previously, we failed to find a significant relationship between risk of arrhythmic events or sudden death and abnormal QT interval dispersion.[20] However, because of the small sample size of the group of ischemic congestive heart failure patients, we cannot conclude that QT interval dispersion does not predict mortality in this subgroup. Recently, Pedretti et al[11] reported also the absence of a significant relationship between the risk of arrhythmic events and QT interval dispersion in patients with low left ventricular ejection fraction after myocardial infarction. In contrast, in postinfarct patients, Perkiömäki et al[5] reported a significantly increased QT dispersion in patients with a history of arrhythmic events or inducible ventricular tachycardia compared with those without susceptibility to arrhythmias, and Glancy et al[4] demonstrated a relation between increased QT dispersion measured more than 4 weeks after myocardial infarction and subsequent all cause mortality. In patients with congestive failure secondary to ischemic heart disease, Barr et al[8] reported a significant increased QT interval dispersion in patients who died suddenly compared with those who died from progressive congestive heart failure or survivors.

Study Limitations

Although great care was taken to use consistent criteria to define the end of the QT interval by a single experienced observer who was unaware of clinical data, the lack of a uniformly accepted definition of the end of the QT interval and the fact that ECGs were read manually in this study remained a limitation of QT interval dispersion measurement.[2,23] However, recently Glancy et al[24] reported that errors between observers and automatic measurement were less important for QT dispersion than rate-corrected QT dispersion.

Another limit of the present study is the possible impact of treatments on survival data. If in this not-randomized study, no conclusion concerning the effects of the drugs was possible, we must emphasize that the increase of all cause and cardiac mortality associated with the use of amiodarone can be explained by the basal characteristics of patients treated with this drug who had a more severe cardiac failure. In our study, the QT interval dispersion was not significantly different in patients with or without amiodarone (67.0 ± 28.8 ms versus 64.0 ± 27.2 ms), similar to the most recent data,[16,25,26,27] which found no change of QT interval dispersion after amiodarone despite a significant prolongation of QT and rate-corrected QT intervals durations by this drug. Nevertheless, other studies suggested that amiodarone shortened QT interval dispersion.[28]

Conclusion

The present data suggest that QT interval dispersion in patients with congestive heart failure is not significantly related to other arrhythmogenic markers, and is the sole independent predictor of arrhythmic events in multivariate analysis.

References

1. Zabel M, Portnoy S, Franz MR. Electrocardiographic indices of dispersion of ventricular repolarization: An isolated heart validation study. J Am Coll Cardiol 1995;25:746-752.
2. Statters DJ, Malik M, Ward DE, Camm JA. QT dispersion: Problems of methodology and clinical significance. J Cardiovasc Electrophysiol 1994;5:672-685.
3. Priori SG, Napolitano C, Diehl L, Schwartz PJ. Dispersion of the QT interval: A marker of therapeutic efficacy in the idiopathic long QT syndrome. Circulation 1994;89:1681-1689.
4. Glancy JM, Garratt CJ, Woods KL, de Bono DP. QT dispersion and mortality after myocardial infarction. Lancet 1995;354:945-948.
5. Perkiömäki JS, Koistinen J, Yli-Mayry S, Huikuri HV. Dispersion of QT interval in patients with and without susceptibility to ventricular tachyarrhythmias after previous myocardial infarction. J Am Coll Cardiol 1995;26:174-179.
6. Davey PP, Bateman J, Mulligan IP, et al. QT interval dispersion in chronic heart failure and left ventricular hypertrophy: Relation to autonomic nervous system and Holter tape abnormalities. Br Heart J 1994;71:268-273.
7. Fu GS, Meissner A, Simon R. Repolarization dispersion and sudden cardiac death in patients with impaired left ventricular function. Eur Heart J 1997;18:281-289.
8. Barr CS, Naas A, Freemann M, et al. QT dispersion and sudden unexpected death in chronic heart failure. Lancet 1994;343:327-329.
9. Pye M, Quinn AC, Cobbe SM. QT interval dispersion: A non-invasive marker of susceptibility to arrhythmia in patients with sustained ventricular arrhythmias. Br Heart J 1994;71:511-514.
10. Mortara AL, Priori S, Cantu F, et al. Autonomic nervous system dysfunction but not dispersion of ventricular repolarization has prognostic implication in chronic heart failure. J Am Coll Cardiol 1997;29:175A. Abstract.

11. Pedretti RFE, Catalano OI, Ballardini L, et al. QT interval dispersion is not useful for predicting arrhythmic events in myocardial infarction survivors with left ventricular dysfunction. *Eur Heart J* 1996;30:252. Abstract.

12. Richardson P, McKenna W, Bristow M, et al. Report of the World Health Organization/International Society and Federation of Cardiology Task Force on the Definition and Classification of Cardiomyopathies. *Circulation* 1996;93:841-842.

13. Fei L, Statters DJ, Camm AJ. QT interval dispersion on 12 lead electrocardiogram in normal subjects. Its reproducibility and relation to the T wave. *Am Heart J* 1994;127:1654-1665.

14. Higham PD. Campbell RW. QT dispersion. *Br Heart J* 1994;71:508-510.

15. Grimm W, Steder U, Menz V, et al. QT dispersion and arrhythmic events in idiopathic dilated cardiomyopathy. *Am J Cardiol* 1996;78:458-461.

16. Fei L, Goldman JH, Prasad K, et al. QT dispersion and RR variations on 12-lead ECGs in patients with congestive heart failure secondary to idiopathic dilated cardiomyopathy. *Eur Heart J* 1996;17:258-263.

17. Zaidi M, Robert A, Fesler R, et al. Dispersion of ventricular repolarization in dilated cardiomyopathy. *Eur Heart J* 1997;18:1129-1134.

18. Fei L, Statters DJ, Anderson MH, et al. Is there a prolonged QT interval in sudden cardiac death survivors with a normal QTc? *Am Heart J* 1994;128:73-76.

19. Zabel M, Killer BS, Woosley RL, Franz MR. Frequency-dependent changes in the dispersion of repolarization and recovery time: Implications for the measurement of QT dispersion. *PACE* 1994;17:762. Abstract.

20. Galinier M, Vialette JC, Fourcade J, et al. QT interval dispersion as a predictor of arrhythmic events in congestive heart failure. Importance of aetiology. *Eur Heart J* 1998;19:1054-1062.

21. Davey PP, Bateman J, Mulligan IP, et al. QT interval dispersion in chronic heart failure and left ventricular hypertrophy: Relation to autonomic nervous system and Holter tape abnormalities. *Br Heart J* 1994;71:268-273.

22. Strunk-Mueller C, Gietzen F, Kuhn H. QTc dispersion in dilated cardiomyopathy—a new method for stratifying the risk of sudden cardiac death? *Eur Heart J* 1996;276:1534. Abstract.

23. Day CP, McComb JM, Campbell RWF. QT dispersion in sinus beats and ventricular extrasystoles in normal hearts. *Br Heart J* 1992;67:39-41.

24. Glancy JM, Weston PJ, Bhullar HK, et al. Reproducibility and automatic measurement of QT dispersion. *Eur Heart J* 1996;17:1035-1039.

25. Hii JT, Wyse DG, Gilles AM, et al. Precordial QT interval dispersion as a marker of torsade de pointe. Disparate effects of class Ia antiarrhythmic drugs and amiodarone.*Circulation* 1992;86:1376-1382.

26. Meierhenrich R, Helguera ME, Kidwell GA, Tebbe U. Effect of amiodarone on QT dispersion and clinical outcome in patients with life-threatening ventricular arrhythmias. *Eur Heart J* 1996;276:1533. Abstract.

27. Grimm W, Steder U, Menz V, et al. Effect of amiodarone on QT dispersion in the 12-lead standard electrocardiogram and its significance for subsequent arrhythmic events. *Clin Cardiol* 1997;20:107-110.

28. Fonseca C, Morais H, Carvalho A, et al. QT interval duration and dispersion in chronic heart failure. Role of amiodarone. *Eur Heart J* 1996;276:465. Abstract.

Dispersion of Ventricular Repolarization and Antiarrhythmic Treatment

Modulation of Dispersion of Ventricular Repolarization by Antiarrhythmic Drugs

Stefan H. Hohnloser

Experimental and clinical data have provided a strong link between the vulnerability of the ventricular myocardium to serious tachyarrhythmias and increased spatial dispersion of ventricular repolarization (DVR).[1-3] Generally speaking, the increase in inhomogeneity of ventricular repolarization is paralleled by an increase in electrical instability favoring the occurrence of reentrant tachyarrhythmias. For instance, the pivotal pathophysiological importance of DVR in the genesis of polymorphous ventricular tachycardia (VT) of the torsade de pointes type has recently been demonstrated by the groups of Antzelevitch[4] and El-Sherif.[5] By three-dimensional mapping of activation and recovery pattern, El-Sherif and coworkers showed that the initial beat of polymorphic VT consistently arose as focal activity from a subendocardial site, whereas subsequent beats were due to successive subendocardial focal activity, reentrant excitation, or a combination of both.[5]

An important principle of the action of Class Ia and Class III antiarrhythmic substances is drug-induced prolongation of repolarization and refractoriness. If these drugs act to not only prolong action potential duration (APD) but also to reduce inhomogeneity of ventricular repolarization, arrhythmia suppression is likely to occur. On the other hand, all of these drugs have the potential to provoke new arrhythmias, particularly those of the torsade de pointes type.[6]

Recent clinical studies have indicated that the interlead variability of the QT interval in the surface electrocardiogram (ECG) may reflect regional differences in ventricular recovery time,[7,8] a hypothesis which was

From Olsson SB, Amlie JP, Yuan S (eds): *Dispersion of Ventricular Repolarization: State of the Art.* ©Futura Publishing Company, Inc., Armonk, NY, 2000.

confirmed by an experimental validation study from our laboratory.[9] The method of analysis of QT dispersion to assess antiarrhythmic drug-associated modifications of DVR would be of particular interest—provided that its clinical utility can be demonstrated beyond doubt—since it is an inexpensive, widely applicable, noninvasive method. It is therefore the purpose of this chapter to summarize the current experimental and clinical evidence of how antiarrhythmic drugs may modify DVR.

Antiarrhythmic–Drug-Induced Modification of DVR: Experimental Findings

Recently a number of carefully conducted experimental studies have evaluated the effects of antiarrhythmic drugs on DVR. In one of these studies, we compared the effects of d-sotalol, quinidine, and amiodarone on DVR in isolated Langendorff-perfused rabbit hearts.[10] DVR was determined in that study by simultaneously recording monophasic action potentials from 6 to 8 different endocardial and epicardial sites at different pacing cycle lengths, with DVR defined as the range of the APD at 90% repolarization (APD$_{90}$). The Class Ia substance increased DVR in a concentration- and rate-dependent manner, as shown in Figure 1. d-Sotalol at a dose of 10^{-6} mol/L produced no significant changes in DVR; but at higher doses, a substantial increase was observed. In contrast to the two other agents, the effects of amiodarone were studied in rabbits that had been fed with the drug for 4 weeks; the results of DVR assessment were compared with those measured in a series of untreated control animals. As depicted in Figure 2, amiodarone was the only drug studied that was absolutely free of a DVR-increasing effect.

On a cellular level, the so-called M cells are thought to play a decisive role in the genesis of inhomogenous ventricular repolarization.[4] M cells, first described by Sicouri and Antzelevitch[11] in dog myocardium, display unique electrophysiological properties different from those of either epi- or endocardium. M cells are distinguished by the ability of their action potentials to prolong disproportionately to those of other ventricular cells at relatively slow rates. It has been demonstrated that blockers of the rapid component of the delayed rectifier current (I_{Kr}) such as erythromycin preferentially act on these M cells, a population of cells largely devoid of I_{Ks}.[12] Accordingly, erythromycin has been shown to provoke a prominent dispersion of repolarization across the ventricular wall, setting the stage for induction of torsade de pointes-like tachyarrhythmias that display characteristics typical of reentry.[12] Similar effects have been demonstrated for quinidine, d-sotalol, and d,l-sotalol: all of these drugs produced prolongation of the action potential and early afterdepolarizations in M cells but not in epicardial or endocardial cells. Opposite findings have been described for chronic amiodarone treatment.[13] Microelectrode studies in

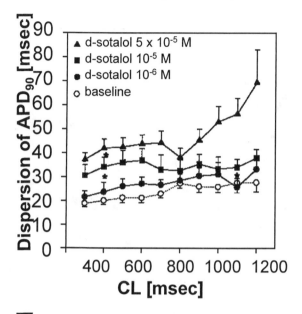

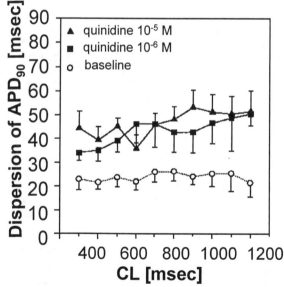

Figure 1. Top: Dispersion of ventricular repolarization (DVR) (mean ± SEM) at various cycle lengths (CLs) during baseline and increasing dosages of d,l-sotalol. Note the increase in DVR particularly at long pacing cycle lengths. **Bottom:** DVR (mean ± SEM) at various CLs during baseline and two different dosages of quinidine. There was a dose-dependent increase in DVR at all driving cycle lengths. APD_{90} = action potential duration measured at 90% depolarization. Modified from Reference 10.

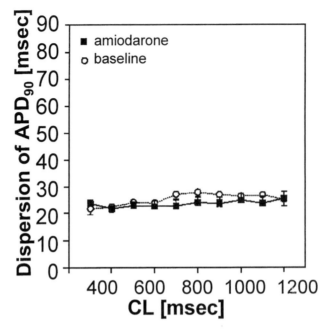

Figure 2. Dispersion of ventricular repolarization (DVR) (mean ± SEM) at various cycle lengths (CLs) in 17 chronically amiodarone-treated hearts and in 18 control preparations. Note the lack of increase in DVR in the amiodarone-treated preparations compared with controls. APD_{90} = action potential duration measured at 90% depolarization. Modified from Reference 10.

transmural strips from the canine left ventricle demonstrated that amiodarone produced a greater prolongation of the APD in epicardium and endocardium, but less of an increase, or even a decrease at slow rates, in the M region. This resulted in a significant reduction of transmural DVR[13] (Fig. 3). These findings are of course in excellent agreement with the above described results using multiple monophasic action potential recordings.

These intrinsic determinants of DVR may further be modified by various pathophysiological factors. Among those, probably the most important ones concern the influence of myocardial ischemia[14] and sympathetic activation.[15] For instance, Opthof and colleagues[15] demonstrated in anesthetized dogs that sympathetic stimulation increases the difference in refractoriness over the border of ischemic and nonischemic myocardium to its opposite effects on normal and ischemic tissue. Dispersion of refractoriness increased up to 59% in individual hearts following sympathetic stimulation during acute, regional ischemia. Given the well-known interactions between ischemia and antiarrhythmic drugs, this interaction may even further enhance DVR.

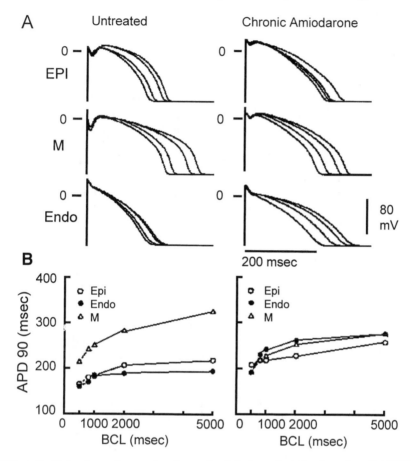

Figure 3. Rate dependence of action potential characteristics in epicardial (EPI), M, and endocardial (Endo) preparations isolated from the hearts of untreated canines and of those exposed to chronic amiodarone administration (**right**). **A.** Simultaneous recording of transmembrane activity in the three different cell types obtained at various basic cycle lengths. **B.** Action potential duration measured at 90% repolarization (APD_{90}) at each site. Note that after exposure to amiodarone the rate dependence of action potential duration is less pronounced in the M cell than in Epi and Endo cells, resulting in less dispersion of action potential durations. Modified from Reference 13.

In summary, there appears to exist a solid line of experimental evidence that antiarrhythmic drugs are potent modifiers of DVR. The M cells play a critical role in drug-induced alterations of transmural dispersion of ventricular recovery due to their relative lack of I_{ks}. From all antiarrhythmic drugs examined so far, only amiodarone could be demonstrated to reduce transmural DVR thereby reducing the likelihood of reentrant arrhythmias such as torsade de pointes.

Antiarrhythmic–Drug-Induced Modification of DVR: Clinical Findings

Most studies evaluating the effects of antiarrhythmic drugs on DVR in the clinical setting have used various methods of assessment of QT dispersion. This interlead difference of QT intervals as determined from the 12-lead surface ECG was proposed in 1990 by Day and coworkers,[7] who suggested that the interlead difference in QT interval may provide a measure of repolarization inhomogeneity which they called "QT dispersion." Advantages and limitations of determination of QT dispersion from the surface ECG are the subject of another chapter of this book. Methodological aspects are therefore not discussed within this chapter.

The first study using QT dispersion to assess antiarrhythmic–drug-induced modification of DVR in the clinical setting was published by Day and colleagues[16] in 1991. These investigators measured rate-corrected QT (QTc) dispersion in 67 infarct survivors randomized to therapy with either sotalol or placebo. Over a 6-month follow-up period they found that QTc dispersion was significantly reduced in patients receiving sotalol compared with placebo, although the maximum QTc was significantly longer in the first group. The authors' interpretation of these observations was that sotalol caused a homogenous prolongation in recovery time in this patient population.[16]

A potentially important application of determination of DVR concerns the occurrence of antiarrhythmic–drug-induced torsade de pointes. As already indicated, the genesis of this particular arrhythmia is largely dependent on increased transmural inhomogeneity of ventricular recovery.[4,5] In support of this, recordings of endocardial monophasic action potentials in selected patients have demonstrated that DVR may indeed facilitate the occurrence of torsade de pointes.[17] However, definite results using this invasive method cannot be expected, simply because it is not suitable for widespread clinical application. Accordingly, it was tempting to test the hypothesis that nonhomogenous prolongation of ventricular repolarization as a consequence of antiarrhythmic drug administration would be manifested by nonhomogenous regional QT interval prolongation. The first study to test this hypothesis was published by Hii and associates[18] in 1992. These authors studied 38 consecutive patients who received both Class Ia therapy and chronic amiodarone treatment. Nine of these patients developed torsade de pointes during exposure to Class Ia drugs. QT dispersion was assessed as the difference between the maximum and the minimum QT interval in the precordial ECG leads. In the 29 patients without torsade de pointes, neither Class Ia drugs nor amiodarone led to significant changes in QT dispersion (50 ± 6 versus 69 ± 7 ms; baseline 54 ± 5 ms). However, there was a striking difference when QT dispersion was analyzed for the nine patients with Class–Ia-induced torsade de pointes. In these patients, therapy with Class Ia drugs was associated with an increase in QT dispersion of 101 ± 37 ms from a baseline value of 44 ± 12 ms (P=0.002). Subsequent amiodarone administration in these nine patients resulted in an average QT dispersion of 49 ± 26 ms, a value which was not significantly different from baseline.[18] Interestingly, none of these patients developed recurrent torsade de pointes while on amiodarone therapy. The main conclusion from that study was that antiarrhythmic–drug-induced torsade de pointes is associated with a pronounced prolongation of QT interval dispersion indicating an increased DVR. These clinical observations are in excellent agreement with the above described experimental findings demonstrating an amiodarone-induced decrease in transmural inhomogeneity in APD.[13]

A study from our institution extended these findings. We were interested in examining changes in DVR in a population of patients with a history of sustained VT or aborted sudden cardiac death treated with d,l-sotalol.[19] Standard 12-lead ECGs at baseline and during sotalol therapy were used to determine QT dispersion (defined as maximum QT minus minimum QT), QTc dispersion, and adjusted QT dispersion (defined as QT dispersion/square root of leads evaluated). Forty-seven patients, 36 males and 11 females, participated in the study. The vast majority of patients (41 of 47; 87%) suffered from coronary artery disease. In the remaining six patients, idiopathic dilative cardiomyopathy was diagnosed as the underlying heart disease. Nine patients presented with a history of prehospital ventricular fibrillation and 38 had experienced at least one episode of sustained VT. An average left ventricular ejection fraction of $34\pm15\%$ was determined by means of either radionuclide angiography or left heart catheterization. Three groups of patients were defined: drug responders (group A; n=17), nonresponders (group B; n=18), and patients who developed torsade de pointes (group C; n=12). There were no significant differences with respect to baseline data among the three predefined patient groups. After exposure to sotalol, the QT interval duration increased to a similar extent in all three groups. Concerning QT dispersion, there were no significant differences among the three groups during drug-free baseline measurements. The QT dispersion averaged 61 ± 18 ms in group A, 58 ± 23 ms in group B, and 57 ± 20 ms in group C. Similarly, QTc dispersion was comparable in all three groups of patients (group A: 65 ± 21 ms; group B: 64 ± 24 ms; group C: 69 ± 21 ms), as was the adjusted QT dispersion (group A: 21 ± 7 ms; group B: 21 ± 7 ms; group C: 23 ± 8 ms).

During oral therapy with sotalol, patients who responded to the drug (group A) showed a small but significant decline in QT dispersion from 61 ± 18 ms to 45 ± 16 ms (P<0.01; Fig. 4). QTc dispersion was reduced from 65 ± 21 ms to 43 ± 14 ms (P<0.005), and the adjusted QT dispersion from 21 ± 7 ms to 14 ± 4 ms (P=0.004). There were no significant changes in QT

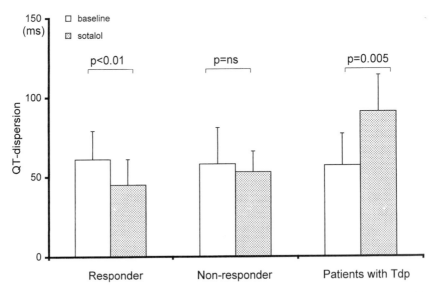

Figure 4. Effects of d,l-sotalol on QT dispersion in three groups of patients with a history of sustained ventricular tachyarrhythmias. There was a small decrease in QT dispersion in patients with sotalol-associated suppression of arrhythmia inducibility compared with baseline. In nonresponders, no significant difference in QT dispersion before and after drug exposure was noted. Most strikingly, patients who developed sotalol-induced torsade de pointes (Tdp) showed a dramatic increase in QT dispersion.

dispersion (58±23 ms versus 53±13 ms), QTc dispersion (64±24 ms versus 53±14 ms), or adjusted QT dispersion (21±7 ms versus 17±4 ms) in those individuals in whom sotalol was ineffective in suppressing the arrhythmia. In contrast, QT dispersion, QTc dispersion, and adjusted QT dispersion increased considerably in those patients who developed an episode of torsade de pointes during exposure to sotalol. In these patients, QT dispersion rose from 57±20 ms during baseline to 91±23 ms during active treatment (P<0.005; Fig. 4). QTc dispersion increased from 69±21 ms to 89±19 ms (P<0.02), and the adjusted QT dispersion from 23±8 ms to 29±7 ms (P=0.04). An increment in QT dispersion of ≥20 ms, a time interval equivalent to one standard deviation of the average QT interval dispersion during drug-free baseline, was noted in 10 of 12 patients. Six group C patients had an on-drug QT dispersion of ≥100 ms, a value that was observed in only one patient from group B and in none of the sotalol responders (group A) (group C versus group B: P=0.02; group C versus group A: P=0.005). Accordingly, the average on-drug QT dispersion was significantly greater in group C patients as compared with group A (P<0.001) or group B patients (P<0.001). From our results, we concluded that an increase in QT dispersion of ≥50% compared with baseline or an absolute value of QT dispersion of 100 ms or more is associated with a high likelihood of development of sotalol-induced torsade de pointes. The decrease in QT dispersion observed in those patients who favorably responded to sotalol therapy, albeit statistically significant, should most likely not be overemphasized.

These conclusions were subsequently supported by a second study from our institution.[20] In that study, 50 patients with persistent atrial fibrillation were randomly assigned to therapy with quinidine or d,l-sotalol in order to restore sinus rhythm. To assess the effects of both antiarrhythmic drugs on DVR, we measured precordial QT dispersion at baseline (i.e., during atrial fibrillation) and during active therapy. There were four cases of proarrhythmia in the quinidine group but none in patients receiving sotalol. In three patients, torsade de pointes was documented during administration of the Class Ia substance. Both antiarrhythmic drugs caused a similar degree of QT interval prolongation (maximal QT interval in quinidine-treated patients 411 ± 39 ms versus 363 ± 38 ms at baseline; $P<0.01$; sotalol: 425 ± 58 ms versus 367 ± 40 ms at baseline; $P<0.01$). QT dispersion as assessed in the precordial ECG leads, however, increased significantly only in the quinidine group: from 34 ± 9 to 44 ± 16 ms ($P=0.02$). Most importantly, however, in all three patients with quinidine-associated torsade de pointes, QT dispersion increased by more than 50% of the control value. Sotalol-treated patients showed no significant changes in the average QT dispersion (36 ± 18 ms versus 40 ± 17 ms; $P=0.44$).

The effects of three different Class III antiarrhythmic agents on DVR were compared in a study by Cui and associates.[21] These investigators studied three groups of patients before and after exposure to amiodarone (n=26), sematilide (n=26), and d,l-sotalol (n=26). Conventional assessment of QT dispersion was performed at baseline and after drug exposure. All three drugs prolonged the maximum QT interval to a similar degree. However, QT dispersion was significantly changed only in the group of patients treated with amiodarone. In this cohort the average QT dispersion declined from 79 ± 13 ms to 49 ± 14 ms ($P<0.001$). In patients treated with sematilide or sotalol, no significant changes in QT dispersion were found, although there was a trend for a decrease in the sotalol group. The main conclusion of that study was that the low incidence of amiodarone-induced torsade de pointes[22] may at least in part be due to the favorable effects of this compound on DVR.[21]

Another line of evidence of how antiarrhythmic drugs may influence DVR was recently provided by Choy et al.[23] These authors treated 12 healthy subjects with quinidine sulfate, and observed significant increases in the maximum QT interval and in QTUc dispersion. Subsequent infusion of KCl (maximum, 40 mE) resulted in a dramatic reduction in QTUc dispersion from 210 ± 62 to 130 ± 75 ms ($P<0.01$). In another cohort of patients suffering from congestive heart failure, KCl infusion led to a similar reduction in QTUc dispersion from a baseline value of 132±68 ms to 84±35 ms (P=0.07). These results not only support the concept of antiarrhythmic–drug-induced modulation of DVR but also indicate that therapeutic means may have a similar potency. The authors concluded that potentially arrhythmogenic QT abnormalities during therapy with I_{Kr} blockers such as quinidine can almost be normalized by elevating extracellular potassium.[23]

Conclusions and Clinical Implications

In summary, there is convincing experimental and clinical evidence that antiarrhythmic drugs can and do modify DVR. Despite the limitations of assessment of QT dispersion from the surface ECG as a surrogate of DVR, the application of this method in various studies has provided potentially relevant findings. Most importantly, there is considerable evidence that an increase in QT dispersion of more than 50% of the baseline value after exposure to antiarrhythmic drugs is associated with a high likelihood of proarrhythmia of the torsade de pointes type. The same applies if a patient demonstrates a QT dispersion of 100 ms or more while receiving a Class Ia or a Class II antiarrhythmic compound. In both circumstances, withdrawal of the drug appears indicated. The second important finding that has emerged from the studies discussed relates to amiodarone. It is probably fair to say that this antiarrhythmic compound appears to be the only one that may favorably alter DVR in the majority of patients. This may be one decisive factor for the well-known low incidence of torsade de pointes tachycardias during therapy with this compound.[22]

The method of QT dispersion measurements is, however, most likely not accurate enough to allow any conclusions about drug effectiveness or ineffectiveness when only small changes are observed. There is substantial hope that technological improvements will, in the future, allow more precise determination of various parameters of ventricular repolarization from the surface ECG (i.e., taking into account the morphology of the T wave, presence or absence of T wave alternans, and so forth). Whether these methods will eventually allow a more accurate assessment of the DVR-modifying effects of antiarrhythmic agents and whether this will eventually translate into increased safety of pharmacological therapy of arrhythmias, remains to be seen.

References

1. Han J, Moe GK. Nonuniform recovery of excitability in ventricular muscle. *Circ Res* 1964;14:44.

2. Kuo CS, Munakata K, Reddy CP, Surawicz B. Characteristics and possible mechanism of ventricular arrhythmia dependent on the dispersion of action potential durations. *Circulation* 1983;67:1356-1367.
3. Vassallo JA, Cassidy DM, Kindwall KE, et al. Nonuniform recovery of excitability in the left ventricle. *Circulation* 1988;78:1365-1372.
4. Antzelevitch C, Sicouri S. Clinical relevance of cardiac arrhythmias generated by afterdepolarizations: The role of M cells in the generation of U waves, triggered activity and torsade de pointes. *J Am Coll Cardiol* 1994;23:259-277.
5. El-Sherif N, Caref EB, Ying H, Restivo M. Electrophysiological mechanism of ventricular arrhythmias in the long QT syndrome. Tridimensional mapping of activation and recovery patterns. *Circ Res* 1996;79:474-492.
6. Hohnloser SH, Singh BN. Proarrhythmia with class III antiarrhythmic drugs: Definition, electrophysiologic mechanisms, incidence, predisposing factors, and clinical implications. *J Cardiovasc Electrophysiol* 1995;6:920-936.
7. Day CP, McComb JM, Campbell RWF. QT dispersion: An indication of arrhythmia risk in patients with long QT intervals. *Br Heart J* 1990;63:342-344.
8. Mirvis DM. Spatial variation of QT intervals in normal persons and patients with acute myocardial infarction. *J Am Coll Cardiol* 1985;3:625-631.
9. Zabel M, Portnoy S, Franz MR. Electrocardiographic indexes of dispersion of ventricular repolarization: An isolated heart validation study. *J Am Coll Cardiol* 1995;25:746-752.
10. Zabel M, Hohnloser SH, Behrens S, et al. Differential effects of d-sotalol, quinidine, and amiodarone on dispersion of ventricular repolarization in the isolated rabbit heart. *J Cardiovasc Electrophysiol* 1997;8:1239-1245.
11. Sicouri S, Antzelevitch C. A subpopulation of cells with unique electrophysiological properties in the deep subendocardium of the canine ventricle. The M cell. *Circ Res* 1991;68:1729-1741.
12. Antzelevitch C, Sun Z-Q, Zhang Z-Q, Yan GX. Cellular and ionic mechanisms underlying erythromycin-induced long QT intervals and torsade de point. *J Am Coll Cardiol* 1996;28:1836-1848.
13. Sicouri S, Moro S, Litovsky S, et al. Chronic amiodarone reduces transmural dispersion of repolarization in the canine heart. *J Cardiovasc Electrophysiol* 1997;8:1269-1279.
14. Mayuga RD, Singer DH. Effects of intravenous amiodarone on electrical dispersion in normal and ischemic tissue and on arrhythmia inducibility: Monophasic action potential studies. *Cardiovasc Res* 1992;26:571-579.
15. Opthof T, Coronel R, Vermeulen JT, et al. Dispersion of refractoriness in normal and ischemic canine ventricle: Effects of sympathetic stimulation. *Cardiovasc Res* 1993;27:1954-1960.
16. Day CP, McComb JM, Matthews J, Campbell RWF. Reduction in QT dispersion by sotalol following myocardial infarction. *Eur Heart J* 1991;12:423-427.
17. Habbab M, El-Sherif N. Drug-induced torsades de pointes: Role of early afterdepolarizations and dispersion of repolarization. *Am J Med* 1990;89: 241-246.
18. Hii JTY, Wyse GD, Gillis AM, et al. Precordial QT interval dispersion as a marker of torsade de pointes. *Circulation* 1992;86:1376-1382.
19. Hohnloser SH, van de Loo A, Kalusche D, et al. Does sotalol-induced alteration of QT-dispersion predict drug effectiveness or proarrhythmic hazards? *Circulation* 1993;88(suppl I):I397.
20. Hohnloser SH, van de Loo A, Baedeker F. Efficacy and proarrhythmic hazards of pharmacological cardioversion of atrial fibrillation: Prospective comparison of sotalol versus quinidine. *J Am Coll Cardiol* 1995;26:852-858.

21. Cui G, Sen L, Sager P, et al. Effects of amiodarone, sematilide, and sotalol on QT dispersion. *Am J Cardiol* 1994;74:896-900.
22. Hohnloser SH, Klingenheben T, Singh BN. Amiodarone-associated proarrhythmic effects: A review with special reference to torsade de pointes tachycardia. *Ann Intern Med* 1994;121:529-535.
23. Choy AM, Lang CC, Chomsky DM, et al. Normalization of acquired QT prolongation in humans by intravenous potassium. *Circulation* 1997;96: 2149-2154.

18

Effect of Class I Drugs on Dispersion of Repolarization

Lennart Bergfeldt

Quinidine, the prototype Class Ia antiarrhythmic drug, has been ascribed several proarrhythmic properties such as slowing of impulse formation and conduction, prolongation of repolarization, which promotes the development of early afterdepolarization, and creation of postrepolarization refractoriness (especially in abnormal tissues). This substance can therefore promote the occurrence of triggered arrhythmias as well as stable reentry, whether the latter is due to a leading circle or spiral wave.[1,2] The other substances belonging to Class I have a similar (Class Ia drugs), or more limited (Class Ib drugs), or different (Class Ic drugs) "repertoire" in this aspect.

The typical "proarrhythmia" torsade de pointes (TdP) ventricular tachycardia has been associated mostly with the Class Ia subgroup, and it is therefore not surprising that the available literature deals mainly with the substances of this subgroup. Salient features of TdP occurring in association with Class Ia antiarrhythmic drugs, as well as with other substances used for cardiac and noncardiac purposes, are the relation to a prolonged QT interval and the bradycardia dependence. The mechanistic discussion has therefore focused on early afterdepolarizations leading to triggered activity, presumably in a myocardial milieu of temporal and spatial heterogeneity of ventricular repolarization.[1,3-6] There is more documentation on early afterdepolarizations, which are not the subject of the present chapter, than on heterogeneity (dispersion) of ventricular recovery of excitability or repolarization. However, dispersion of recovery of ventricular excitability has been assessed in in vitro experiments, either in myocardial strips or in isolated heart preparations, or in vivo in whole

Dr. Bergfeldt is a clinical investigator for the Swedish Heart-Lung Foundation.

From Olsson SB, Amlie JP, Yuan S (eds): *Dispersion of Ventricular Repolarization: State of the Art.* ©Futura Publishing Company, Inc., Armonk, NY, 2000.

animal experiments. Human studies encompass the assessment of mono-phasic action potential duration (MAPD, usually at 90% repolarization and sometimes combined with measurement of activation time, where repolarization time = activation time + MAPD), refractory periods (usually the effective refractory period, ERP), or both, at multiple sites, or noninva-sively by the assessment of the maximum interlead difference of the QT and JT intervals in the surface 12-lead electrocardiogram (ECG) or from body surface maps.

Class Ia Antiarrhythmic Drugs (Quinidine, Procainamide, Disopyramide)

This subgroup of drugs prolongs activation time (decrease conduc-tion velocity) and repolarization through interaction with sodium and potassium channels. Drugs belonging to this subgroup have all been associated with prolongation of the QT interval and the occurrence of TdP ventricular arrhythmias, i.e., the acquired long QT syndrome.[1,4]

The dispersion of ERP between eight different right ventricular *epicar-dial* sites was evaluated in two series of dog experiments, and increased from 16±3 ms and 18±7 ms at baseline to 33±14 ms and 42±10 ms on quinidine.[7,8] In contrast, no change in dispersion was found, despite prolongation of the QRS and QT intervals, when *endocardial* MAPD and ERP were evaluated in dogs at four different right ventricular sites at three doses of quinidine.[9] In line with the above results, it was subse-quently reported that, although quinidine has different effects in vitro on the repolarization of endocardial and epicardial cells in the isolated rabbit heart[10] as well as on endocardial, epicardial, and M cells in the normal dog heart, in vivo experiments in the dog show a uniform prolongation of repolarization in all myocardial cell layers that follows the pattern of the M cells.[11,12] These reports importantly demonstrate the difficulty in predicting the net effect from in vitro studies.

Hii et al[13] compared the effects of Class Ia drugs and of amiodarone on the QT and JT intervals and their dispersion in precordial ECG leads in two groups of patients. Nine (six men) had a documentation of TdP during Class Ia drug therapy, while 29 patients had not had this complica-tion.[13] The majority of these patients had chronic atherosclerotic heart disease and required antiarrhythmic therapy, mostly for ventricular ar-rhythmia. Seven of the nine were treated with quinidine, and one each with disopyramide and procainamide. While taking Class Ia drugs, the group of patients with TdP had a significantly greater dispersion of QT and JT as well as of rate-corrected QT (QTc) and JT (JTc) intervals than the group of patients without TdP; the former group also responded to the drug with a significantly longer QT interval. The group with TdP also had greater dispersion values while taking Class Ia drugs than while taking amiodarone, while the opposite was true for the group without TdP (significant for QT dispersion only). In the drug-free state there was no statistically significant difference between the two groups with regard to the absolute and rate-corrected values of the QT and JT intervals and their dispersion. The baseline QT interval dispersion was on the normal level, and not significantly different in the group that did than in the group that did not develop TdP; 44 ± 12 ms versus 53 ± 29 ms. However, during Class Ia therapy QT dispersion increased to on average 101 ± 37 ms in the TdP group, while it remained on the baseline level in the other group. This study, importantly, demonstrates a relation between the occurrence of TdP and the degree of QT interval dispersion assessed in precordial leads. Baseline dispersion values could not, in this patient cohort, predict the response to drug therapy. Patient characteristics, and data on drug levels, drug exposure time, and serum potassium levels, are provided, but there is no information on concomitant drug therapy or heart rate at the appearance of TdP. Similarly, Hohnloser et al[14] observed a significant increase in QT dispersion in precordial leads in a group of patients with atrial fibrillation who were given quinidine, from 34 ± 9 ms at baseline to 44 ± 16 ms on quinidine (P=0.02). In the parallel group, which was randomized to sotalol, no significant increase in average QT dispersion was seen (36 ± 18ms versus 40 ± 17ms; P=0.44). Three patients in the quinidine group developed TdP, and in all of them the QT dispersion had increased by greater than 50%.

In the *normal human heart* disopyramide prolongs the QT and JT intervals on average 8% to 12% and 7% to 11%, respectively, but the effect on QT dispersion at spontaneous rhythm and at fixed rate atrial pacing (assessed in leads I, II, V_1, V_2, and V_6) is unpredictable.[15] This result might, however, mostly reflect the considerable time-dependent variations (insufficient reproducibility) of QT and JT dispersion, in contrast to the very high reproducibility of the single lead (lead II) assessment of the QT and JT intervals.[15-17] Except for the above mentioned study in healthy subjects and one case in the report by Hii et al,[13] there are no reports on the effects of disopyramide on the dispersion of the recovery of ventricular excitability. A report on TdP during disopyramide therapy,[18] however, presented the speculation that there was a possibility that increased dispersion of repolarization was a crucial element of arrhythmogenicity. From another case report[19] it was clear that the occurrence of such arrhythmias 1) was preceded by uneventful therapy with quinidine, and 2) occurred in relation to additional therapy with negatively chronotropic (and dromotropic) drugs, including verapamil and amiodarone. These observations are even more interesting in light of a recent report on patients with bradycardia-related QT interval prolongation responding with a more pronounced QT prolongation while taking disopyramide than patients with bradycardia not accompanied by QT interval prolongation.[20]

A relation between procainamide administration, TdP, and increased dispersion of repolarization (MAPD and local activation time) as assessed from recordings in the right and left ventricular apices was nicely demonstrated in a case by Habbab and El-Sherif[21] in 1990. They measured the dispersion of repolarization to 180 to 280 ms. In patients without repolarization abnormalities the dispersion of repolarization time between different endocardial sites was 10 to 46 ms,[22] while dispersion of MAPD was 21 to 64 ms.[22,23] In contrast, the dispersion of MAPD was ≤270 ms between different right endocardial sites in patients with the long QT syndrome and TdP of different etiologies.[23] Shechter et al,[24] who studied 12 patients, two with a documentation of TdP, and assessed the ERP at three sites— right ventricular apex and outflow tract plus one left ventricular site (n= 10) or a third right ventricular site (n=2)—did not observe any effect of procainamide on ERP dispersion. They also tried to provoke ventricular arrhythmia by programmed stimulation, and induced nonsustained polymorphic ventricular tachycardia in six cases at baseline (one with previous TdP) and in three after procainamide administration (none with previous TdP). The measurement of ERP is generally made after short runs (8 to 10 beats) at relatively short cycle lengths. This was the case also in this study, where it was measured at a basic cycle length of 500 ms and at sinus rhythm with elevated rate (". . . cycle length was abbreviated, presumably in response to the decreased blood pressure after the infusion."). This might be a limitation of the technique, and against the background of numerous observations of a pattern of short-long cycles preceding the onset of TdP, ERP assessment after short-long cycles might give different and more relevant results. Programmed stimulation with short-long-short cycles has been suggested for the purpose of increasing the sensitivity of the test with regard to ventricular tachycardia induction[25] but, as far as the author knows, this technique has not been used in the present context.

The combined effect of procainamide and ischemia was evaluated in a dog experiment. ERP dispersion was assessed at two sites within the left ventricular myocardium at baseline, after 15 minutes of coronary ligation, creating ischemia in the area of one of the sites, and 10 and 20 minutes after procainamide administration during continuous coronary ligation.[26] At baseline there was no difference in ERP. After 15 minutes occlusion there was a 12.2% dispersion due to shortening of the ERP within the ischemic zone. This difference decreased after procainamide administration, which prolonged ERP more in the ischemic area than in the normal, resulting in a net decrease of the dispersion to 5.5%.

While the report by Hii et al[13] included one case of procainamide-associated TdP with increased QT dispersion on drug, an earlier report[27] on seven cases with TdP during procainamide therapy unfortunately did not include any information on QT or JT dispersion.

Class Ib Antiarrhythmic Drugs

One reference with relation to this topic has been identified. Wolk et al[28] studied the effects of lidocaine (lignocaine) on dispersion of repolarization and refractoriness in a working rabbit heart model of regional ischemia. Suction electrodes for MAPD assessment and separate electrodes for ERP measurement were positioned at one right and two left ventricular sites, one above and one within a region subsequently made ischemic by the tightening of a snare around a coronary artery. The ventricular fibrillation threshold was also assessed. In the area at risk, ischemia induced a shortening of the MAPD and ERP. The resulting dispersion of MAPD between the ischemic area and the area above occlusion was not affected by lidocaine. However, lidocaine augmented the ischemia-induced conduction delay and therefore decreased the dispersion of repolarization (activation time + MAPD) between the two left ventricular sites. In addition, lidocaine significantly decreased the ischemia-induced dispersion of refractoriness. The inducibility of ventricular arrhythmia from the ischemic site was also significantly decreased by the drug, which also abolished the spontaneous occurrence of reperfusion arrhythmias. This experimental study, importantly, underlines the importance of assessing activation time together with the MAP recordings.

Class Ic Antiarrhythmic Drugs

The great interest in the proarrhythmic effects of antiarrhythmic drugs was sparked by the CAST study,[29] and by the negative effects of encainide and flecainide. Some studies on these and the other Class Ic drugs focused more on their effect on conduction velocity and refractoriness per se than on any effect on heterogeneity of ventricular repolarization.[30-33] On the other hand, experimental studies on endocardial and epicardial cell preparations by Krishnan and Antzelevitch[34,35] elegantly showed that flecainide exerts differential effects on these two cell types and thus may lead to transmural dispersion of action potential duration but also to significant dispersion of action potential duration between different epicardial sites. In these studies they also demonstrated reentry—"phase 2 reentry"—related to the occurrence of dispersion of action potential duration and enhanced by changes in cycle length, and slowing of conduction, but found no evidence of enhanced automaticity (afterdepolarizations) and triggered activity. The "proarrhythmic" mechanism was thus different from what has been found for Class Ia drugs. Interestingly, the electrocardiographic abnormalities related to the Brugada syndrome, and the arrhythmia mechanism in this disorder, seem to be associated with disturbances similar to those induced by flecainide.[36-39]

One more reference with relevance for the discussion of Class Ic drugs has been identified. Faber et al[40] randomized 98 patients scheduled for percutaneous coronary angioplasty (PTCA) to pretreatment with either placebo or propafenone. Twelve-lead ECG was recorded (50 mm/s) at baseline 5 minutes before and at the end of 60 seconds occlusion, and QT (QTc) and JT (JTc) intervals and their dispersion were compared between the two groups. In the propafenone group the increase in dispersion was more than twice of that in the placebo group, and the most considerable increase was observed during PTCA of the left anterior descending artery in patients with signs of anterior wall ischemia. There was also a positive correlation with previous anterior wall myocardial infarction and a greater risk for increased dispersion in patients with left ventricular hypertrophy at baseline. The increased dispersion resulting from the combination of ischemia and propafenone was largely generated by a prolongation of the maximal QTc and JTc intervals (rather than shortening of minimum QTc and JTc intervals). This study highlights the importance of the interaction between drug effects, structural abnormalities, and transient events such as ischemia.

QT Interval Dispersion and the Antiarrhythmic Effect on Ventricular Arrhythmia

In a recent report[41] the change in QT dispersion from baseline to steady-state drug therapy was compared in responders (suppressed arrhythmia induction) and nonresponders undergoing electropharmacological testing. Precordial leads recorded at a paper speed of 25 mm/s were used. There was no difference between responders and nonresponders at baseline, while QT dispersion decreased slightly but not statistically significantly during presumed effective therapy, in contrast to a significant increase in QT dispersion in nonresponders. In the quinidine group QT dispersion at baseline and during steady-state treatment, respectively, was 50 ± 24 ms versus 39 ± 14 ms, and 47 ± 22 ms versus 58 ± 28 ms in responders (n=8) and nonresponders (n=48). As judged from Figure 2 in this reference, the individual responses varied considerably; QT dispersion decreased in 5, increased in 2, and did not change in 1 responder, while the corresponding numbers for nonresponders were 12, 24, and 12. Considering also the numerical differences and a probable uncertainty of the visual determination of the QT interval of ±0.5 mm corresponding to 20 ms at paper speed 25 mm/s, these results and their predictive value need confirmation.

Summary

This literature review focusing on Class I antiarrhythmic drug therapy and dispersion of repolarization can be summarized as follows:

1. Class Ia drugs modestly prolong repolarization in the healthy heart but do not seem to increase the dispersion of repolarization.
2. When TdP ventricular tachycardia occurs in patients taking Class Ia drugs it can, noninvasively, be related to an increase in the QT and JT intervals and their dispersion, and, invasively, to dispersion of ventricular repolarization as assessed with MAP recordings at different endocardial sites.
3. The heart rate—instantaneous and/or overall—seems to be crucial, and previously tolerated Class Ia drugs, might become intolerable from proarrhythmic point of view if heart rate decreases, spontaneously or due to concomitant therapy with negatively chronotropic drugs. In contrast, the opposite (rate increase) might be arrhythmogenic in patients taking Class Ic drugs, reflecting different arrhythmia mechanisms.
4. On an individual level, prediction of risk for an adverse drug reaction with regard to increased dispersion of repolarization and proarrhythmia cannot be made if baseline QT and JT intervals are normal.

References

1. Lazzara R, Szabo B, Patterson E, et al. Mechanisms for proarrhythmia with antiarrhythmic drugs. In Zipes DP, Jalife J (eds): *Cardiac Electrophysiology: From Cell to Bedside*. Philadelphia: W.B. Saunders Co.; 1990:402-407.
2. Janse MJ. Functional reentry: Leading circle or spiral wave? *J Cardiovasc Electrophysiol* 1999;10:621-622.
3. Surawicz B. Electrophysiologic substrate of torsade de pointes: Dispersion of repolarization or early afterdepolarizations? *J Am Coll Cardiol* 1989; 14:172-184.
4. Zehender M, Hohnloser S, Just H. QT-interval prolonging drugs: Mechanisms and clinical relevance of their arrhythmogenic hazards. *Cardiovasc Drugs Ther* 1991;5:515-530.
5. Patterson E, Szabo B, Scherlag B, et al. Arrhythmogenic effects of antiarrhythmic drugs. In Zipes DP, Jalife J (eds): *Cardiac Electrophysiology: From Cell to Bedside*. Philadelphia: W.B. Saunders Co.; 1995:496-511.
6. Roden DM. Ionic mechanisms for prolongation of refractoriness and their proarrhythmic and antiarrhythmic correlates. *Am J Cardiol* 1996;78(suppl 4A):12-16.
7. Inoue H, Toda I, Nozaki A, et al. Inhomogeneity of ventricular refractory period in canine heart with quinidine-induced long QT interval: A comparative study on effects of heart rate, isoprenaline, and lignocaine. *Cardiovasc Res* 1985;19:623-630.
8. Inoue H, Toda I, Nozaki A, et al. Effects of bretylium tosylate on inhomogeneity of refractoriness and ventricular fibrillation threshold in canine hearts with quinidine-induced long QT-interval. *Cardiovasc Res* 1985;19:655-660.
9. Brugada J, Sassine A, Escande D, et al. Effects of quinidine on ventricular repolarization. *Eur Heart J* 1987;8:1340-1345.

10. Zabel M, Hohnloser SH, Behrens S, et al. Differential effects of d-sotalol, quinidine, and amiodarone on dispersion of ventricular repolarization in the isolated rabbit heart. *J Cardiovasc Electrophysiol* 1997;8:1239-1245.
11. Sosunov EA, Anyukhovsky EP, Rosen MR. Effects of quinidine on repolarization in canine epicardium, midmyocardium, and endocardium. I. In vitro study. *Circulation* 1997;96:4011-4018.
12. Anyukhovsky EP, Sosunov EA, Feinmark SJ, et al. Effects of quinidine on repolarization in canine epicardium, midmyocardium, and endocardium. II. In vivo study. *Circulation* 1997;96:4019-4026.
13. Hii JTY, Wyse DG, Gillis AM, et al. Precordial QT interval dispersion as a marker of torsade de pointes. Disparate effects of class Ia antiarrhythmic drugs and amiodarone. *Circulation* 1992;86:1376-1382.
14. Hohnloser SH, van de Loo A, Baedeker F. Efficacy and proarrhythmic hazards of pharmacologic cardioversion of atrial fibrillation: Prospective comparison of sotalol versus quinidine. *J Am Coll Cardiol* 1995;26:852-858.
15. Nowinski K, Bergfeldt L. "Normal" response of the QT interval and QT dispersion following intravenous injection of the sodium channel blocker disopyramide: Methodological aspects. *Cardiovasc Drugs Ther* 1995;9:573-580.
16. Kautzner J, Yi G, Camm AJ, et al. Short- and long-term reproducibility of QT, QTc and QT dispersion measurement in healthy subjects. *PACE* 1994;17:928-937.
17. Fei L, Statters DJ, Camm AJ. QT-interval dispersion on 12-lead electrocardiogram in normal subjects: Its reproducibility and relation to the T wave. *Am Heart J* 1994;27:1654-1655.
18. Wald RW, Waxman MB, Colman MJ. Torsade de pointes ventricular tachycardia a complication of disopyramide shared with quinidine. *J Electrocardiol* 1981;14:301-308.
19. Tzivoni D, Keren A, Stern S, et al. Disopyramide-induced torsade de pointes. *Arch Intern Med* 1981;141:946-947.
20. Furushima H, Niwano S, Chinushi M, et al. Relation between bradycardia dependent long QT syndrome and QT prolongation by disopyramide in humans. *Heart* 1998;79:56-58.
21. Habbab MA, El-Sherif N. Drug-induced torsades de pointes: Role of early afterdepolarizations and dispersion of repolarization. *Am J Med* 1990;89: 241-246.
22. Franz MR, Bargheer K, Rafflenbeul W, et al. Monophasic action potential mapping in human subjects with normal electrocardiograms: Direct evidence for the genesis of the T wave. *Circulation* 1987;75:379-386.
23. Bonatti V, Rolli A, Bott G. Recording of monophasic action potentials of the right ventricle in long QT syndromes complicated by severe ventricular arrhythmias. *Eur Heart J* 1983;4:168-179.
24. Shechter JA, Caine R, Friehling T, et al. Effect of procainamide on dispersion of ventricular refractoriness. *Am J Cardiol* 1983;52:279-282.
25. Denker S, Lehmann M, Mahmud R, et al. Facilitation of ventricular tachycardia induction with abrupt changes in ventricular cycle length. *Am J Cardiol* 1984;53:508-515.
26. Levites R, Haft JI, Calderon J, et al. Effects of procainamide on the dispersion of recovery of excitability during coronary occlusion. *Circulation* 1976;53:982-984.
27. Strasberg B, Sclarovsky S, Erdberg A, et al. Procainamide-induced polymorphous ventricular tachycardia. *Am J Cardiol* 1981;47:1309-1314.

28. Wolk R, Cobbe SM, Hicks MN, et al. Effects of lignocaine on dispersion of repolarisation and refractoriness in a working rabbit heart model of regional myocardial ischaemia. *J Cardiovasc Pharmacol* 1998;31:253-261.
29. CAST Investigators. Preliminary report: Effect of encainide and flecainide on mortality in a randomized trial of arrhythmia suppression after myocardial infarction. *N Engl J Med* 1989;321:406-412.
30. Brugada J, Boersma L, Kirchhof C, et al. Proarrhythmic effects of flecainide. Experimental evidence for increased susceptibility to reentrant arrhythmias. *Circulation* 1991;84:1808-1818.
31. El-Sherif N. Experimental models of reentry, antiarrhythmic, and proarrhythmic actions of drugs. Complexities galore! *Circulation* 1991;84:1871-1875. Editorial.
32. Katritis D, Rowland E, O'Nunain S, et al. Effect of flecainide on atrial and ventricular refractoriness and conduction in patients with normal left ventricle. Implications for possible antiarrhythmic and proarrhythmic mechanisms. *Eur Heart J* 1995;16:1930-1935.
33. Stark U, Stark G, Poppe H, et al. Rate-dependent effects of detajmium and propafenone on ventricular conduction and refractoriness in isolated guinea pig hearts. *J Cardiovasc Pharmacol* 1996;27:125-131.
34. Krishnan SC, Antzelevitch C. Sodium channel block produces opposite electrophysiological effects in canine ventricular epicardium and endocardium. *Circ Res* 1991;68:277-291.
35. Krishnan SC, Antzelevitch C. Flecainide-induced arrhythmia in canine ventricular epicardium. Phase 2 reentry? *Circulation* 1993;87:562-572.
36. Fujiki A, Usui M, Nagasawa H, et al. ST segment elevation in the right precordial leads induced with class 1C antiarrhythmic drugs: Insight into the mechanism of Brugada Syndrome. *J Cardiovasc Electrophysiol* 1999;10:214-218.
37. Roden DM, Wilde AAM. Drug-induced J point elevation: A marker for genetic risk of sudden death or ECG curiosity? *J Cardiovasc Electrophysiol* 1999;10:219-223.
38. Alings M, Wilde A. "Brugada" syndrome. Clinical data and suggested pathophysiological mechanism. *Circulation* 1999;99:666-673.
39. Brugada J, Brugada P, Brugada R. The syndrome of right bundle branch block ST segment elevation in V1 to V3 and sudden death—the Brugada Syndrome. *Europace* 1999;1:156-166.
40. Faber TS, Zehender M, Krahnefeld O, et al. Propafenone during acute myocardial ischemia in patients: A double-blind, randomized, placebo-controlled study. *J Am Coll Cardiol* 1997;29:561-567.
41. Gillis AM, Traboulsi M, Hii JTY, et al. Antiarrhythmic drug effects on QT interval dispersion in patients undergoing electropharmacologic testing for ventricular tachycardia and fibrillation. *Am J Cardiol* 1998;81:588-593.

19

Effect of Class III Drugs on Dispersion of Repolarization in Patients with Myocardial Infarction

C.P. Day

Previous chapters have outlined both the clinical and experimental evidence for increased dispersion of ventricular repolarization as a mechanism for ventricular arrhythmogenesis in a range of clinical settings usually characterized by prolongation of the QT interval on the surface electrocardiogram (ECG). In Chapter 10 Professor Janse specifically reviews the role of ventricular recovery time dispersion as a substrate for both ventricular tachycardia and ventricular fibrillation following experimental myocardial infarction.[1,2] Early data from canine experiments, meanwhile, suggested that Class III antiarrhythmic drugs act, at least in part, by differential prolongation of repolarization leading to decreased temporal dispersion of ventricular recovery following infarction and Class I drug induced QT prolongation.[3,4] In addition to providing valuable insights into mechanisms of arrhythmogenesis and the action of Class III drugs, these studies highlighted the need to develop a simple, noninvasive method of measuring recovery time dispersion that could be used in routine clinical practice. Applications of such a method would potentially include the assessment of both arrhythmia risk post infarction and the efficacy of antiarrhythmic drug therapy in reducing this risk.

In 1987, working with the late Professor RWF Campbell, I designed a series of studies to test the hypothesis that the interlead variability in QT interval duration on the standard surface ECG, previously reported by Professor Campbell's group,[5] fulfilled the role of a noninvasive measure

From Olsson SB, Amlie JP, Yuan S (eds): *Dispersion of Ventricular Repolarization: State of the Art.* ©Futura Publishing Company, Inc., Armonk, NY, 2000.

of recovery time dispersion. The strategy adopted in each of these studies was to examine QT dispersion (defined as the difference between the maximum and minimum QT interval recorded in any of 12 ECG leads) in situations where repolarization inhomogeneity was expected to be large and in situations where it was expected to be small. In the first study we showed that QT dispersion was significantly greater in patients with congenital long QT syndromes (CLQTSs) than in patients with similar degrees of QT prolongation due to sotalol, a β-blocker with Class III effects.[6] The evidence for dispersion of repolarization as a mechanism of arrhythmogenesis in CLQTS is reviewed in Chapters 11 and 12. In a second study we showed that QT dispersion was greater following ventricular extrasystoles than after sinus-initiated beats.[7] This was consistent with experimental data obtained in canine hearts that repolarization inhomogeneity was increased after ventricular extrasystoles.[8]

In the third study we examined QT dispersion in patients following myocardial infarction who had been randomized to 1 year's treatment with sotalol or placebo as part of multicenter study of oral sotalol post infarction.[9,10] We hypothesized that, in these two well-matched groups of patients, the Class III effects of sotalol would reduce the increased dispersion of repolarization reported to occur in animal models of infarction,[1,2] and result in decreased QT dispersion. The characteristics of the patients are shown in Table 1. Patients randomized to sotalol or placebo were well matched for age, gender, time from infarction to randomization, and site of infarction. The values of maximum rate-corrected QT (QTc) are shown in Figure 1. As expected, at 1, 3, and 6 month follow up, maximum QTc was significantly greater in the sotalol-treated patients compared with those treated with placebo. In contrast, QTc dispersion (adjusted for the number of measurable leads) was greater in the placebo-treated patients than in those taking sotalol at all stages of follow-up (Fig. 2). In the placebo-treated patients QTc dispersion increased from randomization to 1 month falling to initial levels at 3 and 6 months, while in the sotalol

Table 1
Entry Characteristics of Patients Treated with Sotalol or Placebo

	Sotalol	Placebo
Number	39	28
Sex (%male)	77	79
Site of infarction:		
Anterior (5)	49	46
Inferior (5)	46	54
Age (yrs, mean ± SE)	57±8	57±8
Time from infarct to randomization	7.8±1.9	7.5±2.3
(days, mean ± SE)		

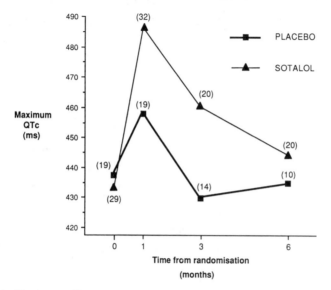

Figure 1. Maximum QTc following randomization to placebo or sotalol. Values shown are means. Number of electrocardiograms in parentheses. Reproduced with permission from *Eur Heart J* 1991;12:423-427.

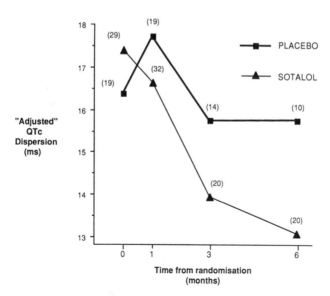

Figure 2. "Adjusted" QTc dispersion following randomization to placebo or sotalol. "Adjusted" QTc dispersion was calculated as the difference between the maximum and minimum QTc in any lead divided by the square root of the number of leads measured. The values shown are means. Number of electrocardiograms in parentheses. Reproduced with permission from *Eur Heart J* 1991;12:423-427.

patients it fell progressively from randomization to 6 months. Sotalol treatment preferentially reduced the QTc dispersion in patients with anterior infarction.

Together with the results of the first two studies, we considered that the results of the postinfarction study provided strong, albeit indirect, evidence that QT dispersion was a simple, noninvasive measure of repolarization inhomogeneity. In each situation where increased dispersion of ventricular recovery was expected, QT dispersion was large, and where dispersion of recovery was expected to be minimal, so too was QT dispersion. We suggested that if validated by invasive methods correlating epicardial monophasic action potentials with surface ECG features, then QT dispersion analysis could have considerable potential for the prediction of arrhythmogenesis and prognosis and for the assessment of antiarrhythmic drug therapy.[10] Nine years after the publication of the last of these papers, it seems timely to assess the progress that has been made toward validating QT dispersion analysis and establishing its utility in clinical practice. In particular, do we now know 1) whether the effect of sotalol on QT dispersion following myocardial infarction in the above study is observed with other drugs with Class III effects; 2) whether this effect truly reflects a reduction in repolarization inhomogeneity; and 3) whether this effect of Class III drugs can be used to reduce the occurrence of serious arrhythmias and sudden death following myocardial infarction? Certainly, it is tempting to speculate that the lower mortality in the sotalol-treated group compared with the placebo-treated group in the sotalol postinfarction study[9] was due to a reduction in repolarization inhomogeneity and associated arrhythmia risk.

Experimental evidence from studies with isolated hearts has now been provided that supports our original hypothesis that QT dispersion reflects regional differences in ventricular recovery time.[11] These studies, reviewed by Drs. Zabel and Franz in Chapter 5, also showed that alternative ECG parameters, including the interval between T wave peak and end (TPE) and T wave area, correlated better with the variability of simultaneously obtained monophasic action potentials than QT dispersion. This may be due to the TPE interval better reflecting the transmural dispersion of repolarization that has been attributed to the delayed recovery of M cells residing in the mid-myocardium.[12] Both before and subsequent to its direct validation, the clinical utility of QT dispersion analysis has been examined and found useful in a wide range of clinical situations reviewed in previous chapters. These have included the prediction of therapeutic efficacy in patients with CLQTS[13] and the prediction of torsade de pointes arrhythmias in patients taking Class Ia antiarrhythmic drugs.[14]

QT dispersion analysis has been most extensively investigated following myocardial infarction. Several studies have shown that increased QT dispersion is associated with an increased risk of late ventricular tachycardia and ventricular fibrillation,[15-17] although this was not observed in the most recent and largest study.[18] As might be expected from these results, increased QT dispersion has also been found to predict mortality following infarction[19] which could be due either to its association with arrhythmia risk or to its recently observed correlation with infarct size.[15,19] This latter observation has been extended to the use of QT dispersion analysis to predict the success of revascularization following infarction.[15,20] If we accept that at least part of the ability of increased QT dispersion to predict postinfarction survival is due to it reflecting repolarization inhomogeneity and associated arrhythmia risk, then it would seem logical to suggest that reducing QT dispersion will reduce this risk and improve survival. Certainly, a reduction in recovery time dispersion may be an added and unexpected benefit of therapy aimed primarily at achieving reperfusion. The remainder of this chapter, however, focuses on the potential use of Class III antiarrhythmic drugs to reduce the dispersion of repolarization and arrhythmia risk following myocardial infarction. Has any progress been made since our original sotalol study was published in 1992?

The Class III antiarrhythmic drug amiodarone has been shown to reduce QT dispersion in patients with postinfarction arrhythmias[21] and in patients with torsade de pointes ventricular arrhythmias induced by Class Ia drugs.[14] In the postinfarction study Cui and colleagues[21] examined QT dispersion in 26 patients with a history of ventricular tachycardia before and after 3 months of treatment with amiodarone, 20 of whom had clinical and ECG evidence of myocardial infarction. Amiodarone significantly reduced both QT and QTc dispersion and the reduction was greatest in those patients with myocardial infarction prior to treatment. Interestingly, sematilide, a selective Class III agent, did not affect QT dispersion in a matched group of patients[21] and dofetilide, a further Class III drug, also had no effect on QT dispersion in 18 patients with ischemic heart disease.[22] No study has been performed in humans to examine whether the effects of amiodarone or sotalol on QT dispersion post infarction correlate with reduced dispersion of repolarization; however, data from animal models of infarction do support this concept. Cardinal and Sasyniuk[3] showed that the Class III drug bretylium tosylate reduced the dispersion of repolarization in infarcted canine hearts by selectively prolonging recovery time in normal compared with infarcted tissue. Similarly, in noninfarcted canine hearts, amiodarone selectively prolonged myocardial repolarization relative to its effect on the slower repolarizing Purkinje fibers, resulting in a reduction in the normal heterogeneity of refractoriness.[23]

Has this effect of Class III antiarrhythmic drugs on QT and repolarization dispersion following infarction been translated into clinical benefit for the patient? The answer is probably yes. As with sotalol,[10] amiodarone has been shown to reduce cardiac mortality in survivors of acute infarction in a placebo-controlled trial.[24] It seems reasonable to suggest that at least part of this benefit is attributable to a reduction in repolarization inhomogeneity and associated arrhythmia risk. More direct evidence that the effect of antiarrhythmic drugs on QT dispersion following myocardial infarction can be used in clinical practice has come from a recent study by Gillis and coworkers.[25] QT dispersion was measured at baseline and during steady state antiarrhythmic drug therapy in 72 patients with documented coronary artery disease and remote infarction, presenting with spontaneous sustained ventricular tachycardia undergoing electropharmacological studies to assess arrhythmia suppression. QT dispersion was similar at baseline in drug responders and nonresponders, whereas during Class III drug therapy QT dispersion was significantly reduced in responders compared with nonresponders. The positive and negative predictive value of QT dispersion during antiarrhythmic therapy to predict a successful response was 32% and 96%, respectively. QT dispersion greater than 50 ms during treatment was associated with ineffective therapy.

In summary, there is now little doubt that QT dispersion on the surface ECG reflects dispersion of ventricular repolarization. Consistent with experimental data showing that repolarization inhomogeneity is a substrate for arrhythmogenesis, increased QT dispersion has been shown to be associated with a risk of serious ventricular arrhythmias in a variety of clinical settings including post myocardial infarction. At least some Class III drugs, including amiodarone and sotalol, reduce QT dispersion following infarction, and data from animal models suggest that this is due to a reduction in the dispersion of ventricular repolarization. This effect may explain, at least in part, the beneficial effect of these drugs on postinfarction survival and has recently been used successfully to predict their efficacy in the treatment of postinfarct ventricular arrhythmias. QT dispersion analysis is therefore close to fulfilling its potential. In the future better surface ECG measures of repolarization inhomogeneity derived from automated recording and analysis technology[26] seem likely to be used increasingly in cardiologic practice as a method of assessing both arrhythmia risk and the efficacy of strategies aimed at reducing this risk.

Acknowledgment None of this work would have been possible without the support and enthusiasm of my late colleague, Professor Ronnie Campbell. He is greatly missed by all of us who were lucky enough to have known him.

References

1. Mandel WJ, Burgess MF, Neville J Jr, et al. Analysis of T wave abnormalities associated with myocardial infarction using a theoretical model. *Circulation* 1968;38:178-188.
2. Lazzara R, El-Sherif N, Scherlag BJ. Electrophysiological properties of canine Purkinje cells in one-day-old myocardial infarction. *Circ Res* 1973;33:722-734.

3. Cardinal R, Sasyniuk BI. Electrophysiological effects of bretylium tosylate on subendocardial Purkinje fibres from infarcted canine hearts. *J Pharmacol Exp Ther* 1978;204:159-174.
4. Inoue H, Toda I, Nozaki A, et al. Effects of bretylium tosylate on inhomogeneity of refractoriness and ventricular fibrillation threshold in canine hearts with quinidine-induced long QT interval. *Cardiovasc Res* 1985;19:655-660.
5. Cowan JC, Yusoff K, Moore M, et al. Importance of lead selection in QT interval measurement. *Am J Cardiol* 1988;61:83-87.
6. Day CP, McComb JM, Campbell RWF. QT dispersion: An indication of arrhythmia risk in patients with long QT intervals. *Br Heart J* 1990;63:342-344.
7. Day CP, McComb JM, Campbell RWF. QT dispersion in sinus beats and ventricular extrasystoles in normal hearts. *Br Heart J* 1992;67:39-41.
8. Kuo CS, Amlie JP, Munakata K, et al. Dispersion of monophasic action potential durations and activation times during atrial ventricular pacing, ventricular pacing and ventricular premature stimulation in canine ventricles. *Cardiovasc Res* 1983;17:152-161.
9. Julian DG, Prescott RJ, Jackson FS, et al. Controlled trial of sotalol for one year after myocardial infarction. *Lancet* 1982;1:1142-1147.
10. Day CP, McComb JM, Matthews J, et al. Reduction in QT dispersion by sotalol following myocardial infarction. *Eur Heart J* 1991;12:423-427.
11. Zabel M, Portnoy S, Franz MR. Electrocardiographic indices of dispersion of ventricular repolarization: An isolated heart validation study. *J Am Coll Cardiol* 1995;25:746-752.
12. Antzelevitch C, Nesterenko VV, Shimizu W, et al. Electrophysiological characteristics of the M cell. In Franz MR, Schmitt C, Zrenner B (eds): *Monophasic Action Potentials.* Berlin/Heidelberg, Germany: Springer Verlag; 1997:212-226.
13. Priori SG, Napolitano C, Diehl L. Dispersion of the QT interval: A marker of therapeutic efficacy in the idiopathic long QT syndrome. *Circulation* 1994;89:1681-1689.
14. Hii JTY, Wyse GD, Gillis AM, et al. Precordial QT interval dispersion as a marker of torsade de pointes. *Circulation* 1992;86:1376-1382.
15. Puljevic D, Smalcelj A, Durakovic J, et al. Effects of postmyocardial infarction scar size, cardiac function, and severity of coronary artery disease on QT interval dispersion as a risk factor for complex ventricular arrhythmias. *PACE* 1998;21:1508-1516.
16. Oikarinen L, Viitasalo M, Toivonen L. Dispersions of the QT interval in postmyocardial infarction patients presenting with ventricular tachycardia or with ventricular fibrillation. *Am J Cardiol* 1998;81:694-697.
17. Perkiömäki JS, Huikuri HV, Koistinen JM, et al. Heart rate variability and dispersion of QT interval in patients with vulnerability to ventricular tachycardia and ventricular fibrillation after previous myocardial infarction. *J Am Coll Cardiol* 1997;30:1331-1338.
18. Zabel M, Klingenheben T, Franz MR, et al. Assessment of QT dispersion for prediction of mortality or arrhythmic events after myocardial infarction. *Circulation* 1998;97:2543-2550.
19. Schneider CA, Voth E, Baer FM, et al. QT dispersion is determined by the extent of viable myocardium in patients with chronic Q-wave myocardial infarction. *Circulation* 1997;96:3913-3920.
20. Moreno FL, Villanueva MT, Karagounis LA, et al. Reduction in QT interval dispersion by successful thrombolytic therapy in acute myocardial infarction. *Circulation* 1994;90:94-100.

21. Cui G, Sen L, Sager M, et al. Effects of amiodarone, sematilide, and sotalol on QT dispersion. *Am J Cardiol* 1994;74:896-900.
22. Sedgwick ML, Rasmussen HS, Cobbe SM. Effects of class III antiarrhythmic drug dofetilide on ventricular monophasic action potential duration and QT interval dispersion in stable angina pectoris. *Am J Cardiol* 1992;70:1432-1437.
23. Gallagher JD, Bianchi J, Gessman LJ. A comparison of the electrophysiologic effects of acute and chronic amiodarone administration on canine Purkinje fibres. *J Cardiovasc Pharmacol* 1989;13:723-729.
24. Ceremuzynski Y, Kleczar E, Kreminska-Pakula M, et al. Effect of amiodarone on mortality after myocardial infarction. *J Am Coll Cardiol* 1992;20:1056-1062.
25. Gillis AM, Traboulsi M, Hii JT, et al. Antiarrhythmic drug effects on QT interval dispersion in patients undergoing electropharmacologic testing for ventricular tachycardia and fibrillation. *Am J Cardiol* 1998;81:588-593.
26. Oikarinin L, Paavola M, Montonen J, et al. Magnetocardiographic QT interval dispersion in postmyocardial infarction patients with sustained ventricular tachycardia: Validation of automated QT measurements. *PACE* 1998;21:1934-1942.

20

Effect of Defibrillation on Dispersion of Repolarization

Paulus Kirchhof, C. Larissa Fabritz, Lars Eckardt,
Günter Breithardt, Wilhelm Haverkamp,
and Michael R. Franz

Summary

Although it has been known for more than 100 years that short, strong electrical shocks can both induce and terminate ventricular fibrillation, the electrophysiological mechanisms underlying these phenomena have not been completely understood. Experimental and clinical data suggest that induction of ventricular fibrillation depends on a critically increased dispersion of repolarization within the ventricles, combined with induction of slowly propagating activation wavefronts. Several observations can be explained by the hypothesis that induction and termination of ventricular fibrillation might depend on similar electrophysiological mechanisms. This chapter reviews the current knowledge on the induction of ventricular fibrillation by a single electrical shock. The possible mechanisms of electrical defibrillation are reviewed, with an emphasis on the common electrophysiological changes that might be involved in both induction and termination of ventricular fibrillation by single electrical field shocks.

Introduction

Application of a strong, short electrical field stimulus to the fibrillating heart is the only safe method of terminating ventricular fibrillation, one of the major causes of death in the industrialized world.[1-3] Although the salutary effects of short, single electrical field stimuli on the fibrillating

From Olsson SB, Amlie JP, Yuan S (eds): *Dispersion of Ventricular Repolarization: State of the Art.* ©Futura Publishing Company, Inc., Armonk, NY, 2000.

heart have been known for more than 100 years,[4,5] the electrophysiological mechanisms by which an electrical shock terminates ventricular fibrillation have still not been fully understood.

The development of the implantable cardioverter-defibrillator (ICD), and the concurrent need to effectively defibrillate the heart with as little energy as possible, has intensified research in the field of defibrillation by an electrical shock, resulting in several improvements in ICD technology.[6-29] An intriguing finding has been the close correlation of the upper limit of vulnerability, the highest shock strength capable of inducing ventricular fibrillation during the vulnerable period, with the defibrillation threshold.[30-35] The development of computerized multisite experimental mapping techniques such as multipolar activation mapping,[36-39] multisite recording of ventricular action potentials during defibrillator shocks,[32,40-42] double-barrel microelectrode recordings of the action potential during defibrillation shocks,[43] and multisite optical mapping of the epicardial action potential[44-47] have enabled the simultaneous measurement of both local activation and repolarization during defibrillation shocks. The abundance of data generated, as well as their complexity, forced investigators to focus on specific effects of defibrillation shocks thought to be critical in the process of defibrillation. Several hypotheses on the mechanism of cardiac defibrillation emanated, and continue to emanate, from this work.[48-51]

This chapter reviews the published data on the induction of ventricular fibrillation and electrical defibrillation, with a special focus on dispersion of repolarization after the electrical shock, and attempts to incorporate most published aspects of electrical defibrillation in this view.

Induction of Ventricular Fibrillation by a T Wave Shock during the Vulnerable Period

Single electrical field shocks can induce ventricular fibrillation during a narrow time window in the cardiac cycle, the so-called "vulnerable period,"[42,52,53] when applied within a certain range of shock strengths.[30,32] Appropriately timed shocks at sufficient shock strength almost inevitably result in ventricular fibrillation.[32,54]

The highest shock strength that induces ventricular fibrillation during this vulnerable period, the so-called "upper limit of vulnerability," correlates closely with the lowest energy that successfully defibrillates the heart, the so-called "defibrillation threshold."[30-33,55,56] After unsuccessful defibrillation shocks, electrically silent intervals are observed.[36,57] This suggests that the electrophysiological changes resulting in electrical defibrillation may be similar to those inducing ventricular fibrillation by T wave shocks.

Correlation of the Vulnerable Period and Dispersion of Ventricular Repolarization

The vulnerable period has long been related to the phase of late ventricular repolarization.[42,52,53,58] Experimental data show that it roughly coincides with the T wave of the surface electrocardiogram (ECG)[53,55,58-61] and closely correlates with the degree of dispersion of repolarization of the ventricular action potential at 70% to 90% repolarization, depending on the shock strength chosen.[32,42] These experimental findings have been confirmed in patients.[62]

Mechanism of Induction of Ventricular Fibrillation during the Vulnerable Period

A short electrical stimulus is capable of exciting cardiac tissue during electrical diastole. The excitability of cardiac tissue is largely determined by its membrane potential: while excitability is maximal during electrical diastole, the stimulus strength needed to induce active depolarization of the membrane increases with more positive membrane potentials.[63-69] During late repolarization, i.e., between levels of 70% to 90% repolarization, a strength-interval relation between excitability and repolarization exists.[66,68,70] During this period of the cardiac action potential, a strong electrical stimulus is capable of inducing either a new action potential or an action potential prolongation, also referred to as a graded response.[40,41,70-72]

A shock can simultaneously induce both forms of action potential modification during the vulnerable period[40,41] (Fig. 1). This is due to dispersed action potential durations and, hence, different degrees of repolarization at the time of the shock, and to inhomogeneous shock strengths in different regions of the heart. Thereby, dispersion of repolarization is increased, while at the same time depolarizations strong enough to propagate are induced.[73] Depolarizations that are strong enough to be propagated at a time when dispersion of repolarization is increased set the stage for reentry around functional block, leading to polymorphic ventricular arrhythmias, possibly in the form of microreentry.[37,73,74] In concordance with this hypothesis, only shocks that induce both graded responses and new action potentials result in ventricular fibrillation during the vulnerable period[41] (Figs. 1 through 3). Comparable conditions exist in experimental models with high transmural dispersion of repolarization prone to polymorphic ventricular arrhythmias.[75-77] Similar electrophysiological phenomena have been observed in experiments that assessed the induction of ventricular tachyarrhythmias by programmed stimulation.[78-81]

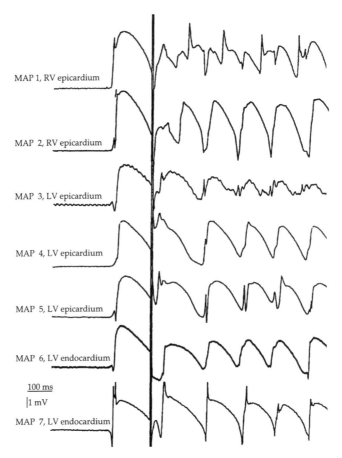

Figure 1. Recording of seven simultaneous endocardial and epicardial monophasic action potentials (MAPs) from an isolated rabbit heart during induction of ventricular fibrillation by an electrical field shock applied in the vulnerable period. The shock induces both new action potentials and graded responses, or action potential prolongations, in different MAPs. In MAPs 1 and 2, a short new action potential is induced. In MAP 3, the action potential is prolonged, followed by early reactivation. In MAP 4, a full new action potential is induced. In MAPs 5, 6, and 7, the action potential is prolonged, followed by almost immediate reactivation in MAP 5, and consecutive reactivation in MAPs 6 and 7. In MAP 6, the shock might have shortened the action potential. LV = left ventricular; RV = right ventricular. See text for details.

Upper and Lower Limit of Vulnerability

Even when timed during the vulnerable period of the heart, electrical field shocks induce ventricular fibrillation only when their shock strength is set between the upper and lower limit of vulnerability.[32,82,83] As shock strength is increased, action potential duration of postshock action potentials decreases while at the same time the duration of graded responses

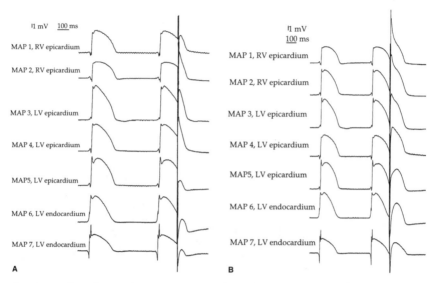

Figure 2. Recording of monophasic action potentials (MAPs) during electrical shocks applied outside of the vulnerable period. Shock strength is sufficient to induce ventricular fibrillation. **A.** Shock applied with a coupling interval too short to fall into the vulnerable period. The shock causes slight action potential prolongation in all MAPs. **B.** Shock applied with a coupling interval too long to fall into the vulnerable period. The shock causes a new action potential in all MAP recordings. In both cases, dispersion of postshock repolarization is low. See text for details.

increases.[32,41,84,85] Thereby, dispersion of postshock repolarization decreases and the substrate for reentry is no longer present. Below the lower limit of vulnerability, shock-induced graded responses are too low to result in propagated wavefronts, and thereby do not induce microreentry.[84]

The shock strength at the upper limit of vulnerability equals the defibrillation threshold (i.e., the lowest energy needed to defibrillate the heart successfully) almost perfectly in experimental and clinical studies.[30,35,56,86,87] Based on this finding, several groups have proposed that the electrophysiological alterations caused by T wave shocks and defibrillation shocks might cause similar electrophysiological effects that finally determine whether ventricular fibrillation will be the sequelae of an electrical shock.[88,89]

Electrophysiology of Ventricular Fibrillation

In contrast to T wave shocks during sinus rhythm, a defibrillation shock is applied during ventricular fibrillation. During ventricular fibrillation, several simultaneous reentrant activation wavefronts meander through the ventricles.[90-93] According to optical mapping studies in isolated hearts, these wavefronts follow a scroll wave pattern.[47,94] Several mathe-

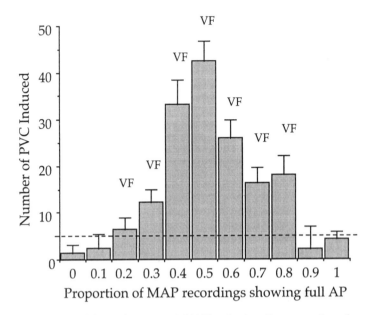

Figure 3. Relation of the action potential (AP) ratio, i.e., the proportion of new APs induced by a shock during the vulnerable period, and the induction of ventricular fibrillation (VF) in the isolated rabbit heart. As a surrogate measure, the number of ventricular activations after a shock is given (y axis). More than five rapid consecutive ventricular activations represent ventricular fibrillation in this model (compare References 42 and 147). An AP ratio of 0 indicates no new AP following the shock, while an AP ratio of 1 indicates new APs in all areas. Induction of VF was most effective when a similar amount of new APs and AP prolongations was induced (i.e., AP ratio = 0.5). PVC = premature ventricular complex. Modified from Reference 41.

matical models, mostly based on nonlinear dynamics, have been applied to describe the activation spread during ventricular fibrillation,[94-99] recently using phase singularities and wavefront curvature to condense the activation sequences during ventricular fibrillation and after defibrillation shocks.[47,48,50,94,96,100] These activation patterns result in early reactivation of excitable tissue, leading to asynchronous, almost instantaneous reactivation of repolarized tissue during ventricular fibrillation.[41,101-104] A defibrillation shock will hence encounter action potentials in many different stages of repolarization (Fig. 4).

Effects of Defibrillation Shocks on the Ventricular Action Potential

Due to their strong electrical field, and probably due to electrotonic influences, defibrillation strength shocks will modify the action potential

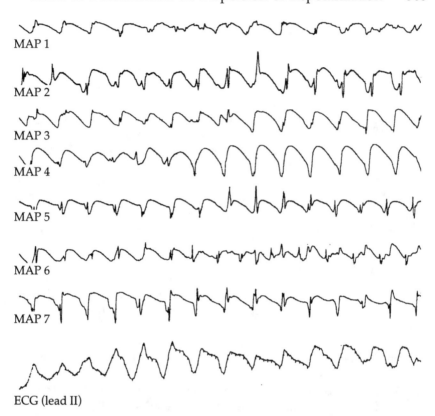

MAP 1

MAP 2

MAP 3

MAP 4

MAP 5

MAP 6

MAP 7

ECG (lead II)

Figure 4. Simultaneous recording of epicardial and endocardial action potentials during ventricular fibrillation. Modified from Reference 41. During ventricular fibrillation, instant reactivation of partially repolarized myocardium results in highly dispersed repolarization time courses in the monophasic action potentials (MAPs). See text for details.

even when they are applied during the plateau of the action potential: both hyperpolarization and depolarization,[102,105-107] resulting in either action potential prolongation or action potential shortening, have been described. Hyperpolarization may occasionally result in action potential shortening, especially so in electrically less coupled isolated tissue preparations, but may result in paradoxical action potential prolongation.[70,105-107] In the overwhelming majority of ventricular myocardium and in a variety of experimental settings, defibrillation shocks prolong repolarization.[44,45,71,72,102,105-108] Differences in the degree of action potential prolongation have been observed. Some authors have distinguished between excitation of graded responses that may or may not be propagated[71] and excitation of new, full action potentials.[44,45,72] Although not strictly proven, there is a consensus among most researchers that the distribution of these phenomena in time and space will determine whether an electrical shock defibrillates the heart or not.[48,49,51,108]

Determinants of Electrical Defibrillation

Termination of ventricular fibrillation may result from halting, critically slowing, or enlarging the curvature of reentrant activity in the ventricles. Many variables influence the effect of a defibrillation shock within the myocardium, including shock strength,[30,109] electrode position and shock field distribution, local repolarization level and timing of the shock,[86,110] fiber orientation and tissue anisotropy,[43,90,111,112] shock waveform,[109,113] and shock-induced virtual electrodes.[50,96,114]

These effects can be divided into two groups: 1) determinants of shock field shape and local shock strength, and 2) determinants of membrane response[51] (Table 1). The first group of effects will determine the local shock strength and voltage gradient distribution, and thereby influence the local response of the membrane potential. The temporal and spatial changes in membrane potential induced by the shock will then determine whether defibrillation is achieved.[51]

Similar to the electrophysiological phenomena resulting in induction of ventricular fibrillation by a T wave shock, electrical defibrillation has mostly been attributed to modification of repolarization and refractoriness: salutary effects of defibrillation shocks that have been associated with successful defibrillation include excitation of a critical mass of ventricular myocardium,[115,116] reduction in postshock dispersion of repolarization,[45,72] extension of postshock refractoriness[117-120] and postshock repolarization,[72,104,119] avoidance of spectral turbulence and shock-induced phase singularities,[50,96,121] and sufficient, "progressive" depolarization of the ventricles.[49]

Table 1
Suggested Factors that Influence Defibrillation Success

Determinants of Shock Strength	Determinants of Membrane Response
Delivered shock strength	Local repolarization level
Electrode position	Shock timing in relation to repolarization
Shock field shape and distribution	
Shock waveform	
Fiber orientation	Tissue anisotropy
Shock-induced virtual electrodes	
Shock strength	Tissue resistance and conductance

All proposed effects have been classified as determinants of local shock strength or local membrane response.

Extension of Refractoriness and Repolarization

Defibrillator shocks are capable of modifying, mainly prolonging, the action potential (see above). The degree of action potential modification depends on local shock strength and shock waveform as well as on local repolarization level. Passive attributes of the myocardium such as tissue resistance, conductance, and anisotropy also influence the local effect of a shock on the local action potential.[70,111,112] Several studies demonstrated an association between extension of refractoriness after defibrillation shocks and successful defibrillation.[36,57,122] On the side of shock strength determinants, a shock field gradient of more than 5 V/cm has been related to successful defibrillation.[74,122] Measurements of action potential durations during defibrillation shocks have demonstrated that this increased postshock refractoriness is paralleled by increased postshock action potential duration.[72,103,104,118,119] Some data suggest that biphasic shocks prolong the action potential more than monophasic shocks; this is a possible explanation for lower defibrillation thresholds with biphasic waveforms.[123] Prolongation of action potential duration appears especially important in regions of low shock field strength[108,110] and adjacent to regions directly depolarized by the shock.[72]

As the local response to a defibrillator shock will be a new action potential in relatively repolarized regions of the heart[63-68] (see above), dispersion of repolarization will be reduced by prolonging action potential durations in all regions of the heart. Therefore, extension of action potential duration, and refractoriness, in regions of low shock strength may reduce dispersion of postshock repolarization.[72,103,104,108,110,119] Indeed, even when the focus of experiments was not on measuring dispersion of repolarization, published recordings[72] show lower dispersion of repolarization after successful than after unsuccessful defibrillation shocks (Fig. 5). Simultaneously measured action potentials from different regions of the heart demonstrated that successful defibrillator shocks reduce dispersion of repolarization[45,113,124-126] (compare Fig. 5).

Mechanism of Defibrillation

Microreentry based on highly dispersed repolarization time courses within a small area of ventricular myocardium has been described during the induction of ventricular fibrillation.[37,41,74] A similar mechanism of induction of polymorphic ventricular tachycardia has been described in an experimental model of torsade de pointes tachycardias, where a high transmural dispersion of repolarization is the substrate for intramural microreentry caused either by inducing propagated responses or by spontaneously occurring afterdepolarizations.[75,77,127-132] Both the substrate for microreentry (i.e., high dispersion of postshock repolarization)[45] and the trigger (i.e.,

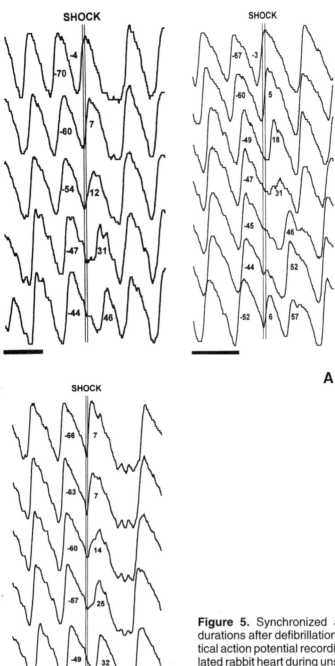

Figure 5. Synchronized action potential durations after defibrillation shocks. **A.** Optical action potential recordings from an isolated rabbit heart during unsuccessful (**top**) and successful (**bottom**) defibrillation shocks. Modified from Reference 72. Continues.

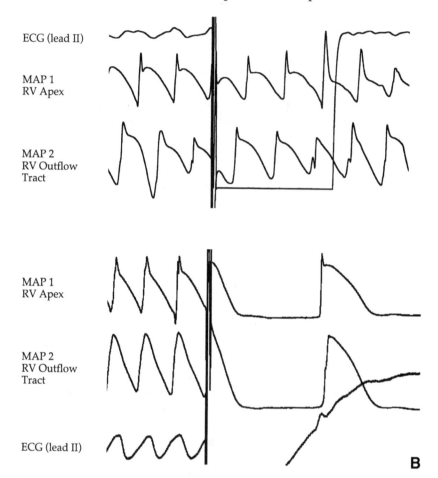

Figure 5 *continued.* **B.** Monophasic action potential (MAP) recordings from the right ventricular apex and outflow tract during unsuccessful (**top**) and successful (**bottom**) shocks of an implantable cardioverter-defibrillator.

propagated activation wavefronts)[36,71] are present after unsuccessful defibrillation shocks[88] (compare Fig. 5). Combined, they will maintain ventricular fibrillation after an unsuccessful defibrillation shock,[48,49] a process that has been described as "reinitiating" ventricular fibrillation.[48,88,133] This hypothesis could also explain that the upper limit of vulnerability correlates closely with the defibrillation threshold, assuming that shocks above the upper limit of vulnerability do not reinitiate ventricular fibrillation.[48,88,134] Figure 5 shows examples of optical action potentials recorded during successful and unsuccessful defibrillation shocks. Comparable to repolarization patterns after T wave shocks, successful shocks are associated with lower dispersion of repolarization than are unsuccessful shocks.

Phase Singularities and Critical Points

Phase singularities, caused by virtual electrodes, have been described as relating to unsuccessful defibrillation.[96,99] While virtual electrodes are part of the determinants of local shock field strength[50] (Table 1), phase singularities may be a different way to look at dispersed repolarization: pivoting points of activation wavefronts[135] and the vortex of an activation scroll wave[47] are characterized by a highly inhomogeneous repolarization time course, resulting from slow, curved activation and repolarization. When regarded in activation maps, these can be described as phase changes, or singularities, within an otherwise homogeneous activation wavefront.[96,136] Phase singularities may hence well represent a more thorough description of microreentry-induced propagated activation wavefronts after defibrillation shocks, and may therefore be related to, or even depend on, high postshock dispersion.

Conclusion

Electrical defibrillation appears to relate to extinguishing the slow, meandering activation wavefronts that form the electrophysiological substrate of ventricular fibrillation. While termination of the reentrant activity existing at the time of the shock is likely related to depolarization of the myocardium and hence to prolongation of repolarization and refractoriness, prevention of new propagated wavefronts may depend on low dispersion of repolarization after the defibrillation shock. The latter could explain the close correlation between the upper limit of vulnerability and the defibrillation threshold observed in clinical and experimental settings.

Outlook

Most studies on the mechanism of defibrillation have been performed in experimental models using isolated tissue or intact, Langendorff-perfused hearts from normal, healthy animals. To test whether modification of postshock repolarization can explain defibrillation success, this hypothesis could be tested in a wider range of conditions, e.g., by measuring in vivo action potential durations during defibrillation shocks or by assessing postshock action potential durations in conditions known to modify action potential duration, such as different temperatures,[137-139] different degrees of ventricular load and stretch,[129,140,141] or addition of action potential modulating drugs[42,129,142] and in diseased myocardium, i.e., after healed myocardial infarction, or in hearts with heart failure, the two main causes of ventricular fibrillation in the clinical setting.

Assessment of defibrillation under these conditions might, for example, identify whether a "suprathreshold" prolongation of repolarization, or a reduction of dispersion of repolarization beyond a critical value, is necessary for successful defibrillation in a given model, thereby broadening our understanding of the electrophysiological changes resulting in electrical defibrillation.

Limitations

Dispersion of repolarization may not always be arrhythmogenic, but especially so when a large dispersion of repolarization is present within adjacent areas of the myocardium.[78-81] Consideration of the spatial distribution of dispersed postshock action potential durations may help explain why defibrillation success is still only partially predictable, even in controlled experimental models.[72,119,133,143,144]

Even the sophisticated action potential mapping techniques available can so far only record from several distinct epicardial and endocardial points[32,41,42,83,119,145,146] or from one epicardial surface of the heart,[45-47] hence, missing action potentials form large intramyocardial and epicardial areas of ventricular tissue.

These considerations may explain that, in rare cases, defibrillation occurs despite a high level of postshock action potential dispersion, lack of postshock action potential prolongation, or persistence of postshock activation, even in controlled experimental settings.[72,119,133,143]

This chapter focuses on the effects of defibrillation shocks on the cardiac action potential. How these effects are exerted most efficiently depends on many factors influencing local shock strength (see Table 1). Modification of these factors may also help to design more efficient ways to effectively defibrillate with low energies.

References

1. Chamberlain DA. Overview of completed sudden death trials: European experience. *Cardiology* 1987;74:10-23.
2. Kannel WB. Some lessons in cardiovascular epidemiology from Framingham. *Am J Cardiol* 1976;37:269-282.
3. Myerburg RJ, Castelanos A. Cardiovascular collapse, cardiac arrest, and sudden death. In Isselbacher KJ, Braunwald E, Wilson JD, et al (eds): *Harrison's Principles of Internal Medicine.* New York: McGraw Hill; 1994:193-198.
4. Batelli F. Le mécanisme de la mort par les courants électriques chez l'homme. *Rev Méd Swiss Romande* 1899;10:605-618.
5. Prevost JL, Batelli F. Sur quelques effets des décharges électriques sur le coeur des mammifères. *Compte Rendu Acad Sc* 1899;129:651.
6. Bardy GH, Dolack GL, Kudenchuk PJ, et al. Prospective, randomized comparison in humans of a unipolar defibrillation system with that using an additional superior vena cava electrode. *Circulation* 1994;89:1090-1093.
7. Bardy GH, Poole JE, Kudenchuk PJ, et al. A prospective randomized comparison in humans of biphasic waveform 60-microF and 120-microF capacitance pulses using a unipolar defibrillation system. *Circulation* 1995;91:91-95.

8. Blanchard SM, Smith WM, Damiano RJ, et al. Four digital algorithms for activation detection from unipolar epicardial electrograms. *IEEE Trans Biomed Eng* 1989;36:256-261.
9. Block M, Breithardt G. Optimizing defibrillation through improved waveforms. *PACE* 1995;18:526-538.
10. Breithardt G, Wichter T, Haverkamp W, et al. Implantable cardioverter defibrillator therapy in patients with arrhythmogenic right ventricular cardiomyopathy, long QT syndrome, or no structural heart disease. *Am Heart J* 1994;127:1151-1158.
11. Cohen TJ, Reid PR, Mower MM, et al. The automatic implantable cardioverter-defibrillator. Long-term clinical experience and outcome at a hospital without an open-heart surgery program. *Arch Intern Med* 1992;152:65-69.
12. Fain ES, Sweeney MB, Franz MR. Improved internal defibrillation efficacy with a biphasic waveform. *Am Heart J* 1989;117:358-364.
13. Guarnieri T, Levine JH, Veltri EP, et al. Success of chronic defibrillation and the role of antiarrhythmic drugs with the automatic implantable cardioverter/defibrillator. *Am J Cardiol* 1987;60:1061-1064.
14. Horowitz L. The automatic implantable cardioverter defibrillator: Review of clinical results, 1980-1990. *PACE* 1992;15:604-609.
15. Jung W, Manz M, Moosdorf R, et al. Clinical efficacy of shock waveforms and lead configurations for defibrillation. *Am Heart J* 1994;127:985-993.
16. Kavanagh KM, Tang AS, Rollins DL, et al. Comparison of the internal defibrillation thresholds for monophasic and double and single capacitor biphasic waveforms. *J Am Coll Cardiol* 1989;14:1343-1349.
17. Kim SG, Fisher JD, Furman S, et al. Benefits of implantable defibrillators are overestimated by sudden death rates and better represented by the total arrhythmic death rate [see comments]. *J Am Coll Cardiol* 1991;17:1587-1592.
18. Kroll MW. A minimal model of the single capacitor biphasic defibrillation waveform. *PACE* 1994;17:1782-1792.
19. Kudenchuk PJ, Bardy GH, Dolack GL, et al. Efficacy of a single-lead unipolar transvenous defibrillator compared with a system employing an additional coronary sinus electrode. A prospective, randomized study. *Circulation* 1994;89:2641-2644.
20. Langer A, Heilman MS, Mower MM, Mirowski M. Considerations in the development of the automatic implantable defibrillator. *Med Instrum* 1976;10:163-167.
21. Manolis AS. Transvenous endocardial cardioverter defibrillator systems. Is the future here? *Arch Intern Med* 1994;154:617-622.
22. Mason P, McPherson C. Implantable cardioverter defibrillator: A review. *Heart Lung* 1992;21:141-147.
23. Mirowski M, Mower MM, Staeven WS, et al. Standby automatic defibrillator: An approach to prevention of sudden coronary death. *Arch Intern Med* 1970;126:158-161.
24. Neuzner J, Pitschner HF, Huth C, Schlepper M. Effect of biphasic waveform pulse on endocardial defibrillation efficacy in humans. *PACE* 1994;17:207-212.
25. Paull DL, Fellows CL, Guyton SW, Anderson RP. Continuing experience with the automatic implantable cardioverter defibrillator. *Am J Surg* 1992;163:502-504.
26. Saksena S, Poczobutt-Johanos M, Castle LW, et al. Long-term multicenter experience with a second-generation implantable pacemaker-defibrillator in patients with malignant ventricular tachyarrhythmias. The Guardian Multicenter Investigators Group. *J Am Coll Cardiol* 1992;19:490-499.

27. Scott BD, Kallok MJ, Birkett C, et al. Transthoracic defibrillation: Effect of dual-pathway sequential pulse shocks and single-pathway biphasic pulse shocks in a canine model. *Am Heart J* 1993;125:99-109.
28. Tchou PJ, Kadri N, Anderson J, et al. Automatic implantable cardioverter defibrillators and survival of patients with left ventricular dysfunction and malignant ventricular arrhythmias. *Ann Intern Med* 1988;109:529-534.
29. Winkle RA, Mead RH, Ruder MA, et al. Long-term outcome with the automatic implantable cardioverter-defibrillator. *J Am Coll Cardiol* 1989;13:1353-1361.
30. Chen PS, Shibata N, Dixon EG, et al. Comparison of the defibrillation threshold and the upper limit of ventricular vulnerability. *Circulation* 1986;73:1022-1028.
31. Fabiato A, Coumel P, Gourgon R, Saumont R. Le seuil de réponse synchrone des fibres myocardiqes. Application à la comparaison expérimentale de l'efficacité des différentes chocs électriques de défibrillation. *Arch Mal Coeur Vaiss* 1967;60:527-544.
32. Fabritz CL, Kirchhof PF, Behrens S, et al. Myocardial vulnerability to T wave shocks: Relation to shock strength, shock coupling interval, and dispersion of ventricular repolarization. *J Cardiovasc Electrophysiol* 1996;7:231-242.
33. Hwang C, Swerdlow C, Kass R, et al. Upper limit of vulnerability reliably predicts the defibrillation threshold in humans. *Circulation* 1994;90:2308-2314.
34. Swerdlow CD, Davie S, Ahern T, Chen PS. Comparative reproducibility of defibrillation threshold and upper limit of vulnerability. *PACE* 1996;19:2103-2111.
35. Swerdlow CD, Kass RM, O'Connor ME, Chen PS. Effect of shock waveform on relationship between upper limit of vulnerability and defibrillation threshold. *J Cardiovasc Electrophysiol* 1998;9:339-349.
36. Chen PS, Shibata N, Dixon EG, et al. Activation during ventricular defibrillation in open-chest dogs. Evidence of complete cessation and regeneration of ventricular fibrillation after unsuccessful shocks. *J Clin Invest* 1986;77:810-823.
37. Frazier DW, Wharton JM, Wolf PD, et al. Mapping the electrical initiation of ventricular fibrillation. *J Electrocardiol* 1989;22:198-199.
38. Harrison L, Ideker RE, Smith WM, et al. The sock electrode array: A tool for determining global epicardial activation during unstable arrhythmias. *PACE* 1980;3:531-540.
39. Ideker RE, Smith WM, Wolf P, et al. Simultaneous multichannel cardiac mapping systems. *PACE* 1987;10:281-292.
40. Behrens S, Li C, Fabritz CL, et al. Shock-induced dispersion of ventricular repolarization: Implications for the induction of ventricular fibrillation and the upper limit of vulnerability. *J Cardiovasc Electrophysiol* 1997;8:998-1008.
41. Kirchhof PF, Fabritz CL, Behrens S, Franz MR. Induction of ventricular fibrillation by T wave field-shocks in the isolated perfused rabbit heart: Role of nonuniform shock responses. *Basic Res Cardiol* 1997;92:35-44.
42. Kirchhof PF, Fabritz CL, Zabel M, Franz MR. The vulnerable period for low and high energy T wave shocks: Role of dispersion of repolarisation and effect of d-sotalol. *Cardiovasc Res* 1996;31:953-962.
43. Zhou X, Rollins DL, Smith WM, Ideker RE. Responses of the transmembrane potential of myocardial cells during a shock. *J Cardiovasc Electrophysiol* 1995;6:252-263.
44. Dillon SM. Optical recordings in the rabbit heart show that defibrillation strength shocks prolong the duration of repolarization and the refractory period. *Circ Res* 1991;69:842-856.

45. Dillon SM. Synchronized repolarization after defibrillation shocks. A possible component of the defibrillation process demonstrated by optical recordings in rabbit heart. *Circulation* 1992;85:1865-1878.

46. Efimov IR, Huang DT, Rendt JM, Salama G. Optical mapping of repolarization and refractoriness from intact hearts. *Circulation* 1994;90:1469-1480.

47. Gray RA, Jalife J, Panfilov A, et al. Nonstationary vortexlike reentrant activity as a mechanism of polymorphic ventricular tachycardia in the isolated rabbit heart. *Circulation* 1995;91:2454-2469.

48. Chen PS, Swerdlow CD, Hwang C, Karagueuzian HS. Current concepts of ventricular defibrillation. *J Cardiovasc Electrophysiol* 1998;9:553-562.

49. Dillon SM, Kwaku KF. Progressive depolarization: A unified hypothesis for defibrillation and fibrillation induction by shocks. *J Cardiovasc Electrophysiol* 1998;9:529-552.

50. Entcheva E, Eason J, Efimov IR, et al. Virtual electrode effects in transvenous defibrillation-modulation by structure and interface: Evidence from bidomain simulations and optical mapping. *J Cardiovasc Electrophysiol* 1998;9:949-961.

51. Walcott GP, Knisley SB, Zhou X, et al. On the mechanism of ventricular defibrillation [see comments]. *PACE* 1997;20:422-431.

52. King B. The Effect of Electric Shock on Heart Action with Special Reference to Varying Susceptibility in Different Parts of the Cardiac Cycle. New York: Columbia University. Aberdeen Press, 1934.

53. Wiggers CJ, Wegren R. Ventricular fibrillation due to single localized induction in condenser shock supplied during the vulnerable phase of ventricular systole. *Am J Physiol* 1940;128:500-505.

54. Sanders WE Jr, Hamrick GL Jr, Herbst MC, et al. Ventricular fibrillation induction using nonsynchronized low energy external shock during rapid ventricular pacing: Method of induction when fibrillation mode of ICD fails. *PACE* 1996;19:431-436.

55. Chen PS, Feld GK, Kriett JM, et al. Relation between upper limit of vulnerability and defibrillation threshold in humans. *Circulation* 1993;88:186-192.

56. Topham SL, Cha YM, Peters BB, Chen PS. Effects of lidocaine on relation between defibrillation threshold and upper limit of vulnerability in open-chest dogs. *Circulation* 1992;85:1146-1151.

57. Sweeney RJ, Gill RM, Reid PR. Refractory interval after transcardiac shocks during ventricular fibrillation. *Circulation* 1996;94:2947-2952.

58. Wiggers CJ. The mechanism and nature of ventricular fibrillation. *Am Heart J* 1940;20:399-412.

59. Axelrod PJ, Verrier RL, Lown B. Vulnerability to ventricular fibrillation during acute coronary arterial occlusion and release. *Am J Cardiol* 1975;36:776-782.

60. Martin DJ, Chen PS, Hwang C, et al. Upper limit of vulnerability predicts chronic defibrillation threshold for transvenous implantable defibrillators. *J Cardiovasc Electrophysiol* 1997;8:241-248.

61. Shibata N, Chen PS, Dixon EG, et al. Influence of shock strength and timing on induction of ventricular arrhythmias in dogs. *Am J Physiol* 1988;255: H891-H901.

62. Swerdlow CD, Martin DJ, Kass RM, et al. The zone of vulnerability to T wave shocks in humans. *J Cardiovasc Electrophysiol* 1997;8:145-154.

63. Costard-Jäckle A, Goetsch B, Antz M, Franz MR. Slow and long-lasting modulation of myocardial repolarization produced by ectopic activation in isolated rabbit hearts. Evidence for cardiac 'memory.' *Circulation* 1989;80:1412-1420.

64. Franz MR, Bargheer K, Costard-Jäckle A, et al. Human ventricular repolarization and T wave genesis. *Prog Cardiovasc Dis* 1991;33:369-384.
65. Franz MR, Costard A. Frequency-dependent effects of quinidine on the relationship between action potential duration and refractoriness in the canine heart in situ. *Circulation* 1988;77:1177-1184.
66. Gettes LS, Shabetai R, Downs TA, Surawicz B. Effect of changes in potassium and calcium concentrations on diastolic threshold and strength-interval relationships of the human heart. *Ann N Y Acad Sci* 1969;167:693-705.
67. Kirchhof PF, Fabritz CL, Franz MRF. Post-repolarization refractoriness versus conduction slowing caused by class I antiarrhythmic drugs—antiarrhythmic and proarrhythmic effects. *Circulation* 1998;97:2567-2574.
68. Michelson EL, Spear JF, Moore EN. Effects of procainamide on strength-interval relations in normal and chronically infarcted canine myocardium. *Am J Cardiol* 1981;47:1223-1232.
69. Michelson EL, Spear JF, Moore EN. Strength-interval relations in a chronic canine model of myocardial infarction. Implications for the interpretation of electrophysiologic studies. *Circulation* 1981;63:1158-1165.
70. Newton JC, Knisley SB, Zhou X, et al. Review of mechanisms by which electrical stimulation alters the transmembrane potential. *J Cardiovasc Electrophysiol* 1999;10:234-243.
71. Gotoh M, Uchida T, Mandel WJ, et al. Cellular graded responses and ventricular vulnerability to reentry by a premature stimulus in isolated canine ventricle. *Circulation* 1997;95:2141-2154.
72. Kwaku KF, Dillon SM. Shock-induced depolarization of refractory myocardium prevents wave-front propagation in defibrillation. *Circ Res* 1996;79:957-973.
73. Gray RA, Jalife J. Effects of atrial defibrillation shocks on the ventricles in isolated sheep hearts. *Circulation* 1998;97:1613-1622.
74. Frazier DW, Wolf PD, Wharton JM, et al. Stimulus-induced critical point. Mechanism for electrical initiation of reentry in normal canine myocardium. *J Clin Invest* 1989;83:1039-1052.
75. Antzelevitch C, Shimizu W, Yan GX, Sicouri S. Cellular basis for QT dispersion. *J Electrocardiol* 1998;30(suppl):168-175.
76. Shimizu W, McMahon B, Antzelevitch C. Sodium pentobarbital reduces transmural dispersion of repolarization and prevents torsades de pointes in models of acquired and congenital long QT syndrome [see comments]. *J Cardiovasc Electrophysiol* 1999;10:154-164.
77. Yan GX, Antzelevitch C. Cellular basis for the normal T wave and the electrocardiographic manifestations of the long-QT syndrome. *Circulation* 1998;98:1928-1936.
78. Han J, Moe GK. Nonuniform recovery of excitability in ventricular muscle. *Circ Res* 1964;14:44.
79. Kuo CS, Amlie JP, Munakata K, et al. Dispersion of monophasic action potential durations and activation times during atrial pacing, ventricular pacing, and ventricular premature stimulation in canine ventricles. *Cardiovasc Res* 1983;17:152-161.
80. Kuo CS, Munakata K, Reddy CP, Surawicz B. Characteristics and possible mechanism of ventricular arrhythmia dependent on the dispersion of action potential durations. *Circulation* 1983;67:1356-1367.
81. Surawicz B, Gettes LS, Ponce ZA. Relation of vulnerability to ECG and action potential characteristics of premature beats. *Am J Physiol* 1967;212:1519-1528.

82. Behrens S, Li C, Franz MR. Timing of the upper limit of vulnerability is different for monophasic and biphasic shocks: Implications for the determination of the defibrillation threshold. *PACE* 1997;20:2179-2187.

83. Behrens S, Li C, Kirchhof P, et al. Reduced arrhythmogenicity of biphasic versus monophasic T-wave shocks. Implications for defibrillation efficacy. *Circulation* 1996;94:1974-1980.

84. Behrens S, Li CL, Franz MR. Effects of myocardial ischemia on ventricular fibrillation inducibility and defibrillation efficacy. *J Am Coll Cardiol* 1997;29:817-824.

85. Tovar OH, Milne KB, Jones JL. Interaction of tilt and stimulus intensity on prolongation of refractory period with monophasic and biphasic defibrillating waveforms. *Proc Ann Int Conf IEEE Eng Med Biol Soc* 1993;15:846-847.

86. Chen PS, Feld GK, Mower MM, Peters BB. Effects of pacing rate and timing of defibrillation shock on the relation between the defibrillation threshold and the upper limit of vulnerability in open chest dogs. *J Am Coll Cardiol* 1991;18:1555-1563.

87. Hwang C, Swerdlow CD, Kass RM, et al. Upper limit of vulnerability reliably predicts transvenous DFT in humans. *PACE* 1994;17:789.

88. Chen PS, Wolf PD, Melnick SD, et al. Comparison of activation during ventricular fibrillation and following unsuccessful defibrillation shocks in open-chest dogs. *Circ Res* 1990;66:1544-1560.

89. Ideker RE, Chen PS, Zhou XH. Basic mechanisms of defibrillation. *J Electrocardiol* 1990;23:36-38.

90. Cha YM, Birgersdotter-Green U, Wolf PL, et al. The mechanism of termination of reentrant activity in ventricular fibrillation. *Circ Res* 1994;74:495-506.

91. Ideker RE, Frazier DW, Krassowska W, et al. Experimental evidence for autowaves in the heart. *Ann N Y Acad Sci* 1990;591:208-218.

92. Worley SJ, Swain JL, Colavita PG, et al. Development of an endocardial-epicardial gradient of activation rate during electrically induced, sustained ventricular fibrillation in dogs. *Am J Cardiol* 1985;55:813-820.

93. Zipes DP. Electrophysiological mechanisms involved in ventricular fibrillation. *Circulation* 1975;52:120-130.

94. Gray RA, Pertsov AM, Jalife J. Spatial and temporal organization during cardiac fibrillation [published erratum appears in *Nature* 1998 May14;393(6681):191]. *Nature* 1998;392:75-78.

95. Cabo C, Pertsov AM, Davidenko JM, et al. Vortex shedding as a precursor of turbulent electrical activity in cardiac muscle. *Biophys J* 1996;70:1105-1111.

96. Efimov IR, Cheng Y, Van Wagoner DR, et al. Virtual electrode-induced phase singularity: A basic mechanism of defibrillation failure. *Circ Res* 1998;82:918-925.

97. Jalife J, Gray R. Drifting vortices of electrical waves underlie ventricular fibrillation in the rabbit heart. *Acta Physiol Scand* 1996;157:123-131.

98. Winfree A. Sudden cardiac death: A problem in topology. *Sci Am* 1983;248:144-161.

99. Winfree AT. Electrical turbulence in three-dimensional heart muscle. *Science* 1994;266:1003-1006.

100. Garfinkel A, Chen PS, Walter DO, et al. Quasiperiodicity and chaos in cardiac fibrillation. *J Clin Invest* 1997;99:305-314.

101. Ramdat-Misier A, Opthof T, van Hemel NM, et al. Dispersion of 'refractoriness' in noninfarcted myocardium of patients with ventricular tachycardia

or ventricular fibrillation after myocardial infarction. *Circulation* 1995;91: 2566-2572.

102. Zhou X, Ideker RE, Blitchington TF, et al. Optical transmembrane potential measurements during defibrillation-strength shocks in perfused rabbit hearts. *Circ Res* 1995;77:593-602.
103. Zhou X, Wolf PD, Rollins DL, et al. Effects of monophasic and biphasic shocks on action potentials during ventricular fibrillation in dogs. *Circ Res* 1993;73:325-334.
104. Zhou XH, Knisley SB, Wolf PD, et al. Prolongation of repolarization time by electric field stimulation with monophasic and biphasic shocks in open-chest dogs. *Circ Res* 1991;68:1761-1767.
105. Knisley SB, Blitchington TF, Hill BC, et al. Optical measurements of trans-membrane potential changes during electric field stimulation of ventricular cells. *Circ Res* 1993;72:255-270.
106. Knisley SB, Hill BC. Optical recordings of the effect of electrical stimulation on action potential repolarization and the induction of reentry in two-dimensional perfused rabbit epicardium. *Circulation* 1993;88:2402-2414.
107. Knisley SB, Smith WM, Ideker RE. Prolongation and shortening of action potentials by electrical shocks in frog ventricular muscle cells. *Am J Physiol* 1994;266:H2348-H2358.
108. Jones JL, Tovar OH. The mechanism of defibrillation and cardioversion. *Proc Ann Int Conf IEEE Eng Med Biol Soc* 1996;84:392-403.
109. Dixon EG, Tang AS, Wolf PD, et al. Improved defibrillation thresholds with large contoured epicardial electrodes and biphasic waveforms. *Circulation* 1987;76:1176-1184.
110. Jones J, Noe W, Tovar O, et al. Can shocks timed to action potentials in low-gradient regions improve both internal and out-of-hospital defibrillation? *J Electrocardiol* 1998;31(suppl):41-44.
111. Fishler MG, Sobie EA, Tung L, Thakor NV. Modeling the interaction between propagating cardiac waves and monophasic and biphasic field stimuli: The importance of the induced spatial excitatory response. *J Cardiovasc Electrophysiol* 1996;7:1183-1196.
112. Fishler MG, Vepa K. Spatiotemporal effects of syncytial heterogeneities on cardiac far-field excitations during monophasic and biphasic shocks. *J Cardiovasc Electrophysiol* 1998;9:1310-1324.
113. Tovar OH, Jones JL. Biphasic defibrillation waveforms reduce shock-induced response duration dispersion between low and high shock intensities. *Circ Res* 1995;77:430-438.
114. Lin SF, Roth BJ, Wikswo JP Jr. Quatrefoil reentry in myocardium: An optical imaging study of the induction mechanism. *J Cardiovasc Electrophysiol* 1999;10:574-586.
115. Chapman PD, Sagar KB, Wetherbee JN, Troup PJ. Relationship of left ventricular mass to defibrillation threshold for the implantable defibrillator: A combined clinical and animal study. *Am Heart J* 1987;114:274-278.
116. Witkowski FX, Penkoske PA, Plonsey R. Mechanism of cardiac defibrillation in open-chest dogs with unipolar DC-coupled simultaneous activation and shock potential recordings. *Circulation* 1990;82:244-260.
117. Sweeney RJ, Gill RM, Reid PR. Characterization of refractory period extension by transcardiac shock. *Circulation* 1991;83:2057-2066.
118. Tovar OH, Bransford P, Moubarak J, et al. Correlation between shock induced response duration and defibrillation. *IEEE/BMSC* 1994;16:21-22.

119. Tovar OH, Jones JL. Relationship between "extension of refractoriness" and probability of successful defibrillation. *Am J Physiol* 1997;272:H1011-H1019.
120. Usui M, Callihan RL, Walker RG, et al. Epicardial sock mapping following monophasic and biphasic shocks of equal voltage with an endocardial lead system. *J Cardiovasc Electrophysiol* 1996;7:322-334.
121. Winfree AT. Electrical instability in cardiac muscle: Phase singularities and rotors. *J Theor Biol* 1989;138:353-405.
122. Zhou X, Daubert JP, Wolf PD, et al. Epicardial mapping of ventricular defibrillation with monophasic and biphasic shocks in dogs. *Circ Res* 1993;72:145-160.
123. Jones JL, Jones RE, Balasky G. Improved cardiac cell excitation with symmetrical biphasic defibrillator waveforms. *Am J Physiol* 1987;253:H1418-H1424.
124. Dillon SM. Homing in on the coupling between defibrillation shocks and the cardiac membrane potential [comment]. *J Cardiovasc Electrophysiol* 1995;6:264-267. Editorial.
125. Moubarak J, Behrens S, Fabritz CL, et al. Post-shock dispersion of repolarization: A common mechanism underlying T wave shock induced ventricular fibrillation and unsuccessful defibrillation. *PACE* 1996;19(II):102. Abstract.
126. Wang T, Kwaku KF, Dillon SM. Repolarization resynchronization may underlie the efficacy of biphasic shocks. *Circulation* 1994;90:I446. Abstract.
127. Antzelevitch C, Sun ZQ, Zhang ZQ, Yan GX. Cellular and ionic mechanisms underlying erythromycin-induced long QT intervals and torsade de pointes. *J Am Coll Cardiol* 1996;28:1836-1848.
128. Eckardt L, Haverkamp W, Borggrefe M, Breithardt G. Experimental models of torsade de pointes. *Cardiovasc Res* 1998;39(1):178-193.
129. Eckardt L, Haverkamp W, Gottker U, et al. Divergent effect of acute ventricular dilatation on the electrophysiologic characteristics of d,l-sotalol and flecainide in the isolated rabbit heart. *J Cardiovasc Electrophysiol* 1998;9:366-383.
130. Johna R, Mertens H, Haverkamp W, et al. Clofilium in the isolated perfused rabbit heart: A new model to study proarrhythmia induced by class III antiarrhythmic drugs. *Basic Res Cardiol* 1998;93(2):127-135.
131. Shimizu W, Antzelevitch C. Cellular and ionic basis for T-wave alternans under long-QT conditions. *Circulation* 1999;99:1499-1507.
132. Zabel M, Hohnloser SH, Behrens S, et al. Electrophysiologic features of torsades de pointes: Insights from a new isolated rabbit heart model. *J Cardiovasc Electrophysiol* 1997;8:1148-1158.
133. Shibata N, Chen PS, Dixon EG, et al. Epicardial activation after unsuccessful defibrillation shocks in dogs. *Am J Physiol* 1988;255:H902-H909.
134. Chen PS, Wolf PD, Ideker RE. Mechanism of cardiac defibrillation. A different point of view. *Circulation* 1991;84:913-919.
135. Konings KT, Smeets JL, Penn OC, et al. Configuration of unipolar atrial electrograms during electrically induced atrial fibrillation in humans. *Circulation* 1997;95:1231-1241.
136. Wiener N, Rosenblueth A. The mathematical formulation of the problem of conduction of impulses in a network of connected excitable elements, specifically in cardiac muscle. *Arch Inst Cardiol Mex* 1946;16:205-265.
137. Bjornstad H, Tande PM, Lathrop DA, Refsum H. Effects of temperature on cycle length dependent changes and restitution of action potential duration in guinea pig ventricular muscle. *Cardiovasc Res* 1993;27:946-950.
138. Jacobsen EA, Mortensen E, Refsum H, Klow NE. The effect of the temperature of contrast media on cardiac electrophysiology and hemodynamics during coronary arteriography. *Invest Radiol* 1992;27:942-946.

139. Sprung J, Laszlo A, Turner LA, e al. Effects of hypothermia, potassium, and verapamil on the action potential characteristics of canine cardiac Purkinje fibers. *Anesthesiology* 1995;82:713-722.
140. Lab MJ, Taggart P, Sachs F. Mechano-electric feedback . *Cardiovasc Res* 1996;32:1-2. Editorial.
141. Zabel M, Portnoy S, Franz MR. Effect of sustained load on dispersion of ventricular repolarization and conduction time in the isolated intact rabbit heart. *J Cardiovasc Electrophysiol* 1996;7:9-16.
142. Sicouri S, Moro S, Litovsky S, et al. Chronic amiodarone reduces transmural dispersion of repolarization in the canine heart. *J Cardiovasc Electrophysiol* 1997;8:1269-1279.
143. Chattipakorn N, KenKnight BH, Rogers JM, et al. Locally propagated activation immediately after internal defibrillation. *Circulation* 1998;97:1401-1410.
144. Deale OC, Wesley R Jr, Morgan D, Lerman BB. Nature of defibrillation: Determinism versus probabilism. *Am J Physiol* 1990;259:H1544-H1550.
145. Shimizu W, Antzelevitch C. Cellular basis for the ECG features of the LQT1 form of the long-QT syndrome: Effects of beta-adrenergic agonists and antagonists and sodium channel blockers on transmural dispersion of repolarization and torsade de pointes. *Circulation* 1998;98:2314-2322.
146. MacConaill M. Ventricular fibrillation thresholds in Langendorff perfused rabbit hearts: all or none effect of low potassium concentration. *Cardiovasc Res* 1987;21:463-468.

Index

Action potential
    antiarrhythmic drugs and, 268
    effect of ischemia on, 213-214,
        215
    effects of defibrillation on, 302-
        304
    heart failure and, 157-158
    heterogeneous repolarization of,
        4
    mechanism of induction of ven-
        tricular fibrillation and, 299
    in normal heart, 145
Action potential duration, 145-146
    antiarrhythmic drugs and, 267
    cardiac agents and, 5-7
    cardiac hypertrophy and, 242
    effect of smoking on, 154
    ischemia and, 156, 214, 216-219
    local repolarization time and,
        112
    spatial coupling between activa-
        tion and activation-recovery
        interval and, 115-117
    spatial heterogeneity of repolar-
        ization and, 85
    transepicardial gradients of re-
        polarization and, 24-25
Action potential duration restitu-
    tion, 25
Activation time, MAP analysis
    and, 125, 131, 133, 134
Activation-recovery interval, elec-
    troanatomical mapping of, 110-
    115
Alternans correlation index, 98
Amiodarone, 268-271, 280-281,
    293-294
Angiotensin-converting enzyme in-
    hibitors, 246
Anthopleurin-A, 179-189

Antiarrhythmic agents, 267-278
    Brugada syndrome and, 9-10
    Class I drugs, 279-287
    Class II drugs, 289-296
    electrophysiological distinctions
        among myocardial cells and,
        5-7
Antihypertensive medications,
    245-246
Apoptosis, right ventricular ar-
    rhythmogenic dysplasia and,
    158
Arrhythmia
    after myocardial infarction, 165-
        173
    electrical heterogeneity and, 3-
        21
        Brugada syndrome and, 8-10
        in heart, 4-8
        long QT syndrome and, 10-
            13, 14
        torsade de pointes and, 13-16
    increased dispersion of repolar-
        ization and, 143-163
        autonomic activity and, 152-
            153
        congenital defects of ionic
            channels and, 158
        extrasystoles and dispersion
            of refractoriness, 150-151
        heart rate and, 151-152
        left ventricular hypertrophy
            and, 154-155
        left ventricular pressure load
            and, 155-156
        myocardial failure and, 157-
            158
        myocardial infarction and,
            156-157
        myocardial ischemia and, 156

319

right ventricular degeneration, necrosis, and apoptosis and, 158
right ventricular overload and, 158
smoking and, 154
ventricular pacing and, 153
mechanism in long QT syndrome, 200
prediction via measurement of QT dispersion, 61
repolarization inhomogeneities in ventricular myocardium and, 23-37
restitution kinetics in normal heart and, 25-32
role of repolarization alternans in formation of arrhythmogenic substrates, 32-35
transepicardial gradients of repolarization and, 24-25
Arrhythmogenic substrates
congestive heart failure and, 254-255, 257
modulated dispersion effect on susceptibility to ventricular fibrillation and, 30-32
role of repolarization alternans in formation of, 32-35
ATX-11
action potential duration and, 7
long QT syndrome and, 11-13
torsades de pointes and, 179-189
Automated QT dispersion measurement, 70-71
Automatic analysis of spatial dispersion of repolarization, 87-94
principal components analysis in, 90-91
repolarization-duration[n]based methods, 88-90
T wave loop analysis, 91-93
wavelet-based technique, 93-94
Autonomic activity
cardiac hypertrophy and, 243

effect on dispersion of repolarization, 152-153
long QT syndrome and, 193-195

Basic cycle length, action potential duration and, 25
Beat-to-beat changes in repolarization, 99-101, 102
Beat-to-beat QT variability, 99, 100
Beta-blockers, 153
Brugada syndrome
defect in ionic channels in, 158
mechanisms for arrhythmia development in, 16
transmural dispersion of repolarization and, 8-10

CARTO system, 121-139
implications of, 133-136
limitations of, 136
methodological aspect of, 123-126, 127, 128
preliminary findings in, 126-133, 134
Chromanol 293B
action potential duration and, 5, 7
long QT syndrome and, 11
Circus movement reentry, torsade de pointes and, 13
Class I antiarrhythmic drugs, 279-287
encainide and flecainide, 283-284
lidocaine, 283
QT interval dispersion and, 284
quinidine, procainamide, and disopyramide, 280-282
Class II antiarrhythmic drugs, 289-296
Complex demodulation method of spectral analysis of T wave alternans, 97
Complexity of repolarization, 204-205
Computerized analysis of ventricular repolarization, 45-48, 49, 50

Conduction velocity
    changes affecting dispersion of
        repolarization of premature
        impulses, 150
    hypothermia and, 148, 149
    ischemia and, 214-216, 217
Congenital defects of ionic chan-
    nels, 158
Congestive heart failure, 253-264
Coronary artery disease, QT dis-
    persion and, 221-222
Correlation method of spectral
    analysis of T wave alternans,
    97-98
Coupling interval dependence
    modulated dispersion, 30-32, 35

Defibrillation, 297-317
    correlation of vulnerable period
        and dispersion of repolariza-
        tion, 299
    determinants of, 304
    effects on ventricular action po-
        tential, 302-304
    electrophysiology of, 301-302,
        303
    extension of refractoriness and
        repolarization, 305, 306-307
    induction by T wave shock dur-
        ing vulnerable period, 298
    mechanism of induction, 299-
        300, 301, 302
    mechanisms of, 305-307
    phase singularities and critical
        points, 308
    upper and lower limit of vulner-
        ability, 300-301
Defibrillation threshold, 298, 301
Delayed afterdepolarization, elec-
    trophysiological distinctions
    among myocardial cells and, 6
Delete-only strategy in electrocar-
    diography, 48, 49, 50
Depolarization contour maps, 28
Diastolic interval, action potential
    duration and, 25-27
Differential threshold method of T
    wave offset detection, 65-68

Digital computerized electrocardi-
    ology, 44-52
    computerized analysis of ven-
        tricular repolarization, 45-48,
        49, 50
    fundamentals and projection ef-
        fect in, 51-52
    repolarization variables and, 48-
        51
    technical aspects of ECG re-
        cordings and storage, 45
Dilated cardiomyopathy, 229-238
Discordant alternans, 35
Disopyramide, 280-282
Dispersion of refractoriness, 239-
    240
    after myocardial infarction, 165-
        173
    extrasystole and, 150-151
    ischemia and, 223
    sympathetic stimulation and,
        270
Dispersion of repolarization; see
    Repolarization
Drug-induced torsade de pointes,
    178-179

Early afterdepolarization
    electrophysiological distinctions
        among myocardial cells, 6
    genesis of torsade de pointes
        and, 13, 15, 175
Effective refractory period
    Class Ia antiarrhythmic drugs
        and, 280-282
    Class Ib antiarrhythmic drugs
        and, 283
Eigen analysis, 90
Electrical heterogeneity, 3-21
    Brugada syndrome and, 8-10
    in heart, 4-8
    long QT syndrome and, 10-13,
        14
    torsade de pointes and, 13-16
Electroanatomical mapping of ven-
    tricular activation-recovery cou-
    pling, 109-119
    activation pattern and, 112, 113

activation-recovery interval pattern and, 112-114
local activation time and, 114, 115
mechanisms of spatial coupling, 115-117
nonfluoroscopic, 110, 111
repolarization pattern and, 114-115
Electrocardiography
correlations between monophasic action potential recordings and, 75-83
QT dispersion and, 44-52, 59-73
computerized analysis of ventricular repolarization, 45-48, 49, 50
effects of T wave in, 64-68
fundamentals and projection effect in, 51-52
heart rate correction in, 63-64
ischemia and, 219-223
lead adjustment and number of valid leads in, 61-63
lead selection in, 63
principal components analysis in, 90-91
repolarization variables and, 48-51
repolarization-duration[n]based methods of measurement, 88-90
reproducibility of QT dispersion in, 69-71
T wave loop analysis, 91-93
technical aspects of ECG recordings and storage, 45
wavelet-based technique, 93-94
use in Marburg Cardiomyopathy Pilot Study, 230-235
Electrophysiological mechanism
of torsades de pointes, 175-198
autonomic nervous system and, 193-195
ionic basis of, 176-179
paradigm of, 179-189

QT/T wave alternans and, 189-193
short-long cardiac sequence and, 189, 190, 191, 192
of ventricular fibrillation, 301-302, 303
Electrotonic interactions, 116-117
Encainide, 283-284
End of repolarization map, 131, 132
Endocardial cell
action potential of, 3, 85
repolarization characteristics of, 5, 6
Epicardial cell
action potential of, 3, 85
ischemia and, 216-219
repolarization characteristics of, 5, 6
Epicardial restitution heterogeneity, 27-30
Extrasystole
dispersion of refractoriness and, 150-151
duration of action potential of, 145
as triggering factor in ventricular fibrillation, 148

Felodipine, 245
Flecainide, 283-284

Gene mutation
in Brugada syndrome, 8
in long QT syndrome, 10-11, 176-177, 199
Global dispersion of ventricular repolarization mapping, 121-139
implications of, 133-136
limitations of, 136
methodological aspect of, 123-126, 127, 128
preliminary findings in, 126-133, 134

Heart
electrical heterogeneity in, 4-8

repolarization inhomogeneities in ventricular myocardium, 24
restitution kinetics in, 25-32
Heart failure
  action potentials and, 157-158
  prognostic value of QT interval dispersion in, 261-262
Heart rate
  correction in measurement of QT dispersion, 63-64
  effect on dispersion of repolarization, 151-152
Heterogeneity of repolarization, 85-107
  automatic analysis of, 87-94
  combined three-dimensional approach to, 101-103
  temporal, 95-101
  transmural, 94-95
Hypertension, 239-252
Hypopotassemia, 157
Hypothermia, 148, 149

Implantable cardioverter defibrillator, 229-230, 298
Ionic mechanisms
  of left ventricular hypertrophy, 241-242
  of long QT syndrome, 176-179
Ischemia, 211-227
  action potential duration and, 156
  assessment of dispersion of repolarization changes in, 211-213
  cardiac hypertrophy and, 242
  dispersion of repolarization as measure of dispersion of refractoriness, 223
  effect on action potential repolarization, 213-214, 215
  influence of local conduction on action potential repolarization, 214-216, 217
  lateral or transmural repolarization gradients and, 216-219
  QT dispersion during, 219-223

Jervell and Lange-Nielsen syndrome, 177

Leads for measurement of QT dispersion, 61-63
Least-square fitting method of T wave offset detection, 68
Left ventricular activation mapping, 110-115
Left ventricular hypertrophy
  effect on dispersion of repolarization, 154-155, 240-246
  hypertension and, 239
Left ventricular pressure load, 155-156
Lidocaine, 283
Lignocaine, 283
Limb leads, 51
Local activation time, 112, 113
  relationship with activation-recovery interval, 114, 115
Local dispersion of repolarization
  global *versus*, 125
  in small areas, 131, 132
Local repolarization time, 112-114
Long QT syndrome
  defect in ionic channels in, 158
  proposed cellular and ionic mechanisms for, 13-15, 16
  repolarization-duration[n]based methods of dispersion measurement in, 88-90
  spatial dispersion of ventricular repolarization in, 199-207
  torsade de pointes in, 175-198
    autonomic nervous system and, 193-195
    ionic basis of, 176-179
    mechanisms of, 179-189
    QT/T wave alternans and, 189-193
    short-long cardiac sequence and, 189, 190, 191, 192
    transmural dispersion of repolarization and, 10-13, 14
Lower limit of vulnerability, 300-301

M cell
  action potential of, 3, 85
  antiarrhythmic drugs and, 268
  repolarization characteristics of,
    5, 6-7
  T wave alternans and, 95-96
MAP mapping; see Monophasic action potential mapping
Marburg Cardiomyopathy Pilot
  Study, 230-235
Marburg Cardiomyopathy Study,
  235-237
Mental stress, QT dispersion and,
  222-223
Microreentry, 305-307
Modulated dispersion, effect on
  susceptibility to ventricular fibrillation, 30-32
Monophasic action potential mapping, 75-83, 121-139, 201-202
  implications of, 133-136
  induction of ventricular fibrilla-
    tion and, 300, 301
  in ischemia, 212, 213-214
  limitations of, 136
  methodological aspect of, 123-
    126, 127, 128
  preliminary findings in, 126-
    133, 134
  proximity effect and, 145-146
Myocardial hypertrophy, 240-246
Myocardial infarction
  dispersion of refractoriness
    after, 165-173
  QT dispersion and, 156-157
Myocardial ischemia, 211-227
  action potential duration and,
    156
  assessment of dispersion of re-
    polarization changes in, 211-
    213
  dispersion of repolarization as
    measure of dispersion of re-
    fractoriness, 223
  effect on action potential repo-
    larization, 213-214, 215

influence of local conduction on
    action potential repolariza-
    tion, 214-216, 217
  lateral or transmural repolariza-
    tion gradients and, 216-219
  QT dispersion during, 219-223
Myocardium
  cells in, 3
  repolarization inhomogeneities
    in, 23-37
    restitution kinetics in normal
      heart and, 25-32
    role of repolarization al-
      ternans in formation of ar-
      rhythmogenic substrates,
      32-35
    transepicardial gradients of re-
      polarization and, 24-25

Navi-Star catheter, 123-124
Neural mechanisms of ventricular
  repolarization, 152-153
Nonfluoroscopic electroanatomical
  mapping of ventricular activation-recovery coupling, 110, 111

Optical mapping technique, 23-37
  restitution kinetics in normal
    heart and, 25-32
  role of repolarization alternans
    in formation of arrhythmo-
    genic substrates, 32-35
  transepicardial gradients of re-
    polarization and, 24-25

Peak slope method of T wave offset detection, 65, 67
Phase singularities in defibrillation, 308
Polymorphic reentrant ventricular
  tachycardia, 175-198
  autonomic nervous system and,
    193-195
  ionic basis of, 176-179
  mechanisms of, 179-189
  QT/T wave alternans and, 189-
    193

short-long cardiac sequence
and, 189, 190, 191, 192
Potassium channel blockers
prolongation of action potential
duration in M cells and, 5-6
torsade de pointes and, 13
Predictive value of QT interval dispersion, 257-259, 261-262
Premature beat
epicardial restitution heterogeneity and, 27-30
extrasystoles and dispersion of
refractoriness and, 150-151
modulated dispersion effect on
susceptibility to ventricular fibrillation, 30-32
Principal components analysis, 90-91, 203-205
Procainamide, 280-282
Projection effect, 51-52
Propafenone, 284
Proximity effect, 145-146, 150
Purkinje fiber, repolarization characteristics of, 5

QT dispersion, 41-58
antiarrhythmic drugs and, 272-276
antihypertensive medications
and, 245-246
automatic analysis of, 87-94
principal components analysis, 90-91
repolarization-
duration[n]based methods,
88-90
T wave loop analysis, 91-93
wavelet-based technique, 93-94
cardiac hypertrophy and, 243-244
Class I antiarrhythmic drugs
and, 284
Class III antiarrhythmic drugs
and, 289-296
clinical significance of, 52-56
congestive heart failure and,
253-264

current status of scalar 12-lead,
42-44
digital computerized electrocardiology and, 44-52
computerized analysis of ventricular repolarization, 45-48, 49, 50
fundamentals and projection
effect in, 51-52
repolarization variables and,
48-51
technical aspects of ECG recordings and storage, 45
dilated cardiomyopathy and,
229-238
genesis of, 80-81
heart failure and, 157-158
hypertension and, 155
during ischemia, 219-223
in long QT syndrome, 202-203
myocardial infarction and, 156-157
myocardial ischemia and, 156
twelve-lead electrocardiogram
and, 59-73
effects of T wave in, 64-68
heart rate correction in, 63-64
lead adjustment and number
of valid leads in, 61-63
lead selection in, 63
reproducibility of QT dispersion in, 69-71
QT duration, 43
QT interval
long QT syndrome and, 200-201
torsade de pointes and, 189-193
QT interval dispersion analysis,
86
Quinidine, 268-271, 280-282

Ramipril, 245
Refractoriness, 239-240
after myocardial infarction, 165-173
defibrillation and, 305, 306-307
extrasystole and, 150-151
ischemia and, 223

sympathetic stimulation and,
270
Repolarization
after myocardial infarction, 165-
173
antiarrhythmic agents and, 267-
278
Class I drugs, 279-287
Class II drugs, 289-296
beat-to-beat changes in, 99-101
computerized analysis of, 45-48,
49, 50
contour maps of, 28
correlations between monophasic action potential recordings
and surface electrocardiograms, 75-83
dilated cardiomyopathy and,
229-238
effects of defibrillation on, 297-
317
correlation of vulnerable period and dispersion of repolarization, 299
determinants of, 304
effects on ventricular action
potential, 302-304
electrophysiology of, 301-302,
303
extension of refractoriness
and repolarization, 305,
306-307
induction by T wave shock
during vulnerable period,
298
mechanism of induction, 299-
300, 301, 302
mechanisms of, 305-307
phase singularities and critical points, 308
upper and lower limit of vulnerability, 300-301
electroanatomical mapping of
ventricular activation-recovery coupling, 109-119
activation pattern and, 112,
113

activation-recovery interval
pattern and, 112-114
local activation time and, 114,
115
mechanisms of spatial coupling, 115-117
nonfluoroscopic, 110, 111
repolarization pattern and,
114-115
hypertension and, 239-252
increased, 143-163
autonomic activity and, 152-
153
congenital defects of ionic
channels and, 158
extrasystoles and dispersion
of refractoriness, 150-151
heart rate and, 151-152
left ventricular hypertrophy
and, 154-155
left ventricular pressure load
and, 155-156
myocardial failure and, 157-
158
myocardial infarction and,
156-157
myocardial ischemia and, 156
right ventricular degeneration, necrosis, and
apoptosis and, 158
right ventricular overload
and, 158
smoking and, 154
ventricular pacing and, 153
inhomogeneities in ventricular
myocardium, 23-37
antiarrhythmic drugs and,
267
restitution kinetics in normal
heart and, 25-32
role of repolarization alternans in formation of arrhythmogenic substrates,
32-35
transepicardial gradients of repolarization and, 24-25
modulation by antiarrhythmic
drugs, 267-278

monophasic action potential
mapping, 121-139
implications of, 133-136
limitations of, 136
methodological aspect of,
123-126, 127, 128
preliminary findings in, 126-
133, 134
myocardial ischemia and, 211-
227
assessment of dispersion of repolarization changes, 211-
213
dispersion of refractoriness
and, 223
effect on action potential repolarization, 213-214, 215
influence of local conduction
on action potential repolarization, 214-216, 217
lateral or transmural repolarization gradients and, 216-
219
QT dispersion during, 219-
223
spatial dispersion in long QT
syndrome, 199-207
spatial heterogeneity of, 85-107
automatic analysis of, 87-94
combined three-dimensional
approach to, 101-103
temporal heterogeneity and,
95-101
transmural heterogeneity and,
94-95
Repolarization alternans, 32-35
Repolarization correlation index,
100, 101
Restitution kinetics, 25-32
modulated dispersion effect on
ventricular fibrillation susceptibility, 30-32
promotion of dispersion of ventricular depolarization and,
27-30
Right ventricular arrhythmogenic
dysplasia, 158
Right ventricular overload, 158

Scalar 12-lead QT dispersion
current status of, 42-44
digital computerized electrocardiology and, 44-52
computerized analysis of ventricular repolarization, 45-
48, 49, 50
fundamentals and projection
effect in, 51-52
repolarization variables and,
48-51
technical aspects of ECG recordings and storage, 45
Short-long cardiac sequence, torsades de pointes and, 189, 190,
191, 192
Single value decomposition, 90
Slope method of T wave offset detection, 65, 67, 68
Smoking effect on dispersion of repolarization, 154
Solid angle theory, 219
Sotalol, 289-296
long QT syndrome and, 11, 14
modification of dispersion of repolarization and, 268-271,
273-275
Spatial coupling between activation and activation-recovery interval, 115-117
Spatial dispersion of ventricular
repolarization, in long QT syndrome, 199-207
Spatial heterogeneity of action potential alternans, 34-35
Spatial heterogeneity of repolarization, 85-107, 144-145
automatic analysis of, 87-94
combined three-dimensional approach to, 101-103
temporal heterogeneity and, 95-
101
transmural heterogeneity and,
94-95
Spectral analysis of T wave alternans, 96-98
Subendocardial ischemia, 219

Sympathetic effects on repolarization, 153

T axis abnormalities, 92, 93
T loop analysis, 53-56
T offset detection, 46-47, 64-68
T wave
    beat-to-beat QT variability detection and, 99, 100
    effect on measurement of QT dispersion, 64-68
    monophasic action potential contact electrode method and, 75-83
    offset detection, 46-47
    predictive value of QT dispersion and, 53-54
    repolarization correlation index and, 101
T wave alternans, 87
    automatic detection of, 95-101
    formation of arrhythmogenic substrates and, 32-34
    torsades de pointes and, 189-193
T wave area method, 68
T wave complexity analysis, 203
T wave loop analysis, 91-93
T wave variability, 87, 95-101
Temporal heterogeneity of repolarization, 95-101
Temporal variability in amplitude, 100
Temporal variability in time, 100
Tetralogy of Fallot, 158
Threshold method of T wave offset detection, 65-68
Time-domain technique of spectral analysis of T wave alternans, 96-97
Torsade de pointes, 175-198
    antiarrhythmic drug-induced, 272-276, 279-287
    autonomic nervous system and, 193-195
    ionic basis of, 176-179
    mechanisms of, 179-189, 200

QT/T wave alternans and, 189-193
short-long cardiac sequence and, 189, 190, 191, 192
transmural dispersion of repolarization and, 13-16
Transepicardial gradients of repolarization, 24-25
Transmural dispersion of repolarization, 3-4
    ischemia and, 216-219
Transmural heterogeneity of repolarization, 86-87, 94-95
Twelve-lead electrocardiogram
    QT dispersion and, 59-73
        effects of T wave in, 64-68
        heart rate correction in, 63-64
        ischemia and, 219-223
        lead adjustment and number of valid leads in, 61-63
        lead selection in, 63
        principal components analysis in, 90-91
        repolarization-duration[n]based methods of measurement, 88-90
        reproducibility of QT dispersion in, 69-71
    use in Marburg Cardiomyopathy Pilot Study, 230-235

U wave, measurement of QT dispersion and, 64
Upper limit of vulnerability, 298, 300-301

Ventricular activation-recovery coupling mapping, 109-119
    activation pattern and, 112, 113
    activation-recovery interval pattern and, 112-114
    local activation time and, 114, 115
    mechanisms of spatial coupling, 115-117
    nonfluoroscopic, 110, 111
    repolarization pattern and, 114-115

Ventricular fibrillation
    after myocardial infarction, 165-173
    effects of defibrillation on dispersion of repolarization, 297-317
        correlation of vulnerable period and dispersion of repolarization, 299
        determinants of, 304
        effects on ventricular action potential, 302-304
        electrophysiology of, 301-302, 303
        extension of refractoriness and repolarization, 305, 306-307
        induction by T wave shock during vulnerable period, 298
        mechanism of induction, 299-300, 301, 302
        mechanisms of, 305-307
        phase singularities and critical points, 308
        upper and lower limit of vulnerability, 300-301
    increased dispersion of repolarization and, 143-163
        autonomic activity and, 152-153
        congenital defects of ionic channels and, 158
        extrasystoles and dispersion of refractoriness, 150-151
        heart rate and, 151-152
        left ventricular hypertrophy and, 154-155
        left ventricular pressure load and, 155-156
        myocardial failure and, 157-158
        myocardial infarction and, 156-157
        myocardial ischemia and, 156
        right ventricular degeneration, necrosis, and apoptosis and, 158

        right ventricular overload and, 158
        smoking and, 154
        ventricular pacing and, 153
    modulated dispersion effect on susceptibility to, 30-32
Ventricular myocardium
    cells in, 3
    repolarization inhomogeneities in, 23-37
        restitution kinetics in normal heart and, 25-32
        role of repolarization alternans in formation of arrhythmogenic substrates, 32-35
        transepicardial gradients of repolarization and, 24-25
Ventricular pacing, 153
Ventricular premature complex, 146-147
Ventricular repolarization, 121-139
    computerized analysis of, 45-48, 49, 50
    contour maps of, 28
    correlations between monophasic action potential recordings and surface electrocardiograms, 75-83
    dilated cardiomyopathy and, 235-236
    increased, 143-163
        autonomic activity and, 152-153
        congenital defects of ionic channels and, 158
        extrasystoles and dispersion of refractoriness, 150-151
        heart rate and, 151-152
        left ventricular hypertrophy and, 154-155
        left ventricular pressure load and, 155-156
        myocardial failure and, 157-158
        myocardial infarction and, 156-157
        myocardial ischemia and, 156

right ventricular degeneration, necrosis, and apoptosis and, 158
right ventricular overload and, 158
smoking and, 154
ventricular pacing and, 153
in long QT syndrome, 199-207
modulation by antiarrhythmic drugs, 267-278
monophasic action potential mapping of, 121-139
implications of, 133-136
limitations of, 136
methodological aspect of, 123-126, 127, 128
preliminary findings in, 126-133, 134
Ventricular tachycardia
after myocardial infarction, 165-173
torsades de pointes, 175-198

autonomic nervous system and, 193-195
ionic basis of, 176-179
mechanisms of, 179-189
QT/T wave alternans and, 189-193
short-long cardiac sequence and, 189, 190, 191, 192
Vulnerable period
correlation with dispersion of repolarization, 299
induction of ventricular fibrillation in, 298
mechanism of induction of ventricular fibrillation during, 299-300, 301, 302

Wavelet transformation method, 100-101
Wavelet-based analysis of repolarization, 93-94